Challenging Diagnosis

Cystic Fibrosis and the Elusive Quest for Certainty

MICHELLE LABONTE

THE UNIVERSITY OF CHICAGO PRESS CHICAGO AND LONDON

The University of Chicago Press, Chicago 60637
The University of Chicago Press, Ltd., London

Published 2026
Printed in the United States of America

35 34 33 32 31 30 29 28 27 26   1 2 3 4 5

ISBN-13: 978-0-226-85360-4 (cloth)
ISBN-13: 978-0-226-85362-8 (paper)
ISBN-13: 978-0-226-85361-1 (ebook)
DOI: https://doi.org/10.7208/chicago/9780226853611.001.0001

Library of Congress Cataloging-in-Publication Data

Names: LaBonte, Michelle, author
Title: Challenging diagnosis : cystic fibrosis and the elusive quest for certainty / Michelle LaBonte.
Description: Chicago : The University of Chicago Press, 2026. | Includes bibliographical references and index.
Identifiers: LCCN 2026015563 | ISBN 9780226853604 cloth | ISBN 9780226853628 paperback | ISBN 9780226853611 ebook
Subjects: LCSH: Cystic fibrosis—Diagnosis | Cystic fibrosis—Diagnosis—Social aspects | Diagnosis—Methodology—Social aspects | Medical technology—Social aspects | Uncertainty
Classification: LCC RC858.C95 L34 2026
LC record available at https://lccn.loc.gov/2026015563

♾ This paper meets the requirements of ANSI/NISO Z39.48-1992 (Permanence of Paper).

Authorized Representative for EU General Product Safety Regulation (GPSR) queries: **Easy Access System Europe**—Mustamäe tee 50, 10621 Tallinn, Estonia, gpsr.requests@easproject.com
Any other queries: https://press.uchicago.edu/press/contact.html

Challenging Diagnosis

TO ANYONE WHO HAS BEEN TOUCHED BY DIAGNOSTIC UNCERTAINTY

Contents

Introduction

By the end of college, friends and family began expressing concern that I looked sick, and people I barely knew often provided me with the unsolicited advice that I should eat more. However, despite eating nearly continuously, I simply could not stop losing weight, and nobody could figure out why. Even with health insurance and access to numerous medical professionals, I went more than a decade with unexplained symptoms before receiving a diagnosis based on laboratory evidence. My experience is not unique.

In the United States alone, an estimated thirty million people are living with an undiagnosed disease, and even those who eventually receive a diagnosis often go through an extended period of diagnostic uncertainty.[1] In addition to the emotional toll on patients and families, a lengthy diagnostic odyssey is associated with delayed access to therapeutics, increased morbidity, and significant medical costs to individuals and health care systems.[2] Aware of the challenges of diagnosis in the setting of rare, novel, or "unusual manifestations of more common diseases," the National Institutes of Health (NIH) launched its Undiagnosed Diseases Program in 2008.[3] After expanding to a network of centers across the country beginning in 2014, the NIH Undiagnosed Diseases Network had evaluated 3,195 people and diagnosed 886 of them by April 2025.[4] However, despite the success of the network in diagnosing these patients, hundreds of millions of people around the world still live with an undiagnosed disease.[5] Why do some individuals, but not others, undergo a prolonged period of diagnostic uncertainty? How do factors such as gender and race impact the diagnostic odyssey? How does the design of diagnostic tests complicate or facilitate diagnosis? My interest in finding answers to these and other questions stems in part from my own experience with diagnostic uncertainty, having gone many years as a child and young adult without access to appropriate therapeutics before being diagnosed with pancreatic insufficiency and refractory gastrointestinal infections.

When my digestive symptoms first began in middle school, I was so embarrassed that I kept them to myself. Initially, I hoped to fix the problem on my own by trying every change in diet that I could imagine. When the seemingly constant need to attend to my digestive challenges made it impossible to fall asleep at night, I would come up with a plan for the next day, convinced that if I just stopped eating ice cream, or alfredo sauce, or unbaked cake batter, my symptoms would resolve. And when changing my diet didn't work, I finally sought medical care, but physicians largely dismissed my concerns. I distinctly remember sitting in a chair as one doctor assured me that my symptoms were due to the stress of being an undergraduate at Princeton. Another physician ordered bloodwork, but when the results came back normal, he told me there was nothing wrong. It didn't take long for me to wonder if the doctors were right. Maybe my digestive problems were "all in my head." Eventually, I gave up on finding a diagnosis and instead became quite skilled at hiding my symptoms. But as my condition worsened, I could no longer pass as healthy, no matter how hard I tried.[6]

Almost ten years after my symptoms began, I finally resumed my search for a diagnosis at age twenty-two while doing PhD research in the biomedical sciences. Working alongside physician-scientists, the concerned inquiries about my health came not just from family, friends, and acquaintances, but from my colleagues with medical training as well. Since I had a new primary care physician, I renewed my search for a diagnosis. What followed were two more years of appointments with doctors, nurses, and nutritionists, who attributed my symptoms to such causes as stress, irritable bowel syndrome, and inadequate diet (despite my assurances that I was eating significantly more than someone twice my weight). It wasn't until I was twenty-four years old that my primary care physician finally referred me to a gastroenterologist, who immediately took my concerns seriously. As he wrote in his clinic note at the time, "I do not have a good diagnosis, but I do not think that her [symptoms are] due to stress."[7] While I didn't read his clinic note until years later, I have a vivid memory of how seriously he took my concerns during that first meeting, and how hopeful I was that I might finally get some answers. As a first step to figuring out what was causing the gastrointestinal symptoms and associated weight loss, my gastroenterologist ordered a series of laboratory tests. Within days, I was diagnosed with several pathogenic gastrointestinal parasites and put on antibiotics to treat the infections; a few months later, I was diagnosed with exocrine pancreatic insufficiency and learned that my pancreas enzymes weren't working properly to digest my food.

Since pancreatic insufficiency is often seen in people with cystic fibrosis (CF), and given my family history of CF, my gastroenterologist wondered if I might also have CF. As he wrote in his clinic note, "I have referred her to Children's Hospital for a sweat test because she may have a variant of cystic fibrosis that gives pancreatic insufficiency."[8] At that time, I already knew that CF was a genetic disease affecting primarily the respiratory and gastrointestinal systems. I also understood that the gene associated with CF coded for a chloride channel and that the gold standard diagnostic test examined sweat for elevated chloride levels. However, I had never suspected that my digestive issues were related to CF because I did not have any respiratory symptoms. In fact, according to a 1994 Cystic Fibrosis Foundation handbook for patients and families that I received several years after one of my relatives had been diagnosed, "virtually every person with CF develops chronic lung disease . . . digestive problems occur in about 85 percent of all people with CF."[9] In other words, CF was described largely as a respiratory disease, with gastrointestinal complications seen in most (but not all) individuals.

Given my lack of respiratory symptoms, it wasn't surprising that my sweat test came back negative, indicating that I did not have CF. However, my gastroenterologist still suspected CF and referred me for genetic testing as well. In fact, even before I had the sweat test, my gastroenterologist wrote in his clinic note that "if [the sweat test] is normal, my suspicion of CF is still high enough that I would refer her . . . for genetic testing for subtle forms of CF."[10] At that time, CF had long been understood as an autosomal recessive genetic disease, meaning that an individual must inherit two mutated copies of the CF gene, one from each biological parent, to have the disease (Figure I.1).[11] While my genetic testing for CF also came back negative, it did indicate that I was a carrier with a single CF gene mutation. At that time, CF carriers were generally described as asymptomatic in the medical and patient education literature, yet that assumption has been increasingly challenged in recent years (as I discuss later in the book). Since the genetic testing I had done only detected a subset of known CF gene mutations, my gastroenterologist suggested more extensive genetic analysis to check for an additional, rare gene mutation. As he noted at the time, "she may have another as yet unidentified

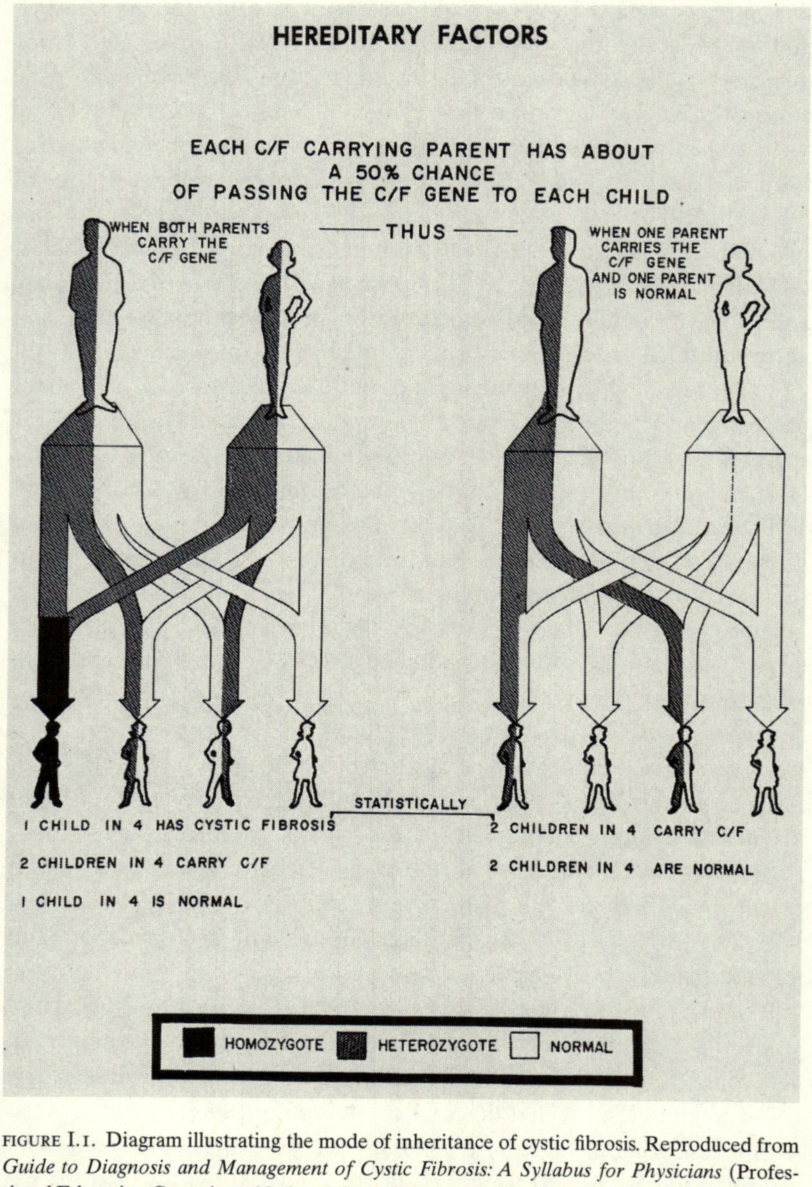

FIGURE I.1. Diagram illustrating the mode of inheritance of cystic fibrosis. Reproduced from *Guide to Diagnosis and Management of Cystic Fibrosis: A Syllabus for Physicians* (Professional Education Committee, National Cystic Fibrosis Research Foundation, 1963). The guide notes that "This syllabus may be reproduced in toto or in part without permission."

mutation that works in concert with the [known mutation] to cause pancreatic insufficiency."[12] My physician's suggestion that I had an additional undetected mutation in the CF gene that might account for my pancreatic insufficiency parallels the assumption that some men with infertility (due to congenital bilateral absence of the vas deferens) also had CF gene mutations that were "yet-to-be-identified," as sociologist Anne Kerr has documented.[13] However, despite the possibility that I had an additional, undetected CF gene mutation, I opted out of further testing because I could not afford to pay for it at that time.

I have never met the diagnostic criteria for CF, yet in the years after I first tested negative for CF, my medical records have included such diagnoses as "pancreatic insufficiency probably due to a cystic fibrosis variant," "pancreatic steatorrhea of unknown etiology," and "atypical CF with pancreatic insufficiency." As historian Charles Rosenberg has noted, to address the inevitable variation in disease presentation between individuals, physicians introduced terms such as "atypical," which served to underscore "the unspoken centrality of such ideal-typical disease models."[14] Furthermore, the term "atypical CF" is no longer favored by many CF professionals, yet people who have been given this label in the medical literature tend not to have the same clinical profile as me.[15] Thus, I still live with the uncertainty of whether there is an underlying diagnosis that might explain why I have pancreatic insufficiency and recurrent and refractory gastrointestinal infections and, more recently, respiratory and other complications that are distinct from those seen in people with CF.[16] However, with my current diagnoses, I now have the benefit of therapeutic interventions that have greatly improved my quality of life. Perhaps more important, physicians no longer suggest that my symptoms are "all in my head," and when new complications arise, my concerns are taken seriously and addressed promptly.[17] My story is not an isolated one. Despite advances in medical knowledge and diagnostic technologies over the past century, why does uncertainty in diagnosis persist?

Challenging Diagnosis examines the sociocultural and scientific factors that have contributed to diagnostic uncertainty in medicine, foregrounding the impact of such uncertainty on patients and families. As numerous scholars have noted, the meaning of "diagnostic uncertainty" has varied across time and in different contexts.[18] My own understanding of the term originally derived from my experiences as a patient, and I came into this project with a working definition of diagnostic uncertainty as the presence of symptoms in the absence of a diagnostic label. In fact, as social scientists

Stefan Timmermans and Mara Buchbinder note, "most of the literature on diagnostic uncertainty draws from people who experience symptoms that evade medical classification."[19] Yet as they and others have pointed out, diagnostic uncertainty can also arise when an individual has "markers of disease in the absence of symptoms."[20] This type of diagnostic uncertainty can occur following a positive newborn screen, when genetic testing indicates the increased risk of disease, or in the setting of "protodiseases" such as high blood pressure or high cholesterol.[21] In this book, I adopt a broad definition of diagnostic uncertainty to mean any case in which there is uncertainty associated with a disease label, whether the presence of symptoms in the absence of a diagnosis, a diagnosis in the absence of symptoms, or test results indicating an increased risk of disease in the future.

Cystic fibrosis is an ideal case for studying the broadly defined concept of diagnostic uncertainty because it is often described in medical and biology texts as a model genetic disease that is straightforward to identify, yet as social scientists and medical professionals have documented, the diagnosis of CF has long been fraught with challenges.[22] Reflecting on the topic of diagnosis in 1957, Yale CF physician Vivian Tappan explained that "it is easy to recognize the extremes of health and disease; it is well nigh impossible to draw a sharp line between them."[23] In the decades before and after Tappan's assertion, medical professionals, patients, and advocates have grappled with how to define cystic fibrosis, how to select and interpret diagnostic and screening tests, and how to ensure that those with the disease are tested in the first place. Ever since the initial comprehensive description of the disease in 1938, the definition of CF has varied over time and in different contexts, ranging from a disease of the pancreas with a life expectancy of less than a year, to a systemic disease affecting primarily the respiratory and gastrointestinal systems, to a disease that can exist in the setting of no overt clinical symptoms in the years following diagnosis. In part because of changing disease definitions and the increasing availability of therapeutic interventions, CF has gradually emerged as a disease of adulthood, with a median predicted age of survival of sixty-five years in the US for those born between 2020 and 2024.[24] In fact, some medical professionals have suggested that we might consider CF and related disorders to exist along a spectrum, further complicating the diagnostic process.[25] Even in people with severe clinical manifestations of the disease in multiple organ systems, or what Tappan might have referred to as the "extreme of disease," diagnosis can still sometimes be elusive.

An examination of diagnostic challenges in the context of CF is broadly applicable and provides important insight into diagnostic uncertainty in medicine more generally. To begin with, numerous diagnostic and screening tests for those with CF have been developed, implemented, and abandoned since the late 1930s to the present day. From invasive tests requiring the skill of a trained physician to those performed at home with nothing more than a bucket of water, CF tests have varied in complexity and in area of focus. For example, tests associated with CF have targeted not only the respiratory and gastrointestinal systems, but also sweat composition, genetics, and lung microbiology, and many of these tests (or their analogues) have been used throughout medicine. Second, cystic fibrosis has been a central point of reference in genomic medicine, with key stakeholders repeatedly looking to CF as a model when reflecting on the application of genetic testing to screening and diagnostic approaches for identifying people with genetic diseases. As just one example, investigators tasked in 1990 with addressing the ethical, legal, and social issues associated with the Human Genome Project highlighted the "recent development of a screening test for cystic fibrosis" following the characterization of the CF gene and concluded that "tracking and examining in detail the cystic fibrosis experience promises to provide an instructive model of the full range of issues of interest to the human genome project."[26] Third, CF provides a model for how assumptions about gender and race can influence diagnostic and screening approaches. As physician Jennifer Taylor-Cousar recently explained, CF "has been described repeatedly as a disease that occurs in white people" such that "people who were Black, brown, they were left out of diagnosis, out of treatment and care for many, many years," an issue that Taylor-Cousar and others have been working to address.[27] Finally, CF is relatively common for a genetic disease, with close to forty thousand people living with CF in the United States alone.[28]

I hope that further deconstructing the layers of diagnostic uncertainty in the case of CF can help social scientists, medical professionals, and patients better understand the challenging diagnostic odyssey of a wide range of diseases, including those that have been contested, such as myalgic encephalomyelitis/chronic fatigue syndrome (ME/CFS), Lyme disease, fibromyalgia, irritable bowel syndrome, multiple chemical sensitivities, and, most recently, long COVID. The history of CF diagnostics also sheds light on the nature and experience of uncertainty associated with markers of disease in the absence of symptoms. Drawing from archival sources, oral history interviews, newspaper accounts, and the medical and scientific literature from the 1930s to the present day, primarily but not exclusively in the United States, *Challenging Diagnosis* demonstrates that technological advances have not led to the level of certainty in diagnosis that many physicians expected. Instead, as the CF case illustrates, diagnostic uncertainty has persisted despite—and because of—new technologies. Each technology, introduced with the hope that it would reduce uncertainty, instead has brought novel forms of uncertainty, such that the diagnosis of CF is no more straightforward today than it was in the mid-twentieth century. These findings are broadly applicable to many diseases beyond CF and demonstrate the significant harms associated with such a heavy reliance on test results that prioritize disease specificity over patient narratives.

* * *

While I didn't appreciate it at the time, my experience following the onset of digestive challenges is characteristic of a particular diagnostic process that has deep historical roots. Within a reductionist biomedical model, a key element of the diagnostic process involves the timely identification of a single, distinct disease entity that best "matches" the patient's symptoms and test results.[29] However, for many people, this ideal diagnostic process is not realized in practice, resulting in confusion and uncertainty about the cause of one's symptoms and expectations for the future.[30] In my own case, I continued to experience diagnostic uncertainty even after the parasitic infection and pancreatic insufficiency diagnoses because of the possibility that my impaired digestion might be one manifestation of a specific disease such as cystic fibrosis. In fact, when New York physician Dorothy Andersen provided the first comprehensive description of CF in 1938, she described it as a pancreas disease that was often, but not always, associated with respiratory complications.[31] In other words, CF was initially, by definition, a specific disease of the pancreas.[32] And while I was *not* ultimately diagnosed with CF, my physicians' (and my own) desire to place my pancreatic insufficiency within the framework of a specific disease can be understood in a broader historical context.

Modern conceptions of disease specificity can be traced to the nineteenth century, when physicians in the Paris hospital setting aimed to link a patient's symptoms during life with a specific lesion within the body on autopsy.[33] In fact, the first test for CF in the late 1930s involved the postmortem detection of specific changes in the pancreas, referred to as "cystic fibrosis of the pancreas."[34] Before diseases were viewed as specific entities, disease concepts emphasized the individual, foregrounding the patient's unique symptoms and progression over time.[35] In addition to the role of pathological anatomy, notions of diseases as "specific, mechanism-based ailments with characteristic clinical courses" were reinforced by physical diagnosis and studies of the chemical and physiological makeup of bodies deemed "normal" and diseased.[36] By the mid-nineteenth century, diseases were increasingly understood to be specific, with a standard progression of symptoms and distinct mechanism of action, such that the course of disease in an individual followed a predictable progression.[37] The notion of disease specificity was further clarified in the setting of the germ theory of disease, in which specific microorganisms could be linked to specific diseases with distinct symptoms and clinical course.[38]

Also in the nineteenth century, the diagnostic process was aided by the introduction of technologies, such as the thermometer and the stethoscope, into medical practice.[39] By the end of the nineteenth century, laboratory-based technologies played a critical role in the diagnosis of specific disease entities. The use of diagnostic technologies expanded further in the hospital setting by the 1920s, such that a physician could make use of the X-ray machine or the blood pressure cuff to arrive at a diagnosis that was assumed to be more objective than one derived without the aid of such technologies.[40] This focus on the objectivity of diagnostic technologies, along with the emphasis on disease specificity and corresponding treatments, was a key component of the biomedical model, which had become the dominant paradigm in the first half of the twentieth century.[41] In fact, the initial diagnostic for CF in living patients in the late 1930s involved the invasive collection and analysis of digestive fluid for the presence of pancreatic enzymes.[42] By the 1950s, once physicians realized that people with CF had elevated chloride levels in their sweat, the diagnosis of CF shifted from pancreatic enzyme analysis to the measurement of sweat electrolyte composition.

This focus on disease specificity continued through the twentieth century, as medical and biological knowledge itself became ever more granular. For example, after World War II, the specificity of disease was further reinforced by attention to individual genes and their protein products.[43] In the case of CF, however, this high level of specificity could not be translated into new diagnostic approaches until after the gene was identified in 1989.[44] Well before genetics-based diagnostics for CF became available, the concept of disease specificity was solidified with the rise of computer-powered diagnostics and associated imaging technologies starting in the 1970s, which allowed for the noninvasive visualization of structures and physiological processes within the body.[45] While imaging technologies have not typically been used in the diagnosis of CF because of their lower specificity for the disease, in some cases imaging results have revealed characteristic changes that prompt the initiation of diagnostic testing.[46]

Stanley Reiser emphasizes how diagnostic technologies, which can give "an appearance of exactness and finality," have come to be prioritized over a physician's own senses or the patient narrative.[47] Not only have results from diagnostic technologies taken priority over other methods of diagnosis, but the use of diagnostic tests within hospitals increased dramatically over the course of the twentieth century.[48] Reflecting on the shift away from the patient narrative and the physician's senses in the diagnosis of disease, Charles Rosenberg notes that "the gradual deployment of an ever-increasing array of seemingly objective tools worked to establish the texture and corporeality as well as the essential unity of disease entities."[49] Thus, within the current biomedical framework, technologies play a fundamental role in the diagnosis and definition of specific disease entities.[50] Reflecting on changes in diagnostic practices since the nineteenth century, Reiser laments that the shift from diagnosis based on "what the patient says" to "what the machine says" has simply "exchanged one partial view of disease for another."[51]

The shift to technology-based diagnostic methods has also meant that it is now possible, even common, to construct new diseases that are not associated with symptoms.[52] Take for example the case of hypertension, which can be diagnosed by the blood pressure cuff during a routine visit to the physician.[53] Once given this label, the newly defined patient may be prescribed medication to lower their blood pressure, and the effectiveness of the medication is measured not by symptoms, but by the numbers generated from a diagnostic technology. Thus, it is possible for an individual to be diagnosed and treated for a disease without ever feeling physically ill, except perhaps because of side effects from the medication. Reflecting on how the reliance on technology makes it possible to diagnose disease in the absence of symptoms, Jacalyn Duffin notes that in some cases, diseases with no symptoms "have much higher status as diseases" than those that have symptoms.[54] This is because diseases such as hypertension have "signs" or "objective indicators of a problem that are detectable to an outsider," whereas diseases such as myalgic encephalomyelitis/chronic fatigue syndrome often do not.[55] Given the existence of an ever-expanding array of predisease diagnostic labels that are not associated with symptoms, and the social legitimacy that such labels come with, the lack of a diagnosis can be especially troubling for patients with unexplained symptoms.[56]

* * *

Due to the prevalence of diagnostic uncertainty in medicine and the challenges (and at times, advantages) it can pose for medical professionals, patients, and families, scholars have taken a range of approaches to examine the topic.[57] In a widely cited study published in 1957, sociologist Renée Fox reflected on medical uncertainty following her participant observation of students training to be physicians at Cornell University Medical College.[58] Based on an analysis of how medical students learn about and respond to uncertainty over their four years of schooling, Fox asserted that uncertainty could arise from three main factors: gaps in student/physician knowledge, limits in medical knowledge, or the inability to distinguish between the two.[59] As Fox noted, this third type of uncertainty was especially salient as students embarked on the physical diagnosis component of their preclinical studies. While the Cornell medical students became more skilled at recognizing and responding to uncertainty over the course of their training, Fox nevertheless pointed to "an irreducible minimum of uncertainty . . . inherent in medicine."[60] Contemplating this persistence of uncertainty, one medical student explained that "studying medicine is a lot like digging a hole in the sand . . . but it seems as though for every shovelful you toss out, some more slides in . . . of course, when you dig *any* hole, you never get to the bottom."[61] Fox's 1957 scholarship on uncertainty reached a wide audience, in part because modified versions of her work were included in *Pre-Med: A National Pre-Medical Journal*, which was made freely available to undergraduate students at 280 colleges across the United States in the early 1960s.[62]

If one focuses on the sources of medical uncertainty that Renée Fox identified, it is possible to attribute delays in diagnosis to knowledge gaps, on the part of either the physician or medicine itself; within this framing is the implicit assumption that diseases are "natural kinds," and diagnosis would be straightforward if these gaps in knowledge could simply be filled.[63] However, as social scientists have documented, the definition of disease is often determined by a combination of social and biological factors, and as such diseases are not stable categories waiting to be discovered or further characterized as new medical knowledge is acquired.[64] In fact, disease definitions do change over time and in different contexts, and this fluidity can be associated with diagnostic uncertainty and related delays in diagnosis. As historian of medicine Keith Wailoo notes, this instability of disease definition can be attributed to such factors as institutional and organizational context, specialists, technology, therapeutic efficacy, cultural context, attitudes regarding race and gender, financial considerations, and government funding.[65] Many other scholars have reinforced the notion that "diagnoses are a way to divide up nature into categories that fit our understanding of the world . . . but that do not ontologically exist."[66] For example, according to physician and geneticist Barton Childs, "although practical necessity requires that we classify, each individual has his or her own disease."[67] Consistent with this view, sociologist Anne Kerr has described CF as "a dynamic entity, whose various meanings and interpretations are shaped by a range of social and material actors, including professionals, patients, technologies and bodies," and other scholars have also documented how the definition of CF has changed over time and in different contexts.[68]

Since Fox's initial scholarship on uncertainty, many social scientists and medical professionals have reflected on uncertainty in diagnostics, with some challenging her work, and others (including Fox herself) reinforcing or expanding on it.[69] In 1979, Donald Light Jr. acknowledged Fox's three sources of uncertainty in the setting of medical education and suggested that additional uncertainties arose "as the young professional takes on actual cases," yet he also argued that Fox placed too great an emphasis on training for uncertainty at the expense of attention to "training for control" in the setting of uncertainties in medicine.[70] Several years later, Paul Atkinson called for a more nuanced treatment of both *certainty* and *uncertainty*, which he felt "should equally be seen as features of the social construction and definition of medical discourse."[71] Despite some debate about the nature and relative importance of uncertainty in medical education and practice, many social scientists and physicians have pointed to uncertainty as inherent in medicine even in the setting of technological advances. Reflecting on Fox's work, Timmermans and Buchbinder note how she highlighted the "recursive nature of uncertainty: while technologies may address some forms of uncertainty, they seem bound, inevitably, to uncover previously unrecognized forms of uncertainty or to produce new ones."[72] In earlier work, Keith Wailoo similarly noted that technologies not only have played a role in "simplifying and resolving our knowledge of disease" but "have been one of many factors *constituting*, *creating*, and *complicating* diseases in our time."[73]

Related to the role of technologies in complicating diagnoses, limitations to the objective ideal of diagnostic technologies have contributed to uncertainty in many contexts. Reflecting on the potential "problems of accuracy, reliability, [and] validity" of diagnostic tests, Dorothy Nelkin and Laurence Tancredi remind us that technology-mediated diagnosis "requires human judgment, and ultimately rests on a set of interpretive assumptions."[74] As one example of the need for human judgment in the context of a diagnostic technology, the initial Wassermann serology test for syphilis required the designation of a somewhat arbitrary threshold to differentiate positive from negative results, with the cutoff based on whether the public health threat of the disease was foregrounded.[75] As another example, a 1947 study of the interpretation of X-ray images noted a significant error rate not only when two different radiologists viewed the same image, but also when the same radiologist viewed the same X-ray image at two different times.[76] Consistent with these examples, human judgment has also been applied to decisions regarding what constitutes a "normal" diagnostic or screening test result for CF. In addition to discrepancies in interpreting a diagnostic test, scholars have noted the flaws inherent in using a test that is not capable of detecting a disease state, especially when a negative result is interpreted as the absence of disease.[77] Furthermore, challenges can arise when contrasting results from two or more diagnostic tests are interpreted, since physicians are more likely to believe evidence that supports their underlying assumptions and disregard conflicting evidence.[78]

Diagnostic uncertainty can also exist at the early stages of diseases with overlapping symptoms or because of variability in the clinical profile of a disease. For example, as documented by patient accounts from the nineteenth century, there was much uncertainty about whether someone had tuberculosis early on in their illness because the initial symptoms were so similar to other diseases, and analogous challenges have been observed in the setting of diphtheria and polio.[79] During the COVID-19 pandemic, confusion about how to interpret symptoms was reflected in widespread patient education materials that provided guidance on how to differentiate the early stages of SARS-CoV-2 infection from influenza or allergies.[80] Similarly, following the first comprehensive description of CF in 1938, many found it difficult to distinguish CF from other diseases with overlapping symptoms, and this challenge has continued to the present day.[81] On a related note, physician Alvan Feinstein suggested in 1963 that diagnostic confusion could be attributed to the wide range of clinical profiles and varying levels of symptom recognition in people with the same disease.[82] He argued that diagnostics was further complicated by the fact that physicians within each medical specialty saw a different population of patients, noting that "Pathologists, at the morgue, see the dead. Epidemiologists, in a field survey, see the asymptomatic. Clinicians see the hospitalized sick as in-patients and the ambulatory or mildly ill as out-patients."[83] This observation is particularly relevant in the case of CF, where many different specialists have been involved in patient care over the years.

In addition to reflecting on how medical professionals have understood and responded to uncertainty, scholars have paid careful attention to the impact of uncertainty on patients and their families. As sociologists Tanya Stivers and Stefan Timmermans point out, diagnostic uncertainty, which they define as "not knowing what causes a patient's symptoms," can take a "social-psychological toll" on patients and families, in which the "cause and legitimacy of symptoms, quality of life, and future plans" are called into question.[84] Highlighting the importance of a diagnostic label in affording social legitimacy, historian of medicine and physician Robert Aronowitz recounted how Alice James (sister of Henry and William James), who had been living undiagnosed as a "chronic invalid" for much of her life, "was dramatically relieved of the stigma and psychological burden of this social role" after she was diagnosed with breast cancer in 1891.[85] This example highlights how significant the stigma associated with undiagnosed disease must have been because cancer was also stigmatized at that time. As another example of the value of a diagnosis in the setting of symptoms, Lorri Devlin spent more than fifty years being told that her symptoms were due to such causes as nervousness, anxiety, or a panic disorder.[86] It wasn't until she had an episode on an airplane, which a passenger later described as a seizure, that she was diagnosed with epilepsy. As Devlin explained, "I literally wept with relief at finally having a diagnosis, an intelligent physician and a drug to manage my symptoms."[87] In this and other cases, the psychogenic label was particularly harmful not only because of the emotional and financial toll of not being believed, but because of the lost opportunity to benefit from effective therapeutics.[88] Furthermore, when a diagnosis comes in the form of a contested illness, in which the actual existence of the disease is debated by physicians and the legitimacy of the diagnosis is questioned, many of the social harms associated with diagnostic uncertainty in the context of unexplained symptoms also exist.[89]

Similar delays in diagnosis due to a psychogenic label have been documented in the case of CF. In just one of many examples, Katie K., born in the late 1980s, "felt sick every day" throughout her childhood, yet even as a young adult she was still seeking a diagnosis that accounted for her digestive issues, coughing, and shortness of breath.[90] By the time she was in her early twenties, she "felt defeated." As Katie recalled, "My doctors had concluded that I was depressed and making up symptoms. It felt like it was time to give up my desperate search and accept a life with an unknown disease."[91] After her ear, nose, and throat specialist became suspicious of lung disease based on the shape of her fingertips, he suggested that she might have cystic fibrosis. In fact, a characteristic feature of more advanced CF is finger or toe clubbing, which can occur in the setting of low oxygen levels.[92] However, her primary care physician disagreed and told her that she "would not be alive right now" if she had CF.[93] Against the advice of her primary care physician, Katie decided to pursue testing and was subsequently diagnosed with CF in 2010, at age twenty-two.[94] In another example, Maryanne O'Hara reflected on her experience with a physician who did not take her seriously before her daughter was diagnosed with CF at age two in the mid-1980s, explaining that "it always bothers me when I see people treated that way, that dismissive way . . . it made me really advocate for Caitlin . . . and if a doctor wasn't ready to take us seriously, then, well, it's time for a new doctor because it's just too important to have somebody who says it's all in your head."[95]

Consistent with accounts from parents and patients about delayed diagnoses, CF physician Lucy Lester recalled that "when I started in 1980 . . . diagnoses were missed all the time . . . because no test was done."[96] As Lester explained, "often, the scenario was such that a mom would bring a baby to a pediatrician or the family doctor and be told, 'oh, the baby just has a cold' . . . so that would be four or five times that mom knew something was wrong, but the doctor just didn't know . . . just kind of blew it off."[97] Lester went on to note that "finally . . . mom would go elsewhere . . . and eventually the sweat test would be done and would be diagnostic" for CF, at which point "the child was usually admitted [to the hospital] to begin a regimen of care."[98] Such delays in testing are just one of many reasons why people experience extended periods of diagnostic uncertainty.

* * *

As highlighted earlier, historians of medicine and technology have documented a wide range of factors that can contribute to diagnostic uncertainty in medicine, ranging from changing definitions of disease to assumptions about race or gender in the design and interpretation of diagnostic tests.[99] Scholars have also noted the increased reliance on technology over the patient narrative in the context of the biomedical model of disease. Furthermore, historians have offered compelling critiques of the presumed objectivity of these diagnostic technologies. *Challenging Diagnosis* builds on this rich historical scholarship and provides novel insight into the diagnostic process by examining a single disease over more than eighty years to document how diagnostic uncertainty persists even when the limitations of specific diagnostic approaches are acknowledged and addressed. As some sources of uncertainty are mitigated, new forms of uncertainty emerge, resulting in iatrogenic harms related to the diagnostic process. Furthermore, *Challenging Diagnosis* highlights the shortcomings of a reductionist biomedical model that relies on diagnostic technologies to identify specific disease entities, an issue that is broadly relevant as access to genetic information has expanded through such avenues as direct-to-consumer genetic testing and the increased use of whole genome sequencing in newborns. Finally, the story of CF diagnostics from the 1930s to the present takes place within the broader historical context of the evolution of postwar scientific funding, debates about health insurance and access to care, increased attention to civil rights and patient advocacy, and the rise of genetic information and related concerns about privacy. However, *Challenging Diagnosis* intentionally stays tightly focused on how diagnostic and screening technologies have been employed in the elusive quest for certainty, trading breadth for depth in the analysis of how stakeholders have grappled with and responded to the persistence of diagnostic uncertainty in medicine.

Chapter 1 sets the stage by looking at early debates about how to define and detect CF, providing an opportunity to examine the fundamental issue of differential diagnosis in medicine and associated uncertainties. Accounts consistent with CF go back hundreds of years or more, but New York physician Dorothy Andersen is often credited with the first comprehensive description of the disease in 1938, which drew in part on the prior work of other physicians, including Swiss pediatrician Guido Fanconi.[100] To characterize what she thought were different underlying causes of celiac disease (long before its association with gluten), Andersen examined autopsy reports and identified a group of patients who had what she termed "cystic fibrosis of the pancreas." Andersen argued in 1938 that "celiac disease is a *clinical picture* 'characterized by arrest of growth, a distended abdomen, and attacks of diarrhoea with large, pale, foul-smelling stools' *rather than a disease entity*," and later suggested that CF was one of several possible disease entities that could lead to symptoms consistent with the celiac syndrome.[101] Although most of the children she and others labeled as having CF by the late 1930s had both respiratory and gastrointestinal symptoms during life, Andersen postulated that all symptoms stemmed from a characteristic pancreatic lesion seen on autopsy. As such, initial diagnostic tests for CF targeted the pancreas. For example, the earliest test used a flexible tube to extract pancreatic fluids from digestive juices to test for the presence of pancreatic enzymes needed for food digestion, which were absent in people with CF. However, in a series of publications beginning in the mid-1940s, Boston physician Sidney Farber, best known for his later work on cancer, suggested that cystic fibrosis should be viewed as a systemic disease involving the mucus-secreting organs. Farber's view was reinforced in the late 1940s when several children with respiratory complications received a postmortem diagnosis of CF even though the disease had been ruled out during life based on a normal pancreatic function test. By the 1950s, physicians increasingly began to view CF as a systemic disease and called for new tests that would reduce diagnostic uncertainty by better identifying those with a wider range of disease manifestations.

The second chapter examines the diagnostic process in CF following the availability of a "better" diagnostic test that could identify patients regardless of their pancreatic function, providing insight into the nature of "gold standard" tests in medical practice. Once physicians realized in the early 1950s that many people with CF had elevated electrolytes in their sweat, a range of diagnostic tests were developed to measure sodium or chloride levels in sweat. To address some of the shortcomings of early sweat tests, in 1959 Johns Hopkins physicians developed a quantitative diagnostic sweat test, later referred to by physicians as the gold standard for CF diagnosis. However, even though this test was often described as the most accurate in medicine, the Gibson–Cooke sweat test for CF was not widely used in practice because some physicians found it too challenging or time-consuming, whereas others didn't even suspect CF in the first place due to physician inexperience, attitudes toward mothers, or assumptions about race. As one example, Terry Wright was born in 1962, three years after the Gibson–Cooke sweat test was developed, yet he was not diagnosed with CF until age fifty-four. As he recalled in 2021, when he was in his thirties, he visited a doctor who told him, "if it wasn't for me being African American, I would have cystic fibrosis."[102] Due to what Dorothy Roberts describes as "medical stereotyping" based on race, Wright went many more years and endured hospitalizations without appropriate treatment before being diagnosed with a sweat test.[103] Thus, even though the sweat test addressed one source of uncertainty stemming from a pancreas-specific test, in that it could diagnose people with a wider range of disease manifestations, diagnostic uncertainty persisted because this highly accurate sweat test was not widely used in practice.

The third chapter examines the development and implementation of screening programs for CF following widespread recognition of missed diagnoses, providing insight into the nature of screening in medicine more broadly. While screening approaches for CF have taken a variety of forms, the chapter focuses on several efforts that began in the 1970s within the broader context of screening programs for a wide range of diseases. At least as early as 1973, individual chapters of the National Cystic Fibrosis Research Foundation (later renamed the Cystic Fibrosis Foundation) enlisted parents to use their own sense of taste to screen for CF through what were termed "Kiss Your Baby" campaigns.[104] Parents were urged to determine whether their baby's skin was salty by means of a kiss and were directed to ask their physician to order a sweat test for CF if this home test was positive. The subjective nature of what constituted "too salty" contributed to challenges in interpreting this home test, but many children were diagnosed following a positive kiss test. Around the time that Kiss Your Baby awareness campaigns began in the United States, a New Zealand physician suggested that "three minutes and a bowl of water might provide a cheap screening test" for cystic fibrosis after he observed rapid skin wrinkling following water exposure in people with the disease.[105] While there was some initial interest in this "bucket test," it temporarily fell out of favor by the late 1970s, in part due to concerns that early skin wrinkling was not specific to CF and because a more promising screening test was being developed around the same time.[106] In 1979, in what one physician would later point to as "the shot heard around the world," physicians in New Zealand described a newborn screening test for CF using blood spots from Guthrie cards that were developed for phenylketonuria (PKU) newborn screening.[107] By 1982, Colorado had become the first US state to implement newborn screening for CF using this method, in which the level of a pancreas enzyme was measured in the blood, and those with a positive screen were referred for a sweat test. While newborn screening addressed issues associated with the sweat test, such as failure to test in the first place, new uncertainty was introduced in the form of false positive and false negative screening results.[108]

By documenting the incorporation of genetic testing into both screening and diagnostic strategies for CF, Chapter 4 provides insight into the benefits and limitations of the use of DNA analysis in medical diagnostics more broadly. As genetic medicine rose to prominence in the 1980s and 1990s, doctors and patients increasingly believed that genetic tests would offer conclusive results and reduce uncertainty. When the CF gene was characterized in 1989, a single mutation was identified in 68 percent of chromosomes studied from people with CF, and academic institutions and biotechnology companies quickly introduced a genetic test that could identify the most common CF gene mutation. With the goal of developing a more comprehensive test, scientists soon attempted to identify what were thought to be four to six additional CF gene mutations. For example, Jeff Pinard, a University of Michigan undergraduate with CF, had only one copy of the most common CF gene mutation, and he worked in the lab of Francis Collins over the summer of 1990 to try to identify the additional mutation that he and his sister with CF had. However, even as scientists characterized additional CF gene mutations, expanded mutation panels were still unable to detect all people with CF because the number of mutations (also referred to as disease-causing variants) in the CF gene vastly exceeded initial estimates.[109] To further complicate matters, a 2004 study documented that the clinical sensitivity of a twenty-five-mutation panel, a measure of how well an individual with CF can be detected, varied dramatically based on how someone was classified according to race or ethnicity, with a low of 23 percent for individuals labeled as "Asian American" and a high of 88.6 percent for those labeled as "Ashkenazi Jewish Caucasian."[110] Today, over two thousand CF gene variants (changes in the gene that may or may not be disease causing) have been described in the Toronto-based Cystic Fibrosis Mutation Database, and a recent study using data from UK Biobank identified more than four thousand CF gene variants.[111] Physicians and scientists have tried to address the problem of false negative results stemming from missing mutations in available screening or diagnostic testing panels by sequencing the CF gene, yet such an approach is also associated with uncertainty because it increases the detection of variants of uncertain clinical significance. Thus, diagnostic uncertainty has persisted, albeit in different forms, following the incorporation of genetic analysis into screening and diagnostic testing approaches. The case of CF raises more general notes of caution as access to genetic information has expanded.

As the fifth chapter illustrates, diagnostic uncertainty in CF has not been limited to tests for the disease itself, providing important insight into how uncertainty manifests in the context of secondary diagnoses.[112] Since people with CF have frequent and often persistent lung infections, they regularly undergo diagnostic testing for the presence of specific microorganisms. This chapter begins by documenting physicians' initial concerns in the late 1970s about the rapid and often fatal decline in health associated with a *Pseudomonas cepacia* (later renamed *Burkholderia cepacia*) diagnosis and subsequent efforts to prevent the spread of the microorganism among people with CF. Beginning in the 1980s, some physicians started to exclude *P. cepacia*–infected people from CF summer camps and other settings to curtail the spread of the microorganism. By the 1990s, however, many physicians had come to believe that people with CF did not always test positive for *P. cepacia* when infected, due in large part to difficulties isolating and identifying the microorganism. These sources of diagnostic uncertainty, coupled with the severe health decline linked to the infection, prompted those in leadership positions in the CF community to eventually consider each person with CF as a potential source of the microorganism, thereby limiting all in-person contact between those with CF by the early twenty-first century. This shift in the framing of CF, prompted by the diagnostic uncertainty associated with a microbe, had an immense impact on the lives of those living with the disease and those who cared for them. The response to concerns about contagion in people with CF has important parallels to infection control measures that have been put in place in the setting of diagnostic uncertainty about other infectious diseases, such as COVID-19.

Finally, the epilogue extends the theme of diagnostic uncertainty to more recent critiques of the notion of the "healthy CF carrier," providing key insights into the potential benefits and harms associated with widespread genetic testing for carrier status. Since CF has long been understood as an autosomal recessive disease, such that someone must have two disease-causing variants of the gene to have CF, brochures and pamphlets with information about carrier screening for CF have traditionally emphasized how carriers have no disease manifestations.[113] Consistent with long-standing descriptions of CF carriers as "healthy," even Gregor Mendel's work with pea plants, widely taught in educational settings, stressed how recessive alleles were completely masked by dominant ones, and that an organism expressed the recessive trait only if two copies of the mutant gene were present.[114] In fact, many have postulated that CF carriers may have a selective advantage, similar to the reduced susceptibility to malaria seen in sickle cell anemia carriers.[115] However, following the 2020 publication of a large-scale case-control retrospective study documenting the increased risk for fifty-seven health conditions in CF carriers, the view of CF carriers as completely healthy has become increasingly untenable.[116] Just as a single *BRCA1* mutation confers an increased risk of breast cancer, the 2020 study provided evidence that a single CF gene mutation is associated with an increased risk of numerous CF-related health conditions, further challenging the strict dichotomy of simple Mendelian genetic diseases versus complex diseases such as cancer, diabetes, and heart disease. Given my status as a CF carrier with pancreatic insufficiency and several other CF-related health conditions, as well as a more recent study suggesting that the risks associated with CF carrier status may be less pronounced, I reflect in the epilogue on how additional uncertainty about the etiology of my own chronic illness has arisen.[117] Furthermore, the type of reframing that has been taking place regarding CF carrier status may extend to other autosomal recessive genetic diseases as well, especially as genetic testing continues to expand and as large-scale studies of the clinical profile of those with common genetic variants become increasingly feasible.[118] These shifts in the understanding of what it means to be a carrier are likely to make it even more challenging to determine whether an individual should be given a disease label, further highlighting the elusive nature of diagnostic certainty in medicine.

Drawing from the history of CF, *Challenging Diagnosis* contributes to a rich body of scholarship focused on the complexity of the diagnostic process, including the fundamental role that technologies have come to play in the diagnosis and definition of disease, as well as the limitations of those technologies. The book documents how, as the constraints of one diagnostic technology for CF were acknowledged and addressed, new challenges arose in their place, such that diagnostic uncertainty remained a constant even after the advent of genetic testing. The book also contributes to scholarship that foregrounds the patient perspective in the history of medicine. In his influential article published in 1985, historian Roy Porter argued that more attention should be placed on presenting historical accounts of the "sufferers" in the history of medicine, and numerous works have since attended to the patient perspective.[119] By examining historical accounts of patients before and after a CF diagnosis over an extended period, the book documents the profound toll that diagnostic uncertainty can take on patients who are eventually labeled with a disease that is not typically associated with uncertainty and stigma in the way that contested diseases are. *Challenging Diagnosis* highlights how pervasive and persistent diagnostic uncertainty is, even for a genetic disease such as CF, and calls into question the validity of a biomedical model that prioritizes the identification of specific and discrete disease entities at the expense of the patient narrative. Furthermore, as the double meaning of the title suggests, *Challenging Diagnosis* not only documents how challenging the act of diagnosis in medicine is, but it also challenges the assumptions that go into making medical diagnoses and, by extension, critiques the stigma and relative lack of access to resources (social, financial, and medical) that result from not having a diagnosis.

CHAPTER ONE

Absent Enzymes

From Localized to Systemic Disease

Byron Bell had been "ill since birth" in Tampa, Florida, in 1951 and "his ailment was variously diagnosed as pneumonia, bronchitis and diarrhea" over the first year and a half of his life.[1] When Byron's mother brought him to the hospital during a visit to Miami in March 1953, the list of possible illnesses expanded to include celiac disease and cystic fibrosis before "tests brought out his true condition" and he was diagnosed with "cystic fibrosis of the pancreas."[2] Around that time, cystic fibrosis was described as an "incurable disease," characterized by a "chronic cough, repeated pneumonias, bulky diarrhea, and a tremendous appetite along with a poor weight gain."[3] Byron's parents soon learned from physicians that their son was unlikely to live to see his second birthday due to the progression of his illness, so they arranged for him to have an early birthday party alongside his sister's fourth birthday celebration.[4] Yet after the *Fort Lauderdale News* ran a story highlighting Byron's short life expectancy in July 1953, his family was contacted by "several mothers" who "tried to cheer the Bells by telling them of similar conditions in their children, who are still living."[5]

One mother called the Bells on the phone and told them about Boston physician Harry Shwachman, who had a track record of "remarkable success . . . with children suffering from cystic fibrosis."[6] Byron's family quickly got in touch with Shwachman, who suggested they bring Byron to Children's Medical Center in Boston for a comprehensive evaluation followed by treatment if the cystic fibrosis diagnosis was confirmed.[7] After arriving in Boston in July 1953, Byron was hospitalized, saw "nearly a dozen specialists," and had numerous tests performed throughout the week.[8] As Byron's mother recalled after seeing him in the hospital during visiting hours, "they put him through a lot of tests and took some fluid out of him, so he was pretty upset" and "didn't look too good."[9] The invasive diagnostic that removed digestive fluid from Byron involved the insertion of a thin, flexible tube into his nose or mouth, past the stomach, and into the initial section of the intestine called the duodenum, from which pancreatic digestive juices were isolated and analyzed.[10]

On completion of this and other tests over several days, the Boston physicians determined that Byron did *not* have cystic fibrosis after all and labeled him with celiac disease instead.[11] In explaining the change in diagnosis, Shwachman noted that "it takes a great deal of specialized laboratory study and analysis to tell the difference" between cystic fibrosis and celiac disease, and he emphasized that "the diseases are frequently confused."[12] After the celiac disease diagnosis, Byron was placed on a special diet and remained in the hospital for close monitoring until he was well enough to return home.[13] As Byron's mother explained of his time in the hospital, "he tells me everyday when I go to see him where the nurses have stuck him with needles," and "he points to the spot and says, 'That hurts'" (Figure 1.1).[14] Despite the challenges associated with his hospitalization, Byron's family was "overjoyed" on hearing that he had celiac disease, as physicians told them that he was expected to make a "complete recovery after a few years' special dietary treatment."[15] In fact, Byron's four-year-old sister, who had been told "before Byron left he might have to go to heaven, . . . whispered to her grandmother" on hearing the news, "Now we can keep him. The angels don't have to take him."[16]

The uncertainty surrounding Byron's diagnosis can be understood within the broader context of widespread concerns about gastrointestinal disease as a significant cause of infant mortality in the late nineteenth and early twentieth centuries and corresponding attempts by physicians to characterize various underlying etiologies of childhood diarrhea.[17] In fact, English physician Samuel Gee's "thorough and vivid description" of celiac disease, which he referred to as the "Coeliac Affection" in 1888, contributed to this wider effort to describe gastrointestinal diseases in children.[18] According to Gee, patients with celiac disease typically began to exhibit gastrointestinal symptoms "during the second year of life," with stools that were "loose, not formed, but not watery; more bulky than the food taken would seem to account for; pale in colour . . . , yeasty, frothy . . . , [and] stinking."[19] Furthermore, children with the celiac label were emaciated due to "failure of digestion" and often had a characteristic distended

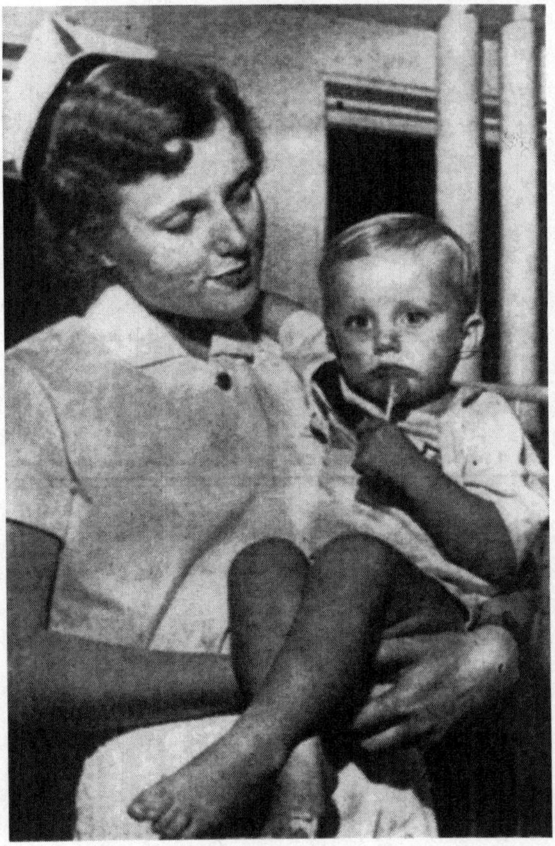

FIGURE 1.1. Photo of Byron Bell with nurse Alice Brown at Children's Medical Center in Boston. Image from Frank Hogan, "'Complete Recovery' Seen for Byron," *Fort Lauderdale News*, July 24, 1953. Copyright orphan.

abdomen.[20] In the decades following Gee's clinical description of the "coeliac affection," numerous physicians attempted to determine the etiology of the disease; by the 1930s, investigators postulated that celiac symptoms were due to several distinct disease entities, one of which was cystic fibrosis.

This chapter looks at early debates about how to define cystic fibrosis and distinguish it from other causes of the celiac syndrome, providing an opportunity to examine the process of differential diagnosis in medicine and the persistence of uncertainty even after the first diagnostic test for cystic fibrosis was introduced. Cystic fibrosis was initially described in the late 1930s as a distinct disease entity that could be distinguished from other causes of the celiac syndrome by a characteristic lesion of the pancreas on autopsy.[21] With the pancreas as the centerpiece of the disease definition, initial diagnostics for CF (including the invasive test that Byron Bell was subjected to) naturally examined pancreas function.[22] However, the pancreas-specific test for CF was limited by technical and theoretical barriers to its use as a diagnostic test. The invasive test to extract digestive juices from the intestine was technically difficult for some physicians to perform, patients didn't always tolerate the procedure, and digestive enzymes could be challenging to analyze once collected. From a theoretical standpoint, challenges also arose to the fundamental definition of CF as a specific disease of the pancreas. Boston physician Sidney Farber, best known for his later work on cancer, called into question the use of a pancreas-specific test when he suggested in the mid-1940s that cystic fibrosis should be viewed as a systemic disease involving the mucus-secreting organs instead of a pancreas disease.[23] Farber's view was reinforced in the late 1940s when several children with respiratory complications, including some of Shwachman's patients, received a postmortem diagnosis of CF even though the disease had been ruled out during life based on a normal pancreatic function test. By the 1950s, physicians increasingly began to view CF as a systemic disease and called for new tests that would reduce diagnostic uncertainty by better identifying those with a wider range of disease manifestations.

As this chapter documents, the pancreas-specific test for CF introduced in the late 1930s reduced some forms of uncertainty by providing a diagnosis for a subset of children with the celiac syndrome, yet the diagnostic technology also contributed to new forms of uncertainty because it was unable to detect all individuals during life who would go on to receive a postmortem diagnosis of CF. As such, uncertainty associated with a CF diagnosis persisted despite the availability of the pancreas-specific test, a theme that we will see repeated throughout the history of attempts to improve the diagnosis of CF by the introduction of new technologies.

From Celiac Disease to Cystic Fibrosis of the Pancreas

Ever since Samuel Gee's comprehensive description of celiac disease, physicians have attempted to determine its underlying etiology.[24] Of relevance to the history of CF, numerous physicians from the late nineteenth

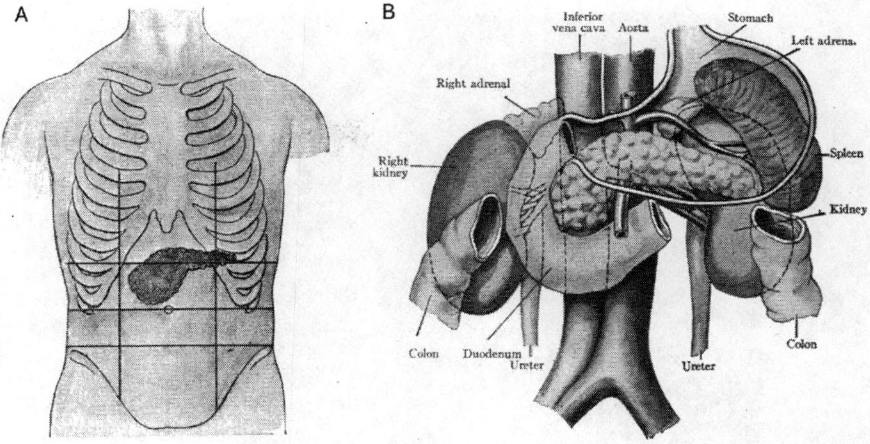

FIGURE 1.2. *A*: "Surface marking of the pancreas." *B*: "Diagram showing the relations of the pancreas." Note that the pancreas is the central unlabeled organ in both diagrams. Images from Robert Coleman Kemp, *Diseases of the Stomach, Intestines, and Pancreas*, 3rd ed. (W. B. Saunders, 1917), figures 403 and 404, respectively. This public domain book was digitized by Google.

century into the 1930s suspected that the pancreas might be involved in celiac disease.[25] Tucked between the stomach and the duodenum (a section of the small intestine), the pancreas is well positioned to empty its enzymes into the intestines to help the body digest food, as illustrated in Figure 1.2.[26] Of note, this *exocrine* function of the pancreas, involved in producing enzymes that aid in food digestion, has been relatively underexplored by historians, who have focused primarily on the hormone-producing, or *endocrine*, capacity of the pancreas in the context of diabetes.[27] Around the same time that physicians were exploring the possible role of the exocrine pancreas in celiac disease, reports began to emerge of patients with gastrointestinal symptoms (often described as celiac-like) "accompanied with frequent bronchitis, terminating sometimes in a fatal broncho-pneumonia."[28] By the mid-1930s, numerous physicians had described cases of celiac-like gastrointestinal symptoms and respiratory disease during life, and several (including Arthur Parmelee and Guido Fanconi) had also noted distinctive changes in the pancreas on autopsy.[29] Within the broader context of debates in the 1930s about the nature of celiac disease and its relationship to respiratory complications, physicians in New York and Boston independently sought to characterize what they thought was a new disease entity, eventually referred to as cystic

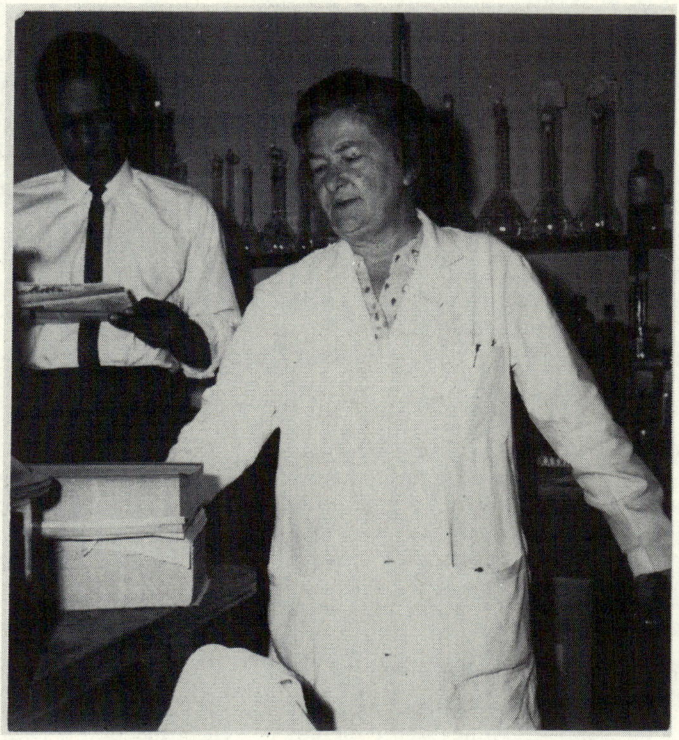

FIGURE 1.3. "Dr. Dorothy Andersen in her Lab." Box 1, folder 13, Dorothy Andersen Papers, Archives & Special Collections, Columbia University Health Sciences Library. Photo not dated. It is unknown who is standing behind Andersen.

fibrosis, that was associated with a characteristic lesion of the pancreas on autopsy.[30]

New York physician Dorothy Andersen is often credited with the first comprehensive description of "cystic fibrosis of the pancreas" in 1938, when she was a pathologist at Babies Hospital of Columbia University (Figure 1.3).[31] According to Andersen, her decision to go into medicine was prompted by the health challenges and early deaths of both of her parents.[32] After completing undergraduate studies at Mount Holyoke College, Andersen attended medical school in the 1920s at Johns Hopkins, where she did laboratory work under the guidance of physician Florence Sabin, the first female to be appointed to the faculty there.[33] Andersen went on to do an internship in surgery, with William Osler as one of her mentors, but she was denied the opportunity to complete training in surgery because of what many have pointed to as gender discrimination.[34] Soon afterward, Andersen began a position as an assistant in pathology at Presbyterian Hospital of Columbia University Medical Center in 1929, and she was affiliated with the Department of Pathology at Columbia for the remainder of her career.[35] Andersen also completed a doctorate in medical science in 1935, and she would later spend many years caring for patients with CF, advocating on their behalf, and corresponding with their parents, all while continuing as a pathologist.[36]

In her role as a pathologist, Andersen's interest in "pancreatic deficiency in infancy and childhood" and its possible relation to a celiac diagnosis was prompted by her autopsy examination of a three-year-old girl with celiac disease in 1935.[37] In the mid- to late 1930s, celiac disease continued to be a general term used to describe patients with severe digestive difficulties associated with diarrhea, characteristic pale stools, a distended abdomen, muscle wasting, reduced height and weight, anorexia, and extreme irritability.[38] The girl, referred to as patient M.D., had improved on a special diet "in which the calories were supplied chiefly by protein milk and bananas," a common regimen for people with celiac disease more than a decade before its association with gluten.[39] However, despite her improvement on the banana diet, the young girl died of bronchopneumonia, which she developed following a neck operation.[40] At that time, pneumonia was the third leading cause of death in the United States and the mortality rate in children was about 75 in 100,000.[41]

As a pathologist, Andersen carried out an autopsy on patient M.D. and observed several abnormalities, including changes in the part of the pancreas involved in food digestion.[42] The focus on autopsy findings to make sense of patients' symptoms during life was a common practice in the hospital setting by the early nineteenth century.[43] At that time, earlier conceptions of "sickness as a general physiological state" had been largely replaced with the view of diseases "as distinct clinical entities, each with a characteristic cause, course, and symptoms."[44] Physicians employed what Michel Foucault has termed the medical gaze, in which they proceeded from a patient's symptoms to the method of autopsy findings to locate diseased entities inside the body, which often manifested as lesions within particular organs.[45] Once located, a pathology that was identified postmortem could be used to explain the symptoms that the patient had experienced during life. As seen explicitly in the clinical case reports in leading medical journals in the United States around the time of Dorothy Andersen's work, the pathology findings were typically prioritized over clinical observations when finalizing a diagnosis.[46] Andersen used this approach to try to make sense of the young girl's symptoms.

While examining patient M.D.'s pancreas on autopsy, Andersen recalled that "a prolonged search for the pancreatic duct revealed only a small duct which . . . was then lost in fibrous tissue."[47] Andersen was aware that pancreatic digestive enzymes were secreted via pancreatic ducts into the initial section of the intestine, where they would act to digest food that had passed through the stomach. Therefore, her inability to find evidence of a duct connecting the pancreas to the intestine suggested that the pancreatic enzymes would not have been able to reach the intestine to aid in M.D.'s digestion. Such whole organ analysis is still practiced by pathologists today, yet physicians were able to extend pathology from the organ to microscopic tissue sections in the mid-nineteenth century, following "improvements in the optics and ease of use of the microscope . . . , the emergence of cell theory . . . , and the application of staining methods for microscopy."[48] In addition to her analysis of the whole organ, Andersen used the microscope to examine tissue sections derived from M.D.'s pancreas and observed "cystic fibrosis of the pancreas," a distinctive change in the tissue structure of the organ located in the part of the pancreas involved in digestive enzyme production.[49] The disease name "cystic fibrosis" is a shortened version of this early description of pancreatic changes visible on autopsy.

To make sense of the pancreatic lesion identified during the autopsy analysis of patient M.D., who in life had been given the celiac disease label based on her symptoms, Andersen sought additional cases of this specific pathology of the pancreas and characterized the clinical profile of these children during life.[50] One might think of Andersen's approach as an inversion of Foucault's medical gaze.[51] As noted earlier, physicians in the mid- to late 1930s were not in agreement about the role of the pancreas in celiac disease, as many patients, but not all, were found to have a normal pancreas on autopsy. Andersen hoped that by describing the clinical profile of individuals with the characteristic pancreatic lesion on autopsy, she might also shed some light on the possible connection between celiac disease and pancreatic disease.[52] In addition, Andersen aimed to compare the identified cases with those of patients with a celiac diagnosis in the absence of pancreatic fibrosis.

To find other examples of children with pancreatic fibrosis, Andersen examined autopsy reports from Babies Hospital at Columbia University, contacted other physicians, and consulted the published literature.[53] In particular, she sought out cases with "extensive lesions of the acinar tissue," known at that time to be responsible for pancreatic enzyme production, and her initial search revealed forty-nine cases of pancreatic fibrosis.[54] In her analysis of the case reports, Andersen explicitly stated that "the disease . . . is not confined to one race, country, or climate," although as subsequent chapters will illustrate, CF would be widely regarded as a "white disease" at other points in time, an erroneous assumption that is reflected throughout the book in archival images of people with CF.[55] Furthermore, because waves of immigrants were coming from Europe to the US in the first half of the twentieth century, "whiteness" as a category was being reconstructed during the period when CF was initially being described.[56] As part of Andersen's attempt to further characterize the disease, she divided the forty-nine cases of cystic fibrosis of the pancreas into three distinct groups based on the clinical features of the patients while living.[57] In other words, she first identified patients by autopsy and then subdivided them based on symptoms. In contrast, as physician and historian of medicine Steven Peitzman notes, patients with Bright's disease, who were initially identified as one group based on their symptoms, were divided into "three distinct pathological variants" based on autopsy findings of the kidney.[58]

Andersen's symptom-based classification system implied a continuum or spectrum of disease, a theme that comes up throughout the history of attempts to define and diagnose CF. As Andersen noted, group I consisted of patients who had died within one week of birth due to bowel obstruction, group II included patients who died between one week and six months from respiratory disease, and group III patients died after six months of age, also from respiratory disease. Many of the group II and group III patients had been given a celiac disease label or had gastrointestinal symptoms consistent with celiac disease before they died.[59] Andersen presented her findings at a joint meeting of the American Pediatric Society and the Society for Pediatric Research in Massachusetts on May 5, 1938, before publishing them in the *American Journal of Diseases of Children* that same year.[60] While many examples of all three categories of patients had been described in the medical literature before 1938, Anderson's contribution was considered significant by physicians because she was able to compile a wide range of cases and put them into a clear framework.[61] Furthermore, many physicians felt that Andersen helped to clarify some of the confusion about celiac disease and provide a much-needed comprehensive description of "cystic fibrosis of the pancreas," or what would become known as cystic fibrosis in the United States and many other regions.[62] In fact, Andersen argued that celiac disease could be considered a "clinical syndrome rather than a disease entity" and suggested that CF was but one cause of celiac symptoms that could be distinguished by the pancreatic abnormality on autopsy.[63]

Andersen's distinction between *syndrome* and *disease* can be placed within the broader history of diagnostics, where a "syndrome" is the label given when a constellation of symptoms cannot be linked to an underlying cause, and a "disease" label is applied when symptoms are accompanied by a proposed mechanism.[64] In the discussion that followed Andersen's 1938 presentation of her work, physician Benjamin Kramer of Brooklyn agreed that cystic fibrosis of the pancreas was a "distinct clinical entity" with symptoms that "may superficially resemble those of celiac disease."[65] However, unlike "true celiac disease, which has been described by Gee and others," Kramer noted that cystic fibrosis of the pancreas was characterized by the "early onset of symptoms, which often begin at birth, the high mortality of this disease, the marked tendency of these patients to contract fatal diffuse bronchopneumonia and the peculiar pancreatic lesion."[66] Consistent with this account, historian of medicine Emily Abel notes that the 1938 characterization of cystic fibrosis "as a distinct clinical entity had removed some very sick children from the celiac label."[67] Of all these features that distinguished CF from celiac disease, the pancreas stood out, contributing to the early characterization of CF as a pancreatic disease that was sometimes, but not always, associated with respiratory complications.

In addition to pondering the relationship between celiac disease and cystic fibrosis of the pancreas, the conversation in response to Andersen's 1938 conference presentation highlighted similar studies that had been carried out in Boston. As one physician in attendance pointed out, Boston pediatricians and pathologists Kenneth Blackfan, S. Burt Wolbach, Sidney Farber, and Charles May had been "engaged in correlating the clinical and pathologic manifestations of infants and children who presented these important changes in the pancreas" over the "past few years."[68] Shortly after Andersen presented her findings in 1938, Boston pediatricians Kenneth Blackfan and Charles May described the "clinical manifestations" of a group of patients at the Infants' and Children's Hospitals in Boston who had been identified by the presence of "an advanced lesion of the pancreas" on autopsy.[69] Based on work that had begun before Andersen's 1938 report and took over fifteen years to complete, they described thirty-five cases of a "well-defined pathologic lesion" of the pancreas, "the existence of which was unsuspected during life."[70] Consistent with Andersen's approach, Blackfan and May used the presence of the pancreatic lesion as a way to identify a distinct group of patients to include in their study, and then characterized the clinical profile of those patients.

Blackfan and May didn't use the term cystic fibrosis of the pancreas, an early indication that the name of the disease would be debated in the years to come, yet they did cite Andersen's 1938 work and provide evidence that the pancreatic lesion and clinical features of the disease were similar across the two studies.[71] In characterizing the clinical course of those with the pancreatic lesion on autopsy, Blackfan and May noted, like Andersen, variation in symptoms during life. Of the thirty-five patients they identified, five "died soon after birth" and thirty had weight loss or difficulty gaining weight, frequent diarrhea, and "a widespread pulmonary infection" leading to death.[72] In addition to the thirty-five cases defined by the presence of a severe pancreatic lesion, the Boston physicians also identified over two hundred patients who had evidence of "early stages of the process" of pancreatic fibrosis on autopsy, a finding that would become especially important in subsequent years as physicians contemplated how best to diagnose the disease during life.[73] Reflecting in 1943 on the early comprehensive descriptions of CF, Boston physician Sidney Farber argued that "these cases had been set apart as a pathologic entity because of the constant occurrence of an obstructive lesion of the pancreas."[74] In other words, despite agreement by many physicians that CF involved the gastrointestinal and respiratory systems, the pancreatic abnormality was a necessary condition for inclusion of cases in this disease category, a diagnostic definition that in the next decade physicians would come to find constraining, and then wholly inadequate, in understanding and diagnosing CF.

A Localized, Pancreas-Specific Test to Diagnose CF in Living Patients

While many physicians agreed that the pancreatic lesion on autopsy defined a newly characterized disease, often referred to as cystic fibrosis of the pancreas or pancreatic fibrosis, this method of diagnosis only allowed for postmortem identification of patients. To identify people with the disease during life, many investigators realized that it would be necessary to employ a diagnostic technology capable of detecting the pancreatic abnormality. In Andersen's initial 1938 report, at a time when many diagnostic

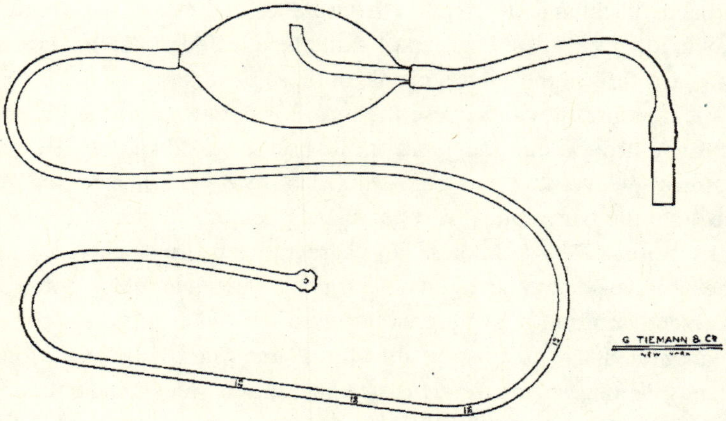

FIGURE 1.4. "Duodenal tube for use in infants, with metal ball and glass bulb, for aspiration and collection of duodenal juice." This public domain image is from Alfred F. Hess, "A Duodenal Tube for Infants," *American Journal of Diseases of Children* 1, no. 5 (1911): 360–65, 361.

technologies were available in the hospital setting, she suggested that it might be possible to distinguish cases of cystic fibrosis of the pancreas from other causes of the celiac syndrome during life by examination of the digestive fluid for the presence of pancreatic enzymes.[75] This focus on diagnosis based on the function of an organ was not unique to CF. By the early twentieth century, as Steven Peitzman points out, there was "enthusiasm for trying to understand disease in terms of what an injured organ could or could not do rather than how it looked."[76] At the time of Andersen's 1938 report, physicians had already developed a technique for the collection and analysis of pancreatic "juice" that could be obtained by duodenal intubation, the same type of invasive procedure that Byron Bell had to remove digestive fluid from the initial section of the intestine (termed the duodenum, as noted earlier).[77] While there is some debate about who first developed the duodenal intubation test as a means to gauge pancreatic function, attempts to obtain duodenal juice in adults, as opposed to stomach contents, had begun by the late nineteenth century.[78]

Of particular importance to CF, physician Alfred Hess described a duodenal tube in 1911 that he had adapted for use in infants.[79] A metal ball was attached to the tube at one end to aid in its movement from the mouth to the stomach and eventually into the duodenum; a glass bulb collected digestive juices (Figure 1.4). Hess argued that the duodenal tube might shed light on the frequent yet "unexplained cases of malnutrition" in infants, which he thought could be due to differences in the pancreatic "ferments" or enzymes.[80] In 1912, in what was later described by Andersen as "pioneer work," Hess documented that the pancreatic enzymes trypsin, lipase, and amylase were present in the duodenal juice in infants.[81] At that time, Hess and others understood that lipase could digest or split fat, amylase was involved in carbohydrate metabolism, and trypsin digested protein.[82] Hess initially used the modified tube shown in Figure 1.4, but then determined that a "simple catheter" worked just as well.[83] While he had expected to see a "deficiency of these ferments" in infants with severe malnutrition, pancreatic enzymes were present in the duodenal juice of all infants he tested.[84] Even though Hess was unable to detect any pancreatic enzyme abnormalities in the duodenal juice of malnourished infants, Andersen noted that several studies in the 1930s, including her own study of children with cystic fibrosis of the pancreas, used the duodenal intubation test to detect decreased enzyme levels in patients with "congenital pancreatic deficiency."[85] Thus, in 1938, when Andersen suggested that the duodenal intubation test could be used to identify patients with cystic fibrosis of the pancreas, numerous studies had already documented that pancreatic enzymes were diminished in the digestive juices of individuals with pancreatic disease.[86]

Andersen and other physicians focused on the pancreas in the diagnosis of CF during life due in large part to the uniqueness of the pancreatic lesion on autopsy. For example, despite acknowledging that the primary presenting symptoms could involve the respiratory system, Boston physicians Kenneth Blackfan and Charles May argued in 1938 that it was necessary to examine the "exocrine function of the pancreas," the part of the pancreas involved in the secretion of digestive enzymes, before establishing a "definite diagnosis" of cystic fibrosis.[87] On a related note, Sidney Farber pointed out that the "roentgen-ray appearance of the pulmonary lesions that are so consistently part of the disease" were not unique to those with cystic fibrosis.[88] As Farber explained, since "these x-ray manifestations of pulmonary disease . . . occur so frequently, . . . studies designed to confirm or exclude this diagnosis, such as analysis of pancreatic-enzyme activity, should be carried out whenever such changes are encountered."[89] Although Farber didn't use terms such as sensitivity and specificity, he had an intuitive sense that the respiratory findings were not diagnostically useful because they were not specific (i.e., someone with lung findings on X-ray might not have CF), whereas the pancreatic findings, though harder to document, were more specific and therefore more useful diagnostically.[90]

As another Boston physician pointed out in 1943, the absence of pancreatic enzymes in duodenal fluid was "almost pathognomonic" (definitive) for pancreatic fibrosis or cystic fibrosis.[91]

From the time of Andersen's 1938 report through the 1940s, physicians stressed the value of the duodenal intubation test, especially as a means to distinguish patients with CF from others with celiac-like symptoms.[92] In fact, the 1940 Boston Infants' Hospital annual report emphasized the importance of this diagnostic test because it used a "clever device" that allowed physicians to determine whether a patient had "true celiac disease, a condition which may be treated with success," or cystic fibrosis, "which so far has been invariably fatal."[93] In the clinicopathological case report of a young boy diagnosed with cystic fibrosis, a Boston physician noted in 1940 that "the absence of duodenal enzymes is a most important finding, and to me points directly at a lesion in the pancreas."[94] During discussion of the pathology of the case, Sidney Farber stressed that pancreatic fibrosis could be distinguished from "true celiac disease" by the absence of pancreatic enzymes in the former.[95] In fact, according to an account in the *Miami Herald* of Byron Bell's time at Children's Medical Center in Boston, "the first indication that the child was not suffering [from] cystic fibrosis came when tests showed 'pancreas fluid looked good.' "[96]

While many physicians, including Sidney Farber, noted the value of the duodenal intubation test in differentiating cystic fibrosis from other causes of celiac-like gastrointestinal symptoms, Farber also argued in 1943 that examination of pancreatic enzyme levels in duodenal fluid "appears to be the most valuable single laboratory aid" in the diagnosis of CF in patients *without* celiac-like symptoms as well.[97] In particular, Farber and his Boston colleagues Harry Shwachman and Charlotte Maddock stressed that the duodenal intubation test allowed for the diagnosis of patients under one year of age with respiratory symptoms that "obscure the nutritional aspect of the disease."[98] In other words, even when physicians acknowledged cases in which the respiratory symptoms of CF were more pronounced than the gastrointestinal symptoms, they still suggested that a pancreatic test be used to diagnose the disease. By the late 1940s, according to a Boston physician, it had "become a very common procedure . . . to intubate any baby or any young child who shows anything that may in any way suggest this pancreatic fibrosis."[99] In fact, reflecting on the duodenal intubation procedure in a 1984 oral history interview, Shwachman recalled that "we got so good at it that we were able to do five procedures in one morning. . . . I think in the years that I did it, I did at least 3,000 intubations."[100]

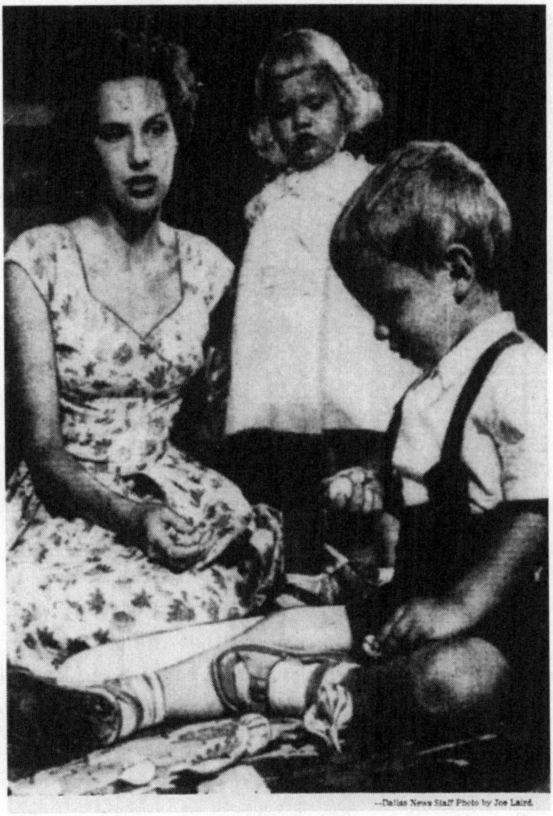

FIGURE 1.5. Photograph of Dr. Wynne Sharples and her two children, Nadya and Sergei, who were diagnosed with cystic fibrosis. Photograph by Joe Laird was included in the article "Her Children Victims: Mother Waging Fight on Disease," by Helen Bullock, *The Dallas Morning News*, May 22, 1955. Permission to reproduce the image granted by *The Dallas Morning News*. © 1955 by The Dallas Morning News.

Several parents pointed to the important role that the duodenal intubation test for pancreas enzymes played in diagnosing their own children with cystic fibrosis in the mid-twentieth century, at a time when the disease was largely viewed as inherited, likely in an autosomal recessive manner.[101] For example, physician Wynne Sharples suspected that her newborn daughter Nadya had CF in the early 1950s, based on the similarity of her symptoms to those of her older brother Sergei, who had already been diagnosed with the disease, and "a test of juices from the child's duodenum . . . confirmed her fears" (Figure 1.5).[102] Sharples would go on to found the Children's Exocrine Research Foundation in 1955, which would eventually be called the Cystic Fibrosis Foundation, "for the single purpose of getting cystic fibrosis cured as fast as possible."[103] (The foundation will be discussed in subsequent chapters.) Similarly, Doris Tulcin, who was president of the Cystic Fibrosis Foundation from 1976 to 1982, recalled that her daughter Ann was "given a duodenal drainage" shortly after her birth in 1953 to "ascertain what enzymes were missing."[104] The results from this test, along with "an intestinal blockage at birth" were "confirmation toward making a diagnosis" of cystic fibrosis.[105] In fact, as Tulcin noted during an interview years later, Ann was diagnosed by physician Dorothy Andersen.[106]

Barriers to Employing the Localized, Pancreas-Specific Test for CF

Despite the importance of the duodenal intubation test for the diagnosis of CF, physicians soon began to recognize both technical and theoretical barriers to its widespread and sustained implementation as a diagnostic. From a technical standpoint related to the "palatability" of the technology, the intubation procedure itself could be difficult for physicians to carry out and for patients to tolerate.[107] Even after the digestive juices were collected from the duodenum, many physicians found it challenging to perform the chemical analysis to detect pancreas enzymes, and false positive (a positive test in the absence of disease) and false negative (a negative test in the presence of disease) results occurred for a variety of reasons. From a theoretical standpoint, some physicians began to question the justification of a localized, pancreas-specific test for a disease that was increasingly being viewed as systemic, especially since the pancreas-specific test failed to detect CF in some children who were not diagnosed until autopsy and had therefore missed out on potentially life-prolonging therapeutic interventions. These challenges would lead many to doubt whether the duodenal intubation test could provide diagnostic certainty.

Technical Challenges Associated with the Duodenal Intubation Test

Although physicians often described the duodenal intubation test as the most definitive diagnostic for CF in the mid-twentieth century, diagnostic uncertainty associated with the test arose in part due to notable variation in how difficult and risky they felt the intubation procedure was.[108] In 1942, Dorothy Andersen stressed that "no untoward effects were observed . . . when the procedure was carried out as described" with the use of a fluoroscopic table to gauge the location of the collection tube as it traveled to the duodenum.[109] However, she did acknowledge "psychic trauma" associated with the test, which was more pronounced in adults compared to infants and children.[110] For infants less than six months old, Andersen and her colleagues typically inserted the tube through the mouth, past the stomach, and into the duodenum, and these "younger infants often appear to consider the tube a fair substitute for a meal, but this illusion decreases with age."[111] For infants and children over six months of age, the tube was typically inserted through the nose. According to Andersen, "older infants object to the passage of the tube, but when it is in place and stationary, they are able to forget about it and sleep or play."[112] In children over two years old, "cooperation can often be obtained throughout the procedure, and after the tube is in place the patient usually becomes engrossed in the crayons and paint books provided."[113]

While Andersen's accounts of the duodenal intubation procedure are generally favorable, not all medical professionals described the technique in such positive terms. For example, Houston physicians characterized the duodenal intubation test as "the most valuable diagnostic procedure" for cystic fibrosis in 1947, yet they used the test to make a diagnosis in only one of the ten patients they described because they found it "difficult to intubate the duodenum" and "technically difficult to perform" the enzyme analysis.[114] In fact, even Dorothy Andersen noted in 1950 that "all of us who have had experience with patients having fibrocystic disease have known trouble in duodenal intubation."[115] Lewis Gibson's experience with the duodenal intubation test while a medical student in the early 1950s suggests that tacit knowledge may have played a role in the challenges that some experienced with the procedure.[116] (Gibson's role in later developing a sweat test for CF will be discussed in Chapter 2.) While working at a hospital in Atlanta during his summer vacations from medical school, Gibson "sometimes encountered considerable difficulty getting a tube . . . into the duodenum," so he sought and received guidance from Andersen.[117] In her response letter to Gibson, Andersen "included a drawing of a small brass dumbbell, about the size of two BB shot, which she tied to the end of the duodenal tube" to "make the tube easier to manipulate." Andersen explained that "she had filed the dumbbell to size and shape herself," which Gibson also did, and "found that it was quite helpful."[118]

Although Andersen's guidance was clearly beneficial to medical professionals in some instances, numerous accounts suggest that the test was not palatable from the perspective of patients.[119] For example, while a Los Angeles physician highlighted the "accuracy" of the duodenal intubation test for the diagnosis of cystic fibrosis in 1948, he also pointed out that the "procedure . . . is a severe ordeal for a baby already exhausted by the disease."[120] Consistent with this description, a young girl from Iowa who was born in 1952 was diagnosed with cystic fibrosis following what was described as a "painful, day-long test for enzymes."[121] Of particular concern, a Melbourne physician noted that the death of two patients "appears to have been precipitated" by the duodenal intubation procedure, highlighting the potentially more serious risks associated with the test.[122] In other words, the diagnostic test itself could place an individual's health, and possibly life, at risk, a concern that contributed to diagnostic uncertainty because the test was not always used in practice.

Some physicians argued that the challenges associated with the duodenal intubation test had contributed to a particularly grim definition of cystic fibrosis that was unwarranted. Describing the duodenal intubation as "disturbing, time-consuming and occasionally unsuccessful," Boston physicians noted that many investigators had been "loath to attempt it unless the clinical features were classical, of long-standing, or extreme in degree," and this approach has "no doubt . . . led to the recognition of the more advanced cases and has, in general, painted a black [*sic*] prognostic picture for the disease."[123] In other words, some physicians suggested that the test was more likely to be used in cases of severe disease, such that those with milder symptoms were unlikely to get tested and continued to experience uncertainty regarding their diagnosis. Following this reasoning, the failure to test and identify people with milder symptoms contributed to a false impression that the prognosis for someone diagnosed with CF was always quite bleak.

Even in cases where the duodenal intubation test was done, physicians noted difficulties in analyzing the pancreatic enzymes in the laboratory setting. As Andersen and her colleague pointed out in 1942, the initial method used to measure enzyme activity in duodenal fluid was too complicated for routine use because it required "fairly elaborate equipment, much of which is not found in a hospital routine laboratory."[124] Even after Andersen and colleagues addressed the lack of widespread access to the needed infrastructure by developing a simpler method of enzyme analysis that was "adequate for diagnostic purposes," concerns about potential sources of error remained.[125] For example, although the pancreas was known to secrete three digestive enzymes, as noted earlier, trypsin alone was often used as a stand-in for the levels of all pancreatic enzymes when carrying out the duodenal intubation test because it was considered to be the "most uniform" and "most reliable index of pancreatic function."[126] However, as Sidney Farber pointed out in 1943, the approach of examining trypsin alone could lead to a false positive diagnosis of cystic fibrosis because "rare exceptions may be encountered" in which a child may have a selective deficiency of trypsin but have normal levels of the other enzymes.[127] Various additional sources of error associated with digestive enzyme analysis following duodenal intubation were identified over the course of the 1940s and into the 1950s.[128]

Questioning the Theoretical Underpinnings of a Pancreas-Specific Test for CF

In addition to grappling with ongoing diagnostic uncertainty due to the unpalatability and technical challenges of the duodenal intubation test in the 1940s and early 1950s, some physicians came to question the theoretical underpinnings of a localized, pancreas-specific test. While many physicians pointed to the pancreatic lesion as a defining feature of cystic fibrosis in the years following Andersen's report, Boston physician Sidney Farber soon found the primary focus on the pancreatic manifestations of the disease to be problematic. As early as 1943, several years before his seminal work on the systemic treatment of childhood leukemia, Farber argued that CF "is unfortunately much more than a lesion of the pancreas, and indeed, the great amount of attention paid to the pancreas in the recent literature, and even in this discussion, may serve to increase the neglect of the respiratory and other changes that emphasize the systemic nature of the process."[129] In fact, Farber clearly felt in 1943 that one could have cystic fibrosis in the absence of pancreatic disease. As he pointed out, "involvement of the lungs and the liver, with no disease in the pancreas, and therefore absence from the clinical picture of those symptoms referable to pancreatic insufficiency, provides further evidence for the systemic nature of the underlying disease process, and places the lesion in the pancreas in its proper setting."[130]

During the pathological discussion of a Massachusetts General Hospital case published in the same year, Farber provided additional context for his view that CF was a systemic disease in which multiple organs could be affected by the same underlying process. In the case of the pancreas, Farber noted that the changes seen on autopsy were caused by inspissated (thickened) pancreatic secretions, leading to obstruction in the regions of the pancreas involved in digestive enzyme secretion. He felt that the obstruction then led to atrophy of these regions, termed the acini, as well as the "formation of new fibrous tissue."[131] Farber went on to explain his view that "the same mechanism responsible for the pancreatic change appears to be responsible for the changes in the respiratory tract," where he noted that the "major bronchi and bronchioles are filled with inspissated material, and these infants may actually die of suffocation."[132] In fact, Farber believed that the lung, pancreas, and other organs were all "affected by a general pathologic process involving secretory structures in many parts of the body."[133] In this model, the secretory structures affected in the setting of CF resulted in the same "fundamental change" in which the "material secreted is more viscid, flows less readily than normal and, by mechanical action, causes obstruction to the duct system or gland system with an eventual fibrous-tissue replacement distal to the point of obstruction."[134]

Consistent with his view of the systemic nature of CF, Farber argued that the disease accounted for a "variety of clinical appearances, the occurrence of which depends on when the obstructive changes occur and which organs are affected."[135] For example, when achylia, or the absence of pancreatic enzyme secretion, occurs before birth, an infant is more likely to develop an intestinal obstruction referred to as meconium ileus. The meconium (the baby's first stool) usually passes within the first day following birth, but when the meconium is especially thick due to the lack of pancreatic digestive enzymes, it can be retained and cause an intestinal obstruction.[136] In those patients who developed achylia after birth, the meconium would be of the proper consistency to pass as the baby's first stool, yet gastrointestinal symptoms would be evident during infancy or later and "the disease picture will be that of the celiac syndrome."[137] In other words, the clinical profile of those diagnosed with CF suggested a spectrum of disease. Furthermore, critiquing the widespread emphasis on the gastrointestinal manifestations of the disease, Farber instead wanted to draw attention to the "possible occurrence in some patients of disease of the lungs, the upper respiratory tract, the liver and the intestinal tract without involvement of the pancreas."[138] Farber felt that cystic fibrosis was characterized by the "widespread involvement of mucus-secreting structures in the body" and postulated that those with the disease might be lacking or deficient in the "mucinase required for the maintenance of mucus in a normal physical state."[139] Almost a decade later, London physician Martin Bodian would point to Farber's work as foundational in the shift to thinking of CF as a systemic disease.[140]

After postulating that the root cause of CF might be a mucus abnormality, Farber suggested in 1945 that the disease be temporarily renamed *muco-viscidosis* because the term was "more inclusive than *pancreatic fibrosis* or *cystic fibrosis* which describes only one feature of the disease."[141] Farber recognized that the disease manifested in the respiratory tract, gastrointestinal system, and salivary glands and noted that "death is produced usually by upper respiratory and pulmonary obstruction and infection."[142] In addition, several years before proposing this name change, Farber highlighted another problem with the term cystic fibrosis, pointing out that there were "no true cysts" in the pancreas of patients with the disease.[143] However, five years after Farber first proposed the new name for the disease, Dorothy Andersen remarked, "I am unable to restrain myself from commenting on the term 'mucoviscidosis,' though I probably should not do so."[144] Andersen was concerned that the name "has the semantic ill effect of giving one the illusion that the basic causation of the disease is known," and she pointed out that "it is possible but not yet proved that the pancreatic and pulmonary lesions rest on the same mechanisms, and until proof is forthcoming I prefer to keep an open mind."[145]

In addition to Farber's critique of the pancreas-centeredness of both the name and the definition of the disease, other physicians came to question the priority placed on pancreatic changes as a means of identifying all patients with CF. About a decade after Andersen's 1938 publication, some physicians started to suspect CF in patients who presented primarily with respiratory symptoms. In 1948, Cleveland physician William Sinclair Jr. described the case history of a male infant who died at five months of age following bronchopneumonia and a history of some gastrointestinal complications.[146] Although the boy had normal pancreas enzyme levels in the duodenal juice and normal fat content in the stools, autopsy analysis revealed that "approximately one-half of the pancreas is the seat of cystic fibrosis while the remainder is approximately normal."[147] Given these findings, Sinclair questioned Andersen's prior claim that one can rule out cystic fibrosis of the pancreas if "appreciable quantities of enzymes are demonstrated in the duodenal juice."[148] In several other well-described cases of patients with CF-like respiratory symptoms, the duodenal intubation test demonstrated normal pancreatic enzyme levels, prompting physicians to rule out CF, yet pancreatic fibrosis was later detected on autopsy.[149] Thus, the recognition that changes in the pancreas could occur before the enzymes in duodenal fluid were significantly reduced reinforced Farber's critique of the pancreas-centeredness of the disease and called into question the value of the duodenal intubation test as a way to diagnose CF.

In his acceptance speech for the 1949 E. Mead Johnson Award for pediatric research, Harry Shwachman described two additional instances of diagnostic uncertainty associated with the test for pancreatic enzymes.[150] One girl had a duodenal intubation test in December 1948, at age two and a half, because she "had sufficient pulmonary symptoms to suggest the possibility of mucoviscidosis," or CF.[151] At that time, the CF diagnosis was "ruled out" because the level of trypsin in her duodenal fluid was normal.[152] Due to the continued suspicion of CF and the finding of increased duodenal fluid viscosity (which was also seen in another patient who was diagnosed postmortem), the duodenal intubation was repeated in November 1949, at which time there was "a slight reduction in the tryptic activity."[153] Reflecting on their "failure to make a correct antemortem [CF] diagnosis" in a different patient with normal pancreatic enzyme levels, Shwachman postulated that some patients could have detectable enzymes in the duodenal fluid "during the early phase of their illnesses."[154] Thus, physicians increasingly came to question the use of duodenal enzyme analysis for the diagnosis of CF, as the test was not sensitive enough to detect the initial damage to the pancreas that was visible on autopsy.

Around the time that the framing of CF was shifting from a pancreatic to a systemic disease, some physicians, including Shwachman, also believed that early diagnosis would lead to better outcomes, in large part because of the increasing availability of therapeutic interventions for the disease.[155] Initial therapeutics for CF focused on the digestive and respiratory complications, with such interventions as oral pancreatic enzyme administration to aid with food digestion, changes in diet, vitamin supplementation, and antibiotics to treat bacterial lung infections.[156] According to Shwachman, "the introduction of the sulfonamides, penicillin and streptomycin marked a signal advance in the management of the pulmonary infection."[157] However, he later recalled in an oral history interview that these early antibiotics "weren't any good" for treating people with CF and instead favored the broad-spectrum antibiotic aureomycin when it became available.[158] As Shwachman explained, "I was the first one to use [aureomycin] in my practice in 1948, and everybody thought I was crazy because I showed that patients did very well . . . that was the first positive step in the treatment, because children would live . . . they were dying much later; they lived through going to school."[159] Expressing a similar sentiment in 1948, Los Angeles physician Lowell Goin argued that "unless recognized fairly early, the disease will be fatal, while with an early diagnosis established and therapy instituted, some of these babies may be saved."[160]

Despite the belief by many physicians that early therapeutic interventions improved outcomes in CF, the ultimately fatal course of the disease was still a significant concern. For example, also in 1948, Boston physician Gertrud Reyersbach noted how "disappointing" it was to treat the respiratory infection in individuals with CF since even when the initial microorganism could be treated, it was often not possible to treat the subsequent infection.[161] She lamented, during the time that physician and historian of medicine Scott Podolsky refers to as the first period of response to antibiotic resistance concerns in the United States, that "often, all the organisms become drug resistant."[162] In other words, antibiotics had introduced hope for better outcomes in CF, but these hopes were tempered because doctors quickly realized that resistance was a problem. However, even with the acknowledgment of such limitations, many physicians still agreed on the value of early diagnosis because of the ability to initiate therapeutics that targeted the respiratory and gastrointestinal systems, and they expressed concern that the duodenal intubation test for pancreas enzymes was not able to identify all people with CF.

Calls for a Systemic-Focused Diagnostic That Would Reduce Uncertainty

By the early 1950s, around the time that Byron Bell was seen at Children's Medical Center in Boston, many physicians thought that the diagnostic criteria for CF should be reevaluated because they had come to believe that it was possible for a patient to have the disease in the absence of clinically detectable gastrointestinal symptoms or reduced pancreatic enzymes.[163] For example, in 1950, physician Gordon Gibbs and colleagues suggested that a different test for CF was needed that was "based perhaps on a defect in some mucolytic system and not dependent on pancreatic insufficiency."[164] Consistent with this view, Shwachman also noted around this time "that this disease is a generalized one and may involve mucus-secreting glands in different degrees and in different parts of the body."[165]

However, not all physicians agreed that the diagnostic criteria for cystic fibrosis should be expanded to include those with subclinical or non-detectable pancreatic disease. As Iowa physician Charles May argued in his 1954 book *Cystic Fibrosis of the Pancreas in Infants and Children*, efforts to "include patients who are assumed to be 'subclinical' or 'partial' manifestations of the definite, fully developed disease" are problematic because the very "existence of such patients is controversial."[166] May was particularly concerned that the inclusion of such patients with milder symptoms would negatively impact diagnostic accuracy "by encouraging too free inclusion of vague digestive disorders or too generous interpretation of minor laboratory findings and pathological changes in the pancreas."[167] Despite these concerns, May did leave open the possibility that these "more frequent minor changes of a similar nature in the pancreas" represented an earlier stage of the same disease process but argued that "considerably more evidence will be required to make it convincing."[168]

In fact, just one year later, Harry Shwachman and colleagues provided the type of evidence that May had called for. In a 1955 publication, the Boston physicians described the history of one patient who had six duodenal intubation tests over three years, from which they were able to "demonstrate progression of the pancreatic lesion from relatively mild involvement to complete enzyme deficiency."[169] They noted that it was therefore "impossible" to make the diagnosis of CF in such patients with "mild" disease manifestations when they are initially seen and that diagnostic certainty can only be established "in retrospect."[170] Based on the finding of progressive pancreatic involvement over time, Shwachman and colleagues reiterated the problem in relying on pancreatic function as a diagnostic metric for the disease, just two years *after* they ruled out CF in Byron Bell in 1953 in part because of the presence of normal levels of pancreatic enzymes in his digestive fluid. As Shwachman and colleagues pointed out in 1955, the "loss of exocrine secreting ability of the pancreas may be gradual" and therefore an individual may have cystic fibrosis in the setting of detectable pancreatic enzymes.[171] In other words, even though the duodenal intubation test was initially favored as a way to allow for the diagnosis of CF during life, it became clear in the 1950s that it was not a decisive test for the disease. Thus, as this chapter has illustrated, diagnostic uncertainty persisted despite the availability of the pancreas-specific test, which addressed some earlier forms of uncertainty while introducing others.

By the mid-1950s, CF had come to be widely understood as a systemic disease as Sidney Farber had initially suggested, and the duodenal intubation test was no longer able to detect all patients who were thought to have the disease. As Harry Shwachman explained in an interview in 1958, CF "isn't a disease of the pancreas."[172] Instead, he described it as "a generalized disease, characterized in most cases by secretion of abnormally thick mucus, which affects many organs."[173] Reinforcing this shift from localized to systemic framing of the disease, a 1965 National Cystic Fibrosis Research Foundation brochure explained that when CF was "first recognized as a separate entity . . . , it was the pancreatic changes and deficiency that attracted attention and led to the name, cystic fibrosis of the pancreas."[174] While the name was "accepted by tradition" at that time, "it is a misnomer."[175] Instead, as the foundation argued, "now we know that the pancreas is not the only part of the body affected—and may not even be the most important part."[176] In another document published at the same time, the foundation stressed that the duodenal intubation test was "not now considered essential, though it may be required in special or doubtful cases."[177]

In contrast to some well-described situations in which the adoption of new technologies led to broader disease definitions, the more systemic reframing of CF occurred before the availability of a new diagnostic test because of the increasing awareness of the disconnect between clinical scenarios, diagnostic testing for pancreas function during life, and post-mortem findings.[178] Although many physicians called for a mucus-based diagnostic test capable of detecting patients with a wider range of manifestations of what was deemed a systemic disease in the 1950s, such a test for CF was not developed and adopted. Instead, a different test (based on the measurement of sweat electrolyte levels) was developed in the 1950s that would serve this purpose and eventually become the "gold standard" for CF diagnosis. In fact, Shwachman and colleagues suggested in 1955 that this newly described "sweat test," which will be discussed in Chapter 2, could be used "to establish a diagnosis in these patients even though there is good enzymatic activity of the duodenal fluid."[179]

Given that Byron Bell's diagnosis changed from CF to celiac disease in 1953 following his normal duodenal intubation test result, one wonders whether Shwachman or another physician reevaluated Byron after the sweat test became available in the mid-1950s. While we know that Byron lived at least until the age of six, it is unclear if he ever received a sweat test or if his diagnosis changed from celiac disease back to CF.[180] As the next chapter will illustrate, the availability of the sweat test, a new diagnostic technology capable of identifying those with a broader range of clinical profiles compared to the pancreas-specific test, would address some previous uncertainties while introducing new ones, such that certainty in diagnosis remained an elusive goal.

CHAPTER TWO

Salty Sweat

Obstacles to Using a Gold Standard Diagnostic Test

Lee Smith Belnap appeared healthy when he was born in 1963, but he nearly died when he was about six weeks old. As his mother described, he choked on what "must have been some mucus in his lungs," and "he was wheezing, . . . losing weight, . . . [and] had several bulky bowel movements a day."[1] Lee was initially diagnosed with a milk allergy by the family doctor, but his failure to improve following a change in diet led his parents to consult a pediatric allergist, who immediately suspected that something more serious was going on.[2]

Without explaining what he was looking for, the physician performed a test on Lee, in which his arm was inserted "into a thin plastic bag" and wrapped "in several towels" to induce sweating.[3] After an hour, Lee's hand was placed "onto a red, gel-like substance in a small dish," and when the doctor removed it from the gel, a "clear, yellowish-white imprint remained."[4] As Lee's mother recalled years later, "the nurse's quick intake of breath and the almost imperceptible sag of Dr. Venning's shoulders told me without words that the test was positive."[5] Lee was given a preliminary diagnosis of cystic fibrosis based on the results of this initial "sweat test" and admitted to the hospital to begin treatment for a serious lung infection. At that time, CF was described as "one of the most common chronic diseases in childhood and adolescence," and clinical profiles could include "chronic pulmonary disease, pancreatic enzyme deficiency, abnormally high sweat electrolytes and, at times, cirrhosis of the liver."[6] The median age of survival was about ten years when Lee was given the CF diagnosis in 1963, an increase from less than one year in the late 1930s, in part due to the availability of antibiotics and pancreatic enzyme replacement therapy.[7]

After a few days in the hospital, Lee was given a "more sophisticated" sweat test for CF, and his mother recalled being "dizzy with relief" when the test turned out to be negative.[8] However, considering Lee's clinical profile, his physician still suspected CF and repeated the sweat test two more times. After three consecutive negative "sophisticated" sweat tests, Lee's doctor remained nonetheless convinced that the boy had CF and sent him for an additional sweat test at a different hospital laboratory.[9] After this fifth sweat test came back positive, Lee's mother kept waiting for his physician to call and tell them that the CF diagnosis was "all a mistake," indicating a lack of faith in the results and highlighting the uncertainty that remained regarding the cause of Lee's medical challenges.[10] However, the CF diagnosis was reinforced when Lee was seen at the Cystic Fibrosis Center in Seattle, where a sixth sweat test came back positive.

The sweat test inconsistencies that Lee experienced can be better understood within the context of mid-twentieth-century concerns about the lack of sufficient regulation of laboratory tests in the US, and efforts to pass legislation to address these regulatory shortcomings.[11] While the regulation of drugs has received a great deal of attention from historians and other scholars, the regulation of clinical testing is relatively underexplored.[12] This chapter examines early attempts to analyze sweat to diagnose CF, providing an opportunity to interrogate the development, regulation, and use of diagnostic tests in the mid-twentieth century. Once physicians realized in the early 1950s that many people with CF had elevated electrolytes in the sweat, they developed a range of screening and diagnostic tests to measure sweat sodium or chloride levels.[13] To address some of the safety and accuracy shortcomings of the early sweat tests, in 1959 Johns Hopkins physicians Lewis "Pete" Gibson and Robert Cooke published a description of a quantitative diagnostic sweat test.[14] However, even with the availability of the highly accurate Gibson–Cooke sweat test, later referred to as the gold standard for CF diagnosis, many people with symptoms were not offered the test for two key reasons. First, some physicians found the Gibson–Cooke sweat test too time-consuming or too challenging, and instead continued to develop and employ new versions of the sweat test, as has been seen with other diagnostic technologies.[15] The corresponding lack of standardization of the sweat test was linked to "erroneous results" and delayed diagnoses.[16] Second, some physicians didn't order the test because they didn't suspect CF in the first place due to attitudes toward mothers, assumptions about race, or physician inexperience, also resulting in missed diagnoses. In light of these concerns, many physicians were calling for better screening methods for CF by the 1970s such that those people with a positive screen would be offered a Gibson–Cooke diagnostic sweat test.

As an analysis of sweat testing for CF from the 1950s through the 1970s makes clear, the idealized diagnostic process, in which all individuals with a disease are given an accurate diagnostic test in a timely manner, was not realized in practice and was a contributing factor to the diagnostic uncertainty that many individuals with CF, including Lee Smith Belnap, experienced. Thus, even though the sweat test addressed one source of uncertainty stemming from the earlier pancreas-specific test, in that it could diagnose people with a wider range of disease manifestations, diagnostic uncertainty persisted in the decades after the Gibson–Cooke sweat test was first described because the "gold standard" diagnostic technology was not widely used.

Early Sweat Tests for Cystic Fibrosis

During a heat wave in New York City in the summer of 1948, ten children were admitted to Babies Hospital in New York over the span of twenty-four hours with symptoms of heat prostration, including vomiting, fever, and unresponsiveness.[17] Of particular note, most of these children had previously been diagnosed with CF based on absent or reduced pancreatic digestive enzymes. As physicians Walter Kessler and Dorothy Andersen pointed out, one such patient was a two-and-a-half-year-old boy who had been diagnosed with CF at ten months with the invasive duodenal intubation test for pancreatic digestive enzymes (described in Chapter 1). Although this patient "was sufficiently well to visit the zoo" on the morning of August 28, he started vomiting while at the zoo and "continued to vomit everything he ingested up to the time of admission."[18] At the hospital, he was "lethargic and dehydrated" and "remained quite unresponsive" for several hours.[19] However, after four days of hospitalization, which included administration of "salt-containing fluids," among other things, he was discharged.[20] The New York physicians postulated that the presence of a "low-grade infection" made children with CF especially susceptible to heat prostration, yet they also acknowledged that a problem with the sweat glands was a possibility.[21]

Although postwar government funding of biomedical research was growing around the time of the heat wave, exploration of the significance of heat prostration in people with cystic fibrosis was privately funded in part by the United Fruit Company.[22] Recall from Chapter 1 that cystic fibrosis was initially described in 1938 as one of several distinct disease entities that could result in the celiac syndrome. Given the connection between CF and celiac disease and the popularity of the "banana diet" for children with these diagnoses in the mid-twentieth century, the United Fruit Company was likely interested in supporting the research for marketing purposes.[23] Drawing in part from United Fruit Company funding, New York physicians provided evidence in the early 1950s that the composition of sweat was altered in individuals with CF, a finding consistent with the increased incidence of heat prostration in this population.[24] The initial study of sweat electrolyte abnormalities in people with CF was published by New York physicians Robert Darling, Paul di Sant'Agnese, George Perera, and Dorothy Andersen.[25] To examine the sweat composition of nine people with cystic fibrosis and eight controls without the disease, gauze was placed on the abdomen and covered with a waterproof adhesive.[26] To induce sweating, individuals were covered with a sheet and a blanket and remained in a room with a constant temperature of 89°F and 50 percent humidity for one to two hours. After the sweat collected by the gauze was weighed, the concentrations of chloride, sodium, and potassium were determined. Noting an increase in sweat electrolytes in people with CF, the investigators concluded that the sweat glands themselves were probably affected, resulting in an increased susceptibility to heat prostration.[27] Shortly after this study, Paul di Sant'Agnese and colleagues found similar results in a larger study (Figure 2.1).[28]

The sweat electrolyte findings reinforced earlier views, first voiced by Sidney Farber as noted in Chapter 1, that CF was a systemic disease that could involve lung manifestations in the setting of normal pancreas enzyme levels. As di Sant'Agnese pointed out in 1955, "varying degrees of involvement of the pancreas, lungs, liver and sweat glands are inherent in this disease," and "complete and incomplete forms of the condition exist."[29] Furthermore, he viewed the sweat test as a reliable diagnostic tool that "may be positive at a time when other findings are not present."[30] In the same year, Boston physician Harry Shwachman and colleagues also expressed enthusiasm for the sweat test, especially in cases without pancreatic insufficiency, yet they still pointed to the pancreas-specific duodenal intubation test discussed in the previous chapter as the "most reliable

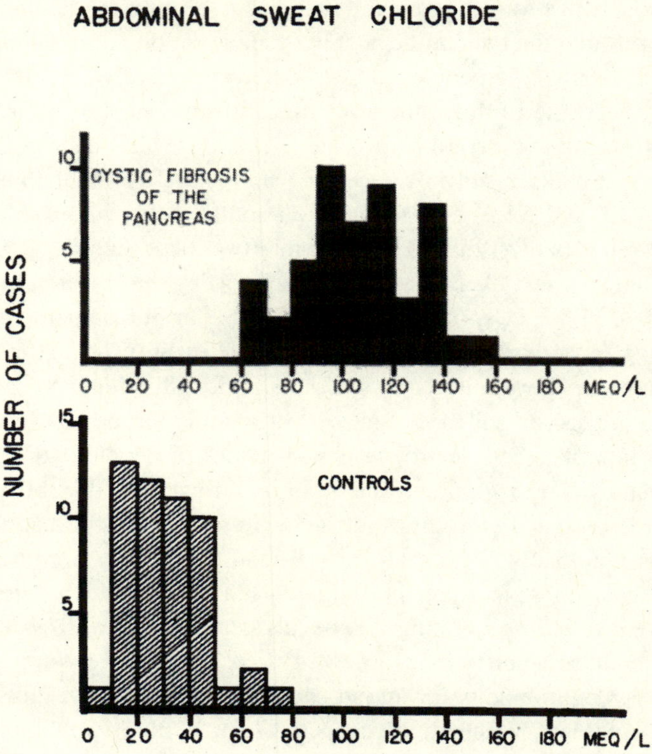

FIGURE 2.1. "Abdominal sweat chloride in 43 patients with cystic fibrosis of pancreas (50 determinations) and 50 controls." Reproduced with permission from Paul A. di Sant'Agnese, Robert C. Darling, George A. Perera, and Ethel Shea, "Abnormal Electrolyte Composition of Sweat in Cystic Fibrosis of the Pancreas: Clinical Significance and Relationship to the Disease," *Pediatrics* 12, no. 5 (1953): 549–63. © 1953 by the AAP.

and direct method of making the diagnosis today."[31] Despite "feel[ing] strongly that no final diagnosis" of CF should be made in the setting of a normal pancreatic function test, the Boston investigators noted that "we are, however, rapidly accumulating evidence to suggest that the detection of the abnormality in the sweat electrolytes may replace the duodenal intubation as a diagnostic procedure."[32] If properly validated, the Boston physicians believed the sweat test was desirable because it could theoretically lead to an earlier diagnosis of CF in people with a wider range of disease manifestations, including those without detectable pancreatic involvement, resulting in the prompt initiation of treatment and more favorable outcomes.

Since the Boston investigators and most other physicians did not have access to the type of heated room used by the New York physicians, variations on the sweat test were devised in the mid-1950s.[33] For example, as described at the 1954 American Academy of Pediatrics conference in Chicago, Shwachman and colleagues placed patients in a plastic bag to induce the sweat production needed to carry out the test.[34] In particular, gauze and plastic sheeting were attached to the patient's back with adhesive and the patient was then "placed in a plastic suit which has an elastic neck and a zipper in front."[35] After being covered with a blanket for 30–90 minutes, the patient was removed from the bag and the electrolyte concentration of the sweat collected by the gauze was recorded. By 1955, the Boston physicians had performed this test on over three hundred people and the bag method was being used in many other locations as well. In an even simpler "'tube' method," described by Philadelphia physicians in 1956, the patient was "placed nude on a plastic sheet and subjected to a moderate thermal stimulus for 20 to 40 minutes," without the need for gauze like the other tests.[36] Sweat was then collected from both the plastic and the patient's back using a syringe, and sweat electrolyte concentrations were determined.[37] In reflecting in 1958 on the Boston and Philadelphia methods that did not require a constant temperature room like that available in her New York hospital, Dorothy Andersen pointed out that "these simpler methods have proved adequate for diagnostic purposes," which highlights how the value of a test is determined to a significant extent by whether it can be broadly disseminated and easily used.[38]

Despite the differences between these initial sweat tests, all required the application of a thermal stimulus to induce sweating. While some researchers were aware of the "theoretical risks" associated with thermal stress, especially for children with chronic health concerns, "no serious ill effects" had been reported in the first several years of the sweat test.[39] However, in 1957, investigators in England reported a fatality in a thirteen-month-old boy who was tested for cystic fibrosis using the gauze method developed by Shwachman and colleagues. In light of their experience, physicians argued that the "bag test should be limited to doubtful cases and when performed due regard must be given to the possibility of hyperthermia."[40] As a Philadelphia physician noted in 1959, "there is a serious caution to be employed in these thermal stimulating tests" because "a small number of children have been reported to have died from sudden acute heat collapse during the procedure."[41] Because of concerns about the iatrogenic or inadvertent harms associated with a thermal stimulus,

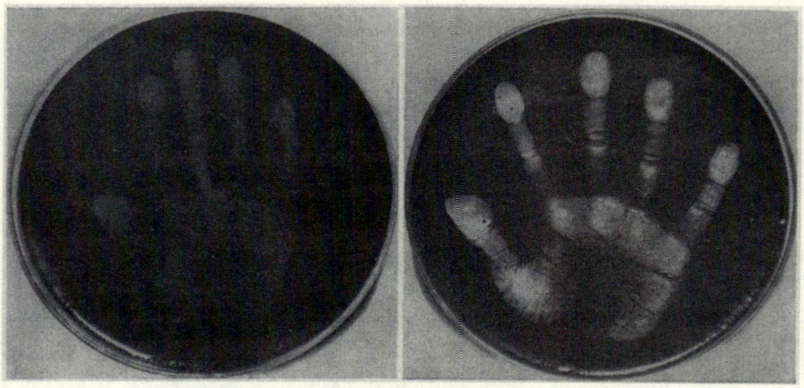

FIGURE 2.2. Results of the chloride plate test. *Left*: "Hand Impression of a Healthy Three-Year-Old Child (Reaction +)." *Right*: "Hand Impression of a Five-Year-Old Child with Cystic Fibrosis of the Pancreas (Reaction +++)." Image from Harry Shwachman and N. Gahm, "Studies in Cystic Fibrosis of the Pancreas: A Simple Test for the Detection of Excessive Chloride on the Skin," *New England Journal of Medicine* 255, no. 21 (November 22, 1956): 999–1001. Reprinted with permission from Massachusetts Medical Society, © 1956.

as well as the technical challenges accompanying such sweat tests, many physicians sought to develop tests for CF in the 1950s that did not include the risk of death associated with a thermal stimulus.

Even before deaths were linked to the bag sweat test, physicians were working to develop simpler and faster methods to detect elevated electrolyte levels in sweat. For example, as detailed in a 1956 report in *The New England Journal of Medicine*, Harry Shwachman and a Harvard College student developed what is often referred to as the chloride plate test.[42] In contrast to the bag sweat test, which took up to one hour and forty minutes to complete, the chloride plate test was described as "an immediate test" that "simplifies the diagnosis of cystic fibrosis from a very complicated one to an instantaneous office procedure," and the agar "chloride test medium" could be made on site in the laboratory setting.[43] To do the test, the patient simply placed their hand on the agar chloride test medium, which looked somewhat like red Jell-O, and the physician noted whether the medium changed color, indicating the presence of chloride.[44] This is likely a variant of the sweat test that was first used on Lee Smith Belnap in 1963.[45] When there is "considerable chloride" in the sweat on the surface of the hand, "an intense whitish-yellowish discoloration occurs immediately," whereas a barely detectable imprint would be noted with low levels of chloride (Figure 2.2).[46] Investigators designated the chemical reactions from "little or no reaction (+)" to "an intense discoloration (+++)" and found that 98.6 percent of their patients with cystic fibrosis had +++ readings, whereas 86 percent of controls had + readings.[47] In the original description of the chloride plate test in 1956, it is unclear whether the investigators viewed it as primarily a screening test, a diagnostic test, or a combination of the two (since they referred to the chloride plate test using both terms), but they did note that the chloride plate test "provides an opportunity of screening large numbers of children for cystic fibrosis."[48] Around that time, the US Commission on Chronic Illness defined screening tests as those that "sort out apparently well persons who probably have a disease from those who probably do not," and noted that a positive screening test should be followed by a diagnostic test.[49]

In the second half of the 1950s, the widely used chloride plate test was variously described as either a screening test or a diagnostic test, and many physicians emphasized the value of such a quick and inexpensive test for CF. Physician Wynne Sharples, the National Cystic Fibrosis Research Foundation president mentioned in Chapter 1 and the parent of two children with CF, described the test as "a timely diagnostic tool."[50] The foundation had been established in 1955 by parents of children with CF to raise awareness and fund research for the disease at a time when other disease-specific foundations were forming and when lay advocacy for a wide range of diseases, including cancer, was growing.[51] Within this broader context, the foundation not only promoted the chloride plate test but also was involved in demonstrating how it worked. For example, on March 10, 1957, the Washington chapter of the foundation met in the "community room of the Washington Post and Times-Herald Building" to demonstrate "the new test . . . on seevral [*sic*] children and their parents" and advertised the event in a local newspaper.[52] Also in 1957, the foundation described the test as "98% accurate," noting that it was "a simple test taking only one second to perform and read!"[53] Furthermore, highlighting how investigators could make the chloride plate test themselves, an Indiana newspaper article explained in 1957 that the test "can be prepared in any hospital laboratory at a cost of about 5 cents and is almost 100% accurate."[54]

In the context of claims about the simplicity, low cost, and accuracy of the chloride plate test, children in traditional school settings were early targets for CF screening in the late 1950s, at a time when screening for tuberculosis was taking place in schools as well.[55] According to Sharples, the US Public Health Service had approved CF screening in schools using the "fingerprint test" on more than 5,000 Philadelphia children in kindergarten through third grade in 1958; by October of that year, 157 children had been tested as part of a pilot study that was deemed a "success" despite some challenges in interpreting the test.[56] Also in 1958, Boston physicians, including Harry Shwachman, screened 3,036 children attending kindergarten through fourth grade in eight schools in Worcester, Massachusetts.[57] Among the eighty-five Worcester schoolchildren who tested positive on the initial screen using the chloride plate test, none were ultimately diagnosed with CF following a quantitative sweat test.[58] Based on these findings, the Boston physicians argued that it might be more effective to target younger children and suggested the use of a "screening test in well-baby clinics where early detection of cystic fibrosis may result in prompt institution of therapy," which many physicians believed would lead to better outcomes.[59] At that time, therapeutics for people with CF fell under three general categories: those that targeted the "obstructive pulmonary lesion" (such as mist tent therapy and postural drainage), antibiotic therapy, and pancreatic enzyme replacement therapy.[60] However, consistent with Dorothy Andersen's concern that the reliability of the chloride plate test had not been established, several cases of misdiagnosis were reported in the 1950s.[61] In these instances, the disease was suspected but incorrectly ruled out due to a false negative chloride plate test, as the CF diagnosis was later established on autopsy.

Despite the challenges associated with the chloride plate test in some instances, it appears that it was used to diagnose a very sick child with CF in 1959. According to an article in the *Chicago Daily Tribune*, Jeannie Wright "seemed charmingly normal until her second birthday," and "then she caught a cold she couldn't seem to shake."[62] After a hospitalization for pneumonia in June 1959, Jeannie eventually improved, yet "her coughing still had her parents up with her every half hour all night, every night."[63] During a heat wave just a few months later, Jeannie "became dangerously dehydrated, . . . went into convulsions," and her temperature rose to 108°F.[64] While hospitalized, "artificial respiration kept her clinging to life even tho [*sic*] her heart stopped at one time."[65] In the words of her mother, Marilyn Wright, "the hospital said it was all over and even asked us what undertaker to call."[66] As she recalled, "you can't imagine how dreadful it is. You have a beautiful baby and all of a sudden she's dying and no one knows why."[67] However, "Jeannie pulled out of it" and was diagnosed with CF in the hospital at age three, likely with the chloride plate test.[68] After her diagnosis, Jeannie began treatment for CF and her health improved dramatically, reinforcing the value of such a "simple, diagnostic test" for the disease.[69]

By the late 1950s, a wide range of sweat tests for CF had been developed, each with distinct advantages and challenges. For example, the chloride plate test was quick, inexpensive, and easy to carry out, yet the interpretation of the test was subjective and prone to error in some settings. In addition to instances of false negative results as discussed earlier, the chloride plate test could produce false positive results, in which a diagnosis of CF was made in the absence of disease. As one physician noted in 1959, "it seems the children often manage to get something salty on their hands, which may be one of the causes for false positives."[70] Furthermore, some physicians used this and other qualitative tests as definitive diagnostics, whereas others treated them simply as screening tests that needed to be followed up with a quantitative test before the diagnosis could be made, indicating that the process of diagnosis was not necessarily consistent across locations.[71] While the quantitative sweat tests, such as the bag test, did provide investigators with a specific sweat chloride or sodium concentration, they introduced an added safety risk to patients due to the need for a thermal stimulus. One quantitative sweat test described in 1956 addressed such safety concerns by injecting a chemical under the skin to induce sweating, but the procedure was painful.[72] Given the limitations of each version of the sweat test in use in the 1950s, physicians continued to try to develop new versions of the test with the hope that a simple and accurate sweat test would allow for prompt diagnosis of the disease.

The Gold Standard Gibson–Cooke Sweat Test

To address some of the concerns associated with early qualitative and quantitative sweat tests, Johns Hopkins physicians Lewis Gibson and Robert Cooke described a new diagnostic variant in 1959 that would eventually be considered the "gold standard" test for CF.[73] According to Stefan Timmermans and Marc Berg, the gold standard in medicine is "the measure against which everything else will be measured: it constitutes the rock bottom to which new candidates for standards are compared, and it defines the truth."[74] An examination of the development and implementation of the Gibson–Cooke sweat test sheds light on the process by which gold standard diagnostics come into being, and the challenges associated with such diagnostics even after the gold standard label has been applied. As David Jones and Scott Podolsky highlight in their analysis of the history of the gold standard in finance and medicine, such standards

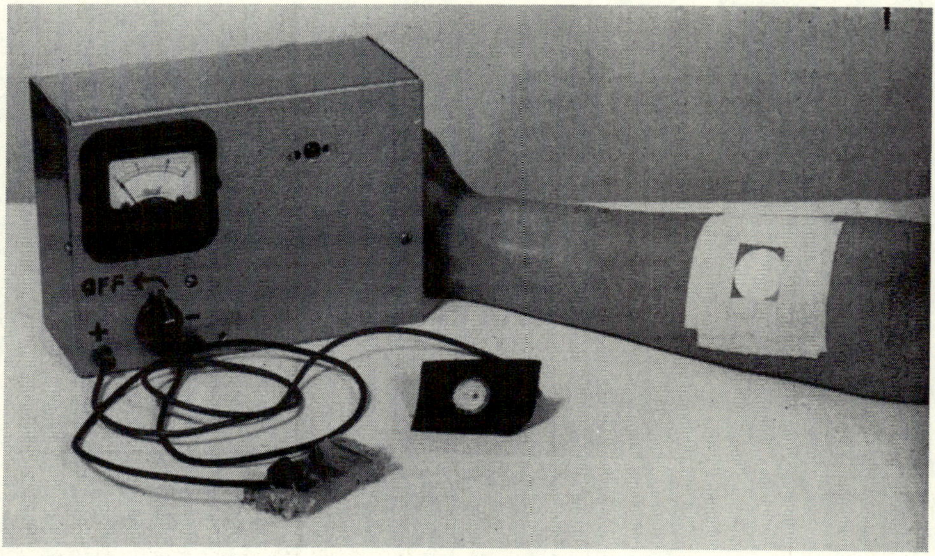

FIGURE 2.3. "Apparatus for delivering electric current; the electrodes; and the collecting system applied to a forearm." Reproduced with permission from L. E. Gibson and R. E. Cooke, "A Test for Concentration of Electrolytes in Sweat in Cystic Fibrosis of the Pancreas Utilizing Pilocarpine by Iontophoresis," *Pediatrics* 23, no. 3 (1959): 545–9. © 1959 by the AAP.

can "represent . . . aspirations toward stability," an assertion reinforced by examining efforts to implement the Gibson–Cooke sweat test.[75]

Referred to as the pilocarpine iontophoresis sweat test, the procedure was described by Gibson and Cooke as rapid, painless, and reliable.[76] Instead of using heat or an injected chemical to induce sweat production, this test stimulated local sweating by the placement of a chemical (pilocarpine) on the skin of the forearm, followed by the administration of an electric current for five minutes to allow the chemical to move into the skin (iontophoresis). In other words, an electric current was used to move a sweat-inducing chemical into the skin. After the electrodes were removed, any remaining chemical was washed off the arm, and a small disc of filter paper was applied to the skin and left in place for thirty minutes to collect sweat (Figure 2.3). Since such a small volume of sweat was produced using this approach, the concentration of chloride collected by the filter paper was then measured with a more sensitive method than that employed with the bag sweat test. Based on analysis of people with CF, their relatives, and controls, Gibson and Cooke determined that all people with CF had chloride concentrations of at least 80 mEq/L, whereas controls had concentrations that were 60 mEq/L or lower.[77] The investigators emphasized the safety, reliability, and convenience of the test, which required only ten minutes of direct patient supervision.

Other physicians reinforced the value of the Gibson–Cooke test as a diagnostic for cystic fibrosis shortly after it was described. For example, Shwachman and his Boston colleagues at the Children's Hospital Medical Center used an "adaptation of" the Gibson–Cooke method to diagnose CF in several infants with meconium ileus, the type of intestinal obstruction described in Chapter 1.[78] Using results from the Gibson–Cooke test, the Boston physicians also highlighted the difference in sweat electrolyte concentrations in babies with CF compared to healthy newborn infants. Consistent with Gibson and Cooke's findings, the babies with CF all had sweat chloride concentrations of 89 mEq/L or greater, whereas controls had concentrations of 49 mEq/L or less. By the early 1960s, numerous hospitals had the ability to carry out the Gibson–Cooke sweat test. For example, the diagnostic sweat test appears to have been used in Kentucky in 1961 to determine whether eleven-month-old Becky Nay had CF (Figure 2.4).[79] That same year, the medical adviser of the Austin chapter of the National Cystic Fibrosis Research Foundation provided a $150 iontophoresis apparatus for sweat testing to Brackenridge Hospital in Texas; as one physician at the hospital noted, "this brings us a long way from having to use plastic sweat bags, furnace rooms, or any other devise [*sic*] to produce sweat."[80] In fact, in the 1960s, many chapters of the National Cystic Fibrosis Research Foundation used money from fundraising efforts to provide hospitals with variants of the Gibson–Cooke sweat test apparatus for the diagnosis of CF.[81]

By 1963, the year that Lee Smith Belnap was born, the National Cystic Fibrosis Research Foundation called the pilocarpine iontophoresis method described by Gibson and Cooke the "preferred procedure" in its *Guide to Diagnosis and Management of Cystic Fibrosis: A Syllabus for Physicians*.[82] While some of the earlier studies noted that those with CF had sweat chloride concentrations of 80 mEq/L or higher, the foundation handbook pointed to a sweat chloride level above 60 mEq/L "in the presence of clinical symptoms" as diagnostic of CF, and physicians would continue to grapple with how to interpret different sweat chloride levels in later decades as well.[83] The foundation also recommended that both chloride and sodium levels be determined as an internal control to ensure that the test had been done properly. Reflecting back on the development of the Gibson–Cooke sweat test nearly three decades later, Harry Shwachman noted that it "became the standard diagnostic procedure" for

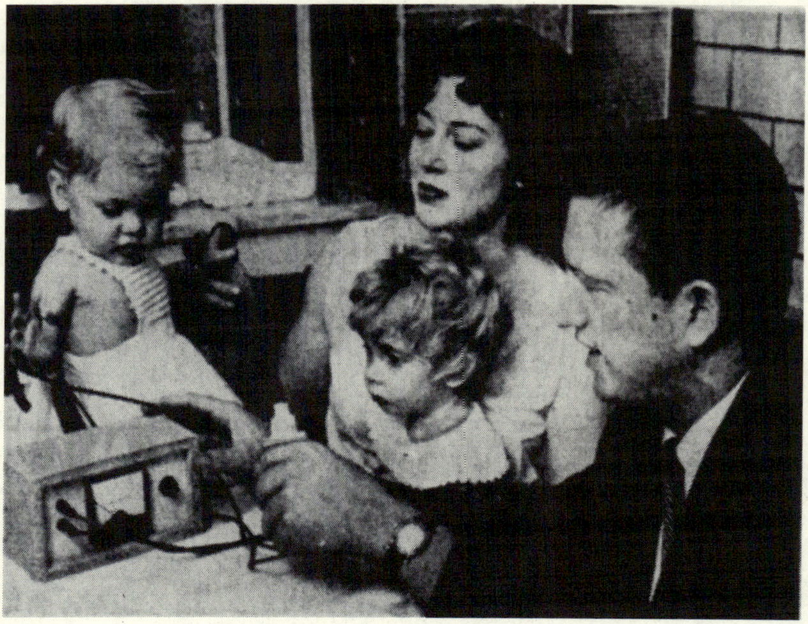

FIGURE 2.4. "CYSTIC FIBROSIS? . . . The sweat test will tell. Analysis of salt in the perspiration of Becky Nay, 11 months, is checked in the Children's Chest Clinic at Children's Hospital. Clinic director Dr. Glenn R. Stoutt, Jr., gets moral support from Elizabeth, 2, and the sisters' mother, Mrs. Frank M. Nay." Image appeared in Robert P. Clark, "Cystic Fibrosis Fund Drive Is Set: Mysterious Disease Kills Many Children," *The Courier-Journal*, September 10, 1961. © The Courier-Journal—USA Today Network via Imagn Images.

CF.[84] To this day, physicians refer to a variant of the Gibson–Cooke sweat test as the "gold standard" diagnostic for the disease.[85] However, despite the availability of the Gibson–Cooke method and its description as "one of the most reliable [tests] in medicine," the next two sections will document how the test was not always used in practice in the decades following its introduction, as some physicians continued to try to develop faster and easier tests for CF, and others didn't even think to test for CF in the first place.[86]

"Supposed Improvements" to the Sweat Test as Obstacles to Standardization

Efforts to improve sweat testing for CF in the 1960s occurred in the setting of broader concerns about the reliability of diagnostic tests in the

US, including evidence of widespread error and fraud.[87] Reflecting on this period years later, microbiologist and physician Morris Schaeffer argued that "nearly everyone involved," including physicians, pathologists, administrators, educators, and legislators, "may be blamed for having accepted the shameful lack of adequate standards and facilities and for permitting obviously incompetent and sometimes overtly dishonest laboratory operations to exist."[88] While the 1965 Medicare regulations stipulated that some laboratories be certified to receive reimbursement, relatively few were covered by this law, and only ten states had laboratory certification programs at that time.[89] To further address such concerns and to expand the federal regulation of laboratory tests, Congress passed the Clinical Laboratory Improvement Act (CLIA) in 1967, which "required federal licensing and inspection of laboratories testing specimens received across state lines."[90] However, even with Medicare and CLIA '67, many laboratories in the US still remained unregulated, and, Congress continued to try to pass new laws to better deal with laboratory error, fraud, and cost.[91]

An examination of how sweat tests were carried out and modified in the mid-twentieth century sheds light on the types of challenges faced by medical professionals, patients, and families as broader efforts to regulate laboratory tests were taking place in the US. Although the Gibson–Cooke sweat test remained in use in the decades following its description in 1959, physicians continued to tinker with, develop, and implement new versions of the sweat test for CF, reflecting both a dissatisfaction with the Gibson–Cooke version and the reduced emphasis on consistency and standardization in medicine more broadly at the time.[92] For example, in 1962 investigators at a Veterans Administration hospital described a variant of the sweat test, in which sweating was stimulated by placing a rubber glove on the patient's hand and immersing it "in a paraffin bath at a constant temperature of 120°F."[93] Using this technique, they diagnosed a forty-one-year-old man with CF because he had elevated chloride and sodium values and a clinical profile consistent with the disease.[94] Of particular note, the investigators pointed out that the patient had sweat electrolyte concentrations "higher than those reported in the literature perhaps because of the different technique employed in sweat collection."[95] In fact, variation in test method was repeatedly pointed to as a challenge to establishing a standardized range of sweat electrolyte concentrations that were indicative of CF.

Similarly, Boston investigators at the Children's Hospital Medical Center were continuing to work on "improving diagnostic techniques for cystic fibrosis" in 1964 despite the existence of the Gibson–Cooke method.[96] In an interview with the *Journal of the American Medical Association* the following year, Harry Shwachman acknowledged that "some might question the need for a new test for cystic fibrosis since the standard sweat test is one of the most reliable in medicine," yet he explained that there was a "need for a rapid screening procedure which can be applied to the newborn and for a test to detect the heterozygote or carrier of the CF gene."[97] Although Shwachman and a colleague had recently described a new test for CF that measured electrolyte concentrations in fingernail and toenail clippings, he acknowledged that this method was "too difficult a procedure at present for use as a screening method."[98]

That same year, Minnesota physician Warren Warwick and his colleague, who also saw a need for a rapid screening test for CF to allow for early therapeutic intervention and improved outcomes, described the silver electrode sweat test.[99] Instead of locally administering a chemical or subjecting the whole body to thermal stress to stimulate sweat production, the silver electrode method used a heated, parafilm-covered aluminum cylinder placed on the forearm or other region of the skin for five minutes. A silver electrode was then positioned directly on the resulting "moist skin surface," and the chloride concentration was determined in situ in a matter of seconds.[100] This method was used to screen preschool children in Minnesota in May 1966 by nurse JoAnn Koroshec, who worked with Warwick.[101] During what was described as a party-like event, children entered the room and immediately their left arms were washed, a "small heated aluminum cylinder" was put in place, and then "the children moved around the room, holding the cylinders to their arms." To allow enough time to induce sweating, the "walk around the room was timed to take exactly five minutes," then nurse Koroshec removed the cylinder and "placed on the child's arm a silver electrode measuring device, connected to an indicator" that provided a sweat chloride value (Figure 2.5).[102] According to Koroshec, eighteen thousand children in Minnesota had been screened with the silver electrode sweat test by 1966.[103] As a note of caution when he first described the test, Warwick emphasized that the silver electrode measurements needed to be done with care to avoid sweat evaporation, which could lead to artificially high chloride readings.[104]

Notes of caution like Warwick's were common in the CF community, as many expressed concerns that the proliferation of new tests for CF (including Warwick's silver electrode test) was contributing to misdiagnosis of the disease through testing errors and the lack of test standardization. In fact,

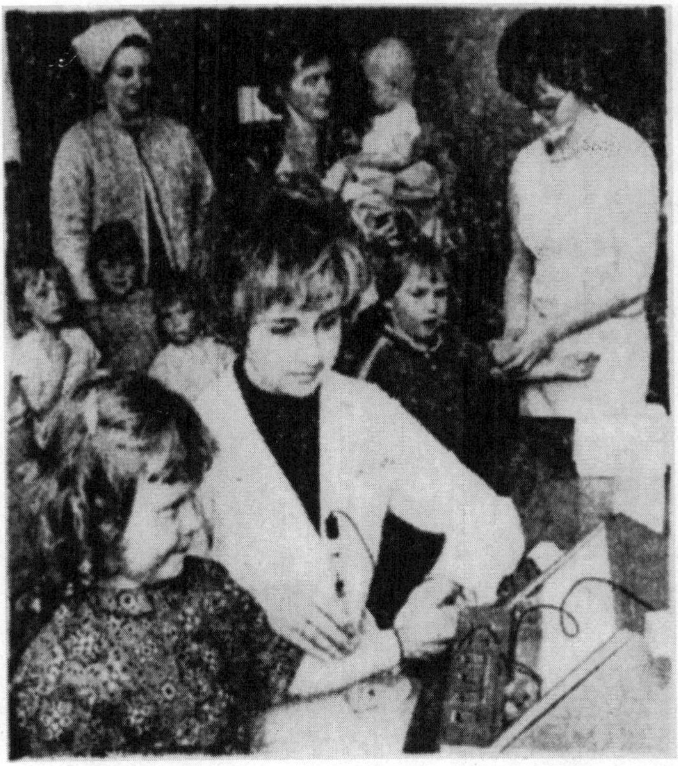

FIGURE 2.5. "A sweat test which rules out cystic fibrosis was given to youngsters in Ely last week. Donna Marie Hoover, 5, watches the indicator with Nurse JoAnn Koroshec. In background, cousin Wanda Hoover, 5 has a test cylinder placed on her arm by Mrs. Ronald Sorjanen, project chairman of Ely's Mrs. Jaycees." Photo appeared in Walter Eldot, "Free Sweat Test for Ely Children Almost Like Party," *Duluth News Tribune*, May 15, 1966. Reproduced with permission from *Duluth News Tribune*.

a film produced for the National Cystic Fibrosis Research Foundation in 1967 stressed the importance of carrying out the Gibson–Cooke pilocarpine iontophoresis test for diagnosis, noting that other tests should only be used for screening purposes.[105] The film, which was produced at the Children's Hospital Medical Center in Boston and the NIH in Bethesda, Maryland, featured physicians Harry Shwachman and Paul di Sant'Agnese and was intended "for showing to physicians, medical students, nurses, physical therapists and technicians throughout the nation."[106] As a Gibson–Cooke sweat test was being carried out in the middle of the film, di Sant'Agnese explained that "several simple screening tests . . . are *not* recommended,

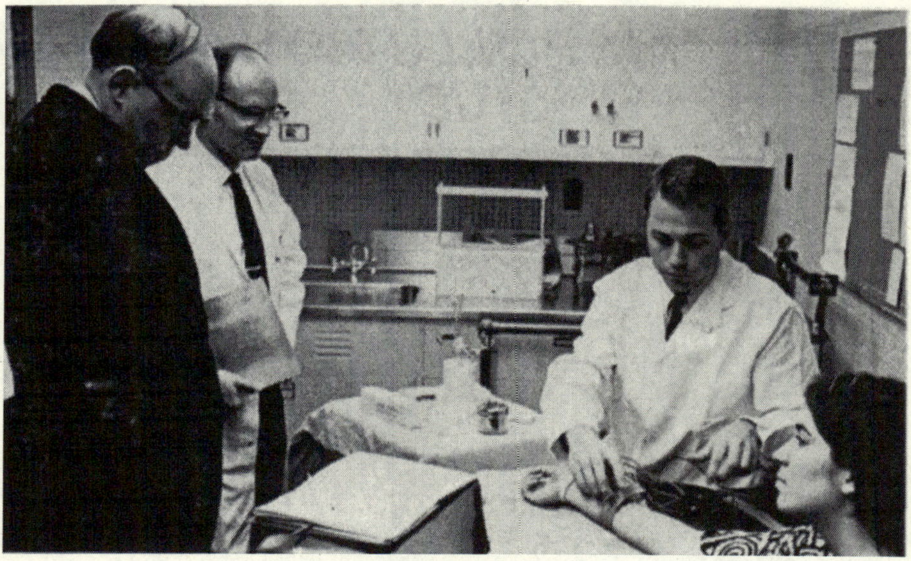

FIGURE 2.6. "SCENE IS SET. Film director John MacKenzie confers with (from left) Dr. Paul di Sant'Agnese and Dr. George Peters on proper angle from which to shoot apparatus used in making sweat test on normal volunteer. The device measures the concentration of salt in patient's sweat after increased sweating has been induced." Reproduced from George J. Mannina, "NIAMD Scientists Featured in Training Film on Cystic Fibrosis," *NIH Record*, April 18, 1967. Photo by Jerry Hecht.

however, except for those skilled in their interpretation, and they should never be used to make a final diagnosis" (Figure 2.6).[107]

Just a few months after film production at the NIH, as efforts to pass CLIA were underway, President Lyndon Johnson visited the NIH Clinical Center to learn about strategies to improve laboratory tests. At the clinical pathology department, President Johnson "saw how NIH specialists have redesigned automatic laboratory analyzers, have married these to a computer and have written computer programs," all changes that the NIH staff hoped would "lead to more accurate, efficient and rapid automatic processing of about 85 percent of daily biochemical analyses."[108] However, despite the passage of CLIA in 1967, caution remained within and outside the CF community about the state of laboratory tests. For example, as sportswriter and novelist Frank Deford recounted, his daughter Alex was diagnosed with CF in 1972 through a sweat test at "Children's Hospital in Boston" after she was brought by ambulance from a hospital in Connecticut that had "botched the sweat test" the first time around.[109]

By 1973, in the context of widespread awareness of continued problems with laboratory tests in the US, Lewis Gibson expressed concern that so many false positive and false negative results had been associated with the sweat test. He was convinced that the high incidence of misdiagnosis was because the "basically sound procedure" that he and Robert Cooke described in 1959 was not being used in practice.[110] Instead, investigators had made numerous modifications to the original test, and Gibson argued that these "*supposed improvements* in my opinion are not improvements at all, but rather introducers of inaccuracies which tend to lead to an undeserved distrust of the whole procedure."[111] In light of the "unnecessary suffering caused by the resulting inaccuracies," Gibson made a "strong plea . . . for the careful performance" of the test as it was originally described.[112] Consistent with Gibson's concerns, the transcript of the 1967 film had a handwritten note from 1974 about the Gibson–Cooke sweat test description in which the word "reliable" was circled and connected by a line to a question mark and the comment "no longer thought to be true."[113]

To address the "unacceptably high" incidence of false positive and false negative sweat test results, which was estimated to be 10–13 percent in the mid-1970s, the Cystic Fibrosis Foundation convened the GAP (Guidance-Action-Projection) Conference on Problems in Sweat Testing in 1975.[114] Gibson and other physicians across the US attended the meeting, which was held in Hilton Head, South Carolina, over two days in February.[115] The consensus among conference participants was that the Gibson–Cooke pilocarpine iontophoresis method was "the most reliable and satisfactory test for the diagnosis of CF," yet it was clear from questionnaire survey results presented at the conference that this test was not necessarily carried out in practice.[116] In fact, only 63 percent of US CF centers responding to a 1974 survey were using the Gibson–Cooke method for the diagnosis of CF. Among all North Carolina hospitals responding in 1974, only 6 percent employed the Gibson–Cooke test.[117] Instead, many facilities used screening tests, such as the chloride plate test, as definitive diagnostics for the disease.[118] As noted in the conference report, "a final and very important conclusion was that *no patient should receive a diagnosis of cystic fibrosis without benefit of a well-done quantitative pilocarpine iontophoresis sweat test*" performed through an experienced laboratory.[119]

In the same year in which the GAP Conference on Problems in Sweat Testing was held, broader reforms to laboratory testing were proposed in Congress. In 1975, Senators Jacob Javits and Edward Kennedy sponsored a congressional bill to amend the Clinical Laboratory Improvement Act of 1967.[120] In this setting of increased government attention to laboratory regulation, a report was published in April 1976 by the Committee for a Study for Evaluation of Testing for Cystic Fibrosis. Established in 1974, the group was sponsored by the National Institute of Arthritis, Metabolism, and Digestive Diseases and the Division of Lung Diseases of the National Heart and Lung Institute, and it received input from the CF Foundation, the US Army and the US Navy.[121] Consistent with the CF Foundation's GAP Conference recommendations, the committee report emphasized the superiority of the Gibson–Cooke test when done by an experienced laboratory. However, given the technical challenges associated with the Gibson–Cooke method, especially when the test was performed only occasionally, the committee report stressed the need for "additional research" to determine the "design characteristics of an ideal instrument" to measure sweat electrolyte concentrations in a wider range of settings.[122] In other words, even when the sweat test was deemed "one of the best diagnostic tests in medicine," experts were still calling for a better sweat test.[123] It simply wasn't enough to have a highly accurate test; it was also pertinent that the test be easy to carry out in practice.

Despite calls in the mid-1970s to address the limitations of CF testing, sweat tests continued to be associated with CF misdiagnoses into the late 1970s.[124] As noted by Johns Hopkins physicians in 1978, sixty-two patients had been referred to them with previous sweat testing between May 1976 and January 1978.[125] After repeating the sweat test using the Gibson–Cooke method, the Johns Hopkins physicians determined that 43.5 percent of the patients had been misdiagnosed.[126] Consistent with the Johns Hopkins findings, a Pennsylvania parent wrote in to *The Atlanta Constitution* health column in 1979, asking, "is it true that one of the diagnostic tests for cystic fibrosis—the sweat test—is not very accurate?"[127] As Mrs. D. L. explained, the CF "diagnosis was made in our local hospital," but "when we went to a large hospital in a nearby city, the test was repeated, and our child was found to be normal."[128] The physician in charge of the newspaper column responded that "your experience is not all that rare" and went on to note that "when sweat tests are done in hospitals or clinics that don't do them often, there is typically a higher rate of false positives than might otherwise be expected."[129] Also in 1979, Nebraska physicians reported on the delayed diagnosis of a boy who had two negative sweat tests, done a year apart "by the general hospital laboratory, using the chloride electrode applied to the skin."[130] When he was finally seen at the CF Center at the University of Nebraska College of Medicine, he tested positive for CF with the Gibson–Cooke method.[131] Pointing to this and other cases of misdiagnosis, the Nebraska physicians emphasized that "no laboratory test is infallible and that the sweat test is particularly fallible if not done by most exacting standards."[132]

In the 1980s, physicians continued to express concern about misdiagnoses associated with the sweat test.[133] While the Gibson–Cooke method was consistently described as the most reliable sweat test for CF, investigators lamented that the test wasn't always done, or done properly, in practice. Since the Gibson–Cooke method required skill and experience, investigators continued to explore other test methods that could be more easily employed in a wider range of clinical settings. For example, in 1982, the Ohio company Wescor promoted the use of its recently developed gel disc for administrating the sweat-stimulating chemical pilocarpine, along with its Macroduct system, a small device with capillary tubing for the collection of sweat that did not require the use of gauze or filter paper.[134] Noting that there had been an "explosive revolution in laboratory technology" in the years since the sweat test was first described, a Wescor employee suggested that it was "a notable anomaly" that the CF Foundation was still recommending a test that had been initially described in 1959.[135] (Lewis Gibson and colleagues would provide evidence more than a decade later that the Macroduct collection system "provides results equally as satisfactory" as the 1959 Gibson–Cooke test, and variants of the original Macroduct system continue to be used in many settings today.[136]) In this context of concern about the state of CF diagnostics and persistent efforts to develop better sweat tests, Johns Hopkins physicians noted in 1986 that four of their patients previously had false negative sweat tests, "resulting in a mean diagnostic delay of 7.3 years."[137] Thus, more than three decades after the sweat electrolyte abnormality in CF had been described, standardization of the sweat test remained an elusive goal. Further compounding the issue, many babies with symptoms consistent with the disease were not being tested in the first place, as the next section illustrates.

Additional Barriers to Testing for CF and Calls for Widespread Screening

Even as physicians attempted to develop faster and easier sweat tests that could be used to screen all children, many individuals were still not being

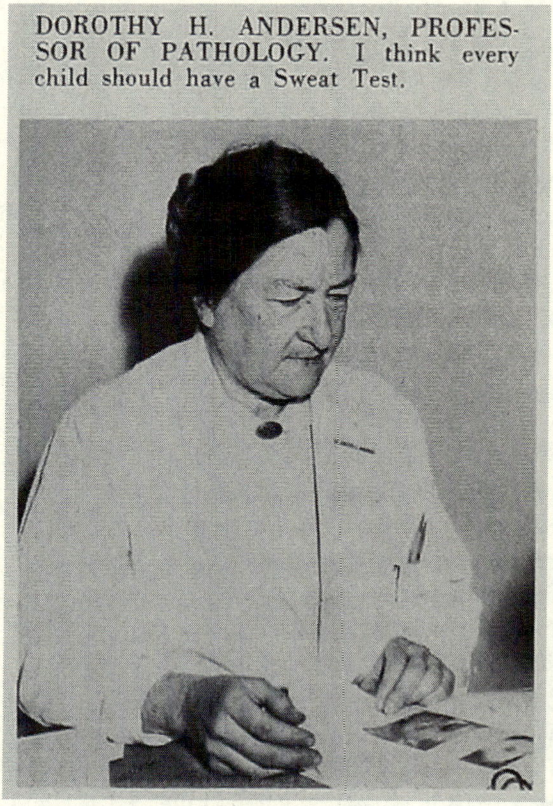

FIGURE 2.7. Image of Dorothy Andersen, including caption stating, "I think every child should have a Sweat Test," which appeared in *P & S: The Yearbook of the College of Physicians and Surgeons*, Columbia University, 1960. Permission to reproduce granted by Archives & Special Collections, Columbia University Health Sciences Library.

diagnosed in a timely manner because they had not been screened or given a diagnostic test for the disease when symptoms first arose. Aware of these missed opportunities, Dorothy Andersen argued in the 1960 yearbook of the College of Physicians and Surgeons at Columbia University that "every child should have a Sweat Test," yet her wish was not realized in the decades that followed (Figure 2.7).[138] In the absence of a screening test that could be widely implemented, numerous reasons were put forth for the failure of physicians to test some children for CF, including biases stemming from attitudes toward mothers, assumptions about race, and physicians' lack of knowledge of CF.

As one example of the dismissal of mothers' concerns about the health of their children, in the late 1960s Ann Hendon "knew something was wrong from the beginning" with her son Kevin since he was "fussy . . . wasn't gaining weight . . . cried constantly," and "when he caught a cold, it would linger for weeks."[139] However, Kevin's physician, as well as their extended family, didn't take Ann's concerns seriously. In fact, the "local doctor" initially thought that Kevin had a "mild case of asthma," but after several visits, "he decided that Kevin's only problem was 'a neurotic mother.'"[140] When Kevin was seen by a different pediatrician who had been recommended by Ann's friend, the physician immediately suspected CF and asked, "does he taste salty when you kiss him?"[141] After Ann answered yes, Kevin received a chloride plate test that came back "weakly positive," followed by a quantitative sweat test at another medical facility, and he was given the CF diagnosis in October 1969 at the age of seventeen months. Kevin's father noted years later that the Cystic Fibrosis Foundation–sponsored "kiss your baby" campaigns (discussed in Chapter 3) to raise awareness of the disease and promote diagnostic testing following a positive home "kiss test" had not yet begun when Kevin was diagnosed.[142]

In the early 1970s, Bill and Susan Kocher had a similar experience when their baby, John, went through a "nightmare of illness" before CF was suspected.[143] After several doctors told them "nothing was wrong," including one doctor who "said that Susan herself was the problem because she was so 'nervous' about the baby," John was finally diagnosed with CF after Susan insisted that he be hospitalized.[144] Accounts of delayed diagnoses due to the dismissal of mothers' concerns had been documented before the Gibson–Cooke test was described. For example, according to a Kansas study published in 1957, one child's health concerns were initially attributed to "maternal anxiety" before the CF diagnosis was made when the child was hospitalized, and similar accounts of the "nervous mother" have been widespread throughout the twentieth and even into the twenty-first century.[145] The dismissive attitude that some physicians have had toward mothers' concerns about the health of their children can be at least partially understood in the context of widespread notions of the "anxious parent" and the "vulnerable child" in the twentieth century.[146]

Another source of delayed or missed diagnoses was the erroneous assumption that CF was restricted to certain racialized groups.[147] In the years following the availability of the sweat test, CF was often described as a "white disease," yet some physicians wondered if such assumptions simply reflected the racial classification of the patient populations "where this disease was given, originally, prominent clinical and research emphasis."[148] For example, physicians at "Boston Children's Hospital" didn't provide care for a single Black person with CF in the late 1950s, and Black individuals made up "a very small percentage" of the patient population seen at the Boston hospital at that time.[149] In an attempt to identify additional Black individuals with CF, physicians at Children's Hospital of DC screened 5,260 Black outpatients, ages three months to sixteen years, between March 1962 and February 1963.[150] While the extensive screening went "without confirmation of a case," they did note that the outcome was "comparable to previous surveys among the white race" done in the Boston area.[151] Based on their awareness of a number of Black people with CF, including three diagnosed on autopsy, physicians at the Children's Hospital of DC concluded in 1969 that "a substantial number" of Black children "are still escaping the diagnosis of cystic fibrosis during their life span."[152]

Keith Wailoo and Stephen Pemberton have documented how descriptions of CF, as either a white disease or a pan-ethnic disease, have changed according to social and cultural contexts, and Dorothy Roberts has illustrated the harms associated with "medical stereotyping" based on race, including in the context of CF.[153] As noted in the introduction, the failure to diagnose CF due to assumptions about race was exactly what happened to Terry Wright, the cofounder and president of the National Organization of African Americans with Cystic Fibrosis.[154] Wright was born in 1962, three years after the Gibson–Cooke test was developed. However, despite having symptoms consistent with CF since childhood, he was not diagnosed until he was fifty-four years old. As Wright recounted in 2021, he visited a doctor when he was in his 30s who told him "if it wasn't for me being African American, I would have cystic fibrosis, and since then I was still going untreated, living with that disease, suffering, not knowing why I was going through all the many things that I was suffering."[155] As his wife Michele explained in an interview for a 2021 *JAMA* article, "Terry has been hospitalized more times than we've been on dates."[156] In fact, after several one-month hospitalizations in 2016 and 2017, it was his wife who located a doctor who suspected CF and ordered a sweat test, which resulted in his diagnosis, highlighting the important role that family members can play in the diagnostic process.[157]

In addition to biases related to attitudes toward mothers and assumptions about race, inadequate knowledge on the part of the physician was another source of delayed or missed diagnoses. Since therapeutic interventions were available for the disease, failure to diagnose CF during life could have dire consequences. As parent James Conniff recalled in 1966, his son died at six weeks of age, on Father's Day, when "we woke to find Bobby suffocated in his crib."[158] Only later did he find out that Bobby had CF, which appears to have been diagnosed on autopsy. Even though his son had "the strange symptoms" consistent with CF since birth, James Conniff explained that "most doctors had not been schooled to suspect this masked killer."[159] Conniff went on to point out that "it hurts more to lose a youngster if you know he need not have died."[160] One wonders whether a similar fate could have befallen Lee Smith Belnap; recall that he had initially been misdiagnosed with a milk allergy in 1963. As Lee's mother explained, he "manifested all the symptoms of cystic fibrosis" as a baby, yet "our family doctor, unfortunately, was not at that time familiar with the disease."[161] Reflecting on the period of misdiagnosis, Lee's mother noted that he "lost a month changing from one formula to another in the mistaken belief the baby had a food allergy," and "that month nearly cost our child his life."[162] When Lee was eventually diagnosed with CF, "his body was not only painfully emaciated, but he had already suffered irreparable lung damage."[163]

Despite the adverse health outcomes associated with Lee's delayed diagnosis, he did benefit early on from seeing a doctor who not only was aware of CF, but who was also persistent in his belief in Lee's CF diagnosis even after several negative sweat test results. Lee's mother soon realized that their experience with faulty sweat tests was not an isolated one, noting that "in 1964, although an accurate, inexpensive test for detecting C-F was common nationally, I found tests given in the local hospital were so often in error that conscientious doctors, suspecting cystic fibrosis, sent their small patients to a C-F clinic elsewhere."[164] Thus, as Lee's case and many others make clear, the existence of a highly accurate test for a disease does not necessarily translate to a timely diagnosis if physicians don't think to use it. Furthermore, as discussed earlier, resistance to using an accurate diagnostic tool such as the Gibson–Cooke sweat test can lead to the proliferation of less accurate tests and result in devastating misdiagnoses.

Delayed or missed diagnoses based on physician inexperience, attitudes toward mothers, and racial bias, as well as growing dissatisfaction with the limitations of available sweat tests, drove physicians and parents to call for a new method that could easily screen for CF in *all* children to identify those who should be referred for diagnostic testing using the gold standard Gibson–Cooke method. As Lee Smith Belnap's mother reflected on the topic in 1969, "reliable as the pilocarpine iontophoresis [Gibson–Cooke test] is in diagnosing a child already suspected of having cystic fibrosis, it is still too time-consuming to be used for mass screening."[165] The next chapter will document how physicians and families tried to address the persistence of diagnostic uncertainty despite the availability of a quantitative diagnostic sweat test by exploring a range of possible screening tests for CF in the 1970s and 1980s, in the hope that all children with the disease would be diagnosed promptly and started on treatment, which many believed would lead to better outcomes.

CHAPTER THREE

Blood, Sweat, and Wrinkled Hands

Screening Tests for Cystic Fibrosis

After losing her first child to a "crib death" at three months of age, Jan Lowman spent endless hours trying to figure out what had happened to the baby.[1] As Jan explained, "when she died, I guess I became kind of paranoid," and "I read a lot of magazines and all types of literature on children's diseases."[2] One night in 1978, at around 11:30, she came across information on a "kiss test" for cystic fibrosis, urging parents to kiss their babies, and if they tasted especially salty to reach out to their doctor for diagnostic testing. At that time, Jan and her husband, Charles, had three living children, a baby daughter, a two-year-old son, and a four-year-old daughter. The night that she learned about the kiss test, Jan kissed each of her children and noticed that her son "Eric appeared to be salty," but "the other two didn't."[3] Following Eric's positive home test, Jan called her pediatrician, whom she described as "a wonderful man."[4] However, as Jan recalled, he "tried to put me off, but I persisted that the children be tested further."[5]

Shortly after Jan performed the kiss test on her children, they were given diagnostic sweat tests for cystic fibrosis at the Children's Medical Center in Dayton, Ohio. Recall from Chapter 2 that the quantitative sweat test measured sweat electrolytes, which were elevated in people with CF. Consistent with the home kiss test results, Eric's sweat test for CF was positive and he was diagnosed with the disease. His older sister Nikki was also diagnosed with CF despite a negative kiss test, and CF was ruled out in the youngest child, Stacy, after a negative sweat test.[6] Around that time, the Cystic Fibrosis Foundation described CF as "a chronic, degenerative disease that primarily attacks the lungs and digestive system" and noted

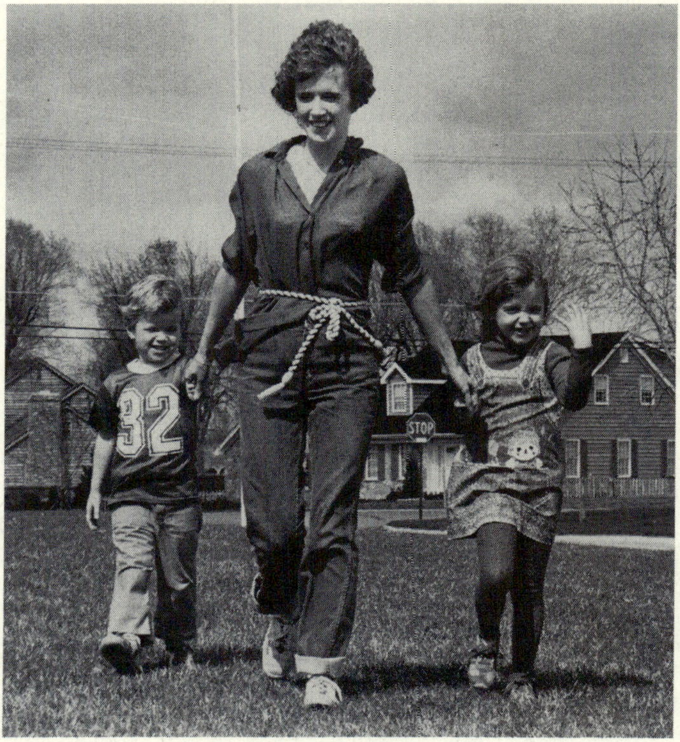

FIGURE 3.1. Jan Lowman with her son Eric (four) and daughter Nikki (six). Both were diagnosed with cystic fibrosis after their mother performed the kiss test on them at home in 1978. Reproduced with permission from Jim Nichols, "Ignorance Isn't Bliss," *Dayton Daily News*, April 20, 1980. Photograph by Wally Nelson. Courtesy of Wright State University, *Dayton Daily News* Archive.

that it was "the number one genetic killer of American young people."[7] Consistent with the wide range of clinical profiles seen in people with CF, Nikki's symptoms were "basically respiratory," whereas Eric's symptoms were "more in the digestive system," requiring him to take pancreatic enzymes with food.[8] Reflecting on the role of the kiss test in the CF diagnoses, Jan remarked that "I guess I am the only person in the area to ever have discovered CF that way."[9] Following the diagnosis of Nikki and Eric, Jan became involved with the Cystic Fibrosis Foundation, taking part in their fundraising and awareness efforts. In fact, an article promoting the kiss test and featuring the Lowman family appeared in the *Dayton Daily News* on April 20, 1980 (Figure 3.1). According to the article, "Mrs. Lowman says mothers should conduct the kiss test (it really is a lick rather than a kiss) just to satisfy any thoughts they might have about their children having Cystic Fibrosis."[10]

Jan Lowman's administration of the home kiss test in 1978 can be placed within a longer history of interest in screening for a wide range of diseases.[11] As Stanley Joel Reiser has documented, screening efforts in the late nineteenth century involved the inspection of "seemingly healthy" children in the school setting for evidence of contagious disease.[12] By the early twentieth century, given problems in population health that were revealed by exams done during the draft for World War I, routine health checkups were promoted as "preventive evaluations."[13] Screening was initially done on a per-disease basis, followed in the late 1940s and early 1950s by "multiphasic screening" for many diseases at once, although the focus on single versus multiple diseases would continue to fluctuate over time.[14] Reflecting on screening in the mid-twentieth century, Reiser explained that it "placed a great burden on the doctor, now required in addition to the normal problems of practice to deal with the anxieties of the false-positive or the marginally pathological finding, and the hollow security of the false negative."[15] While early screening approaches focused on children or adults, screening involving newborns became widespread in the US in the 1960s in the case of PKU, in which early detection allowed for the initiation of a special diet to prevent the cognitive disability seen in individuals with untreated disease.[16] Despite the many benefits of newborn screening, including potentially sparing parents "diagnostic odysseys," the possibility of early therapeutic intervention, and improved outcomes, numerous harms have also been associated with newborn screening, including stigmatization, false positive and false negative results, and overmedicalization.[17]

In discussions about strategies for newborn screening over the past several decades, many scholars have pointed to James M. G. Wilson and Gunnar Jungner's 1968 criteria for disease screening as foundational. Asked by the World Health Organization to develop principles and practices for screening programs, Wilson and Jungner noted that "the object of screening for disease is to discover those among the apparently well who are in fact suffering from disease" so that preventive measures could be put in place.[18] In discussing how one should evaluate the results of a screening test, Wilson and Jungner focused on a number of metrics, the first of which was the validity of a test, defined as "the measure of the frequency with which the result of that test is confirmed by an acceptable diagnostic

Screening result	True disease classification of apparently well population	
	Diseased persons	Persons without disease
Positive	With disease and with positive test (true positives)	Without disease but with positive test (false positives)
Negative	With disease but with negative test (false negatives)	Without disease and with negative test (true negatives)
Total	Total unknown cases of disease	Total persons without disease

$$\text{Sensitivity}^a = \frac{\text{Diseased persons with positive test}}{\text{All persons in population with disease}}$$

$$\text{Specificity}^a = \frac{\text{Non-diseased persons with negative test}}{\text{All persons in population without disease}}$$

FIGURE 3.2. "The Efficiency of a Screening Test." Reproduced from James Maxwell Glover Wilson and Gunnar Jungner, *Principles and Practice of Screening for Disease*, World Health Organization, https://iris.who.int/handle/10665/37650. © 1968.

procedure."[19] To illustrate this point, Wilson and Jungner explained that one needed to first determine the number of true positives (those who have the disease and receive a positive screening test) and true negatives (those who do not have the disease and receive a negative screening test) and then use that information to calculate the sensitivity and specificity of the screening test, respectively (Figure 3.2). In "an ideal test," the sensitivity and specificity would be high, and the false negative and false positive results would be correspondingly low.[20] In addition to reflecting on how to evaluate the results of screening, Wilson and Jungner laid out ten principles of early disease detection, "perhaps the most important" of which stipulated that "there should be an accepted treatment for patients with recognized disease."[21] However, as Diane Paul and Jeffrey Brosco have noted, Wilson and Jungner's tenet that a therapeutic intervention be available "was being described by some as outmoded" by the 1990s.[22] In fact, as efforts to implement newborn screening for CF were contemplated in the last third of the twentieth century, one can detect a consistent tension between efforts to implement screening to reduce delays in diagnosis, debates about the validity of screening tests, and uncertainty about whether early detection would actually lead to better health outcomes.

This chapter examines the development and implementation of screening programs for CF in the 1970s and 1980s following the widespread recognition of missed diagnoses despite the availability of the sweat test, providing insight into the nature of screening in medicine more broadly. Screening approaches for CF have taken a variety of forms in terms of who was doing the screening (ranging from medical professionals to parents), where the screening was taking place (such as the home, the school, the laboratory, or the physician's office), and what was being measured (including electrolytes in sweat, hair, or nails, skin wrinkling following water exposure, or proteins in the meconium, stool, or blood).[23] In the setting of widespread interest in screening for CF, the Committee for a Study for Evaluation of Testing for Cystic Fibrosis was established in the US in 1974 to evaluate, among other things, the "various screening tests for the diagnosis of cystic fibrosis in the newborn infant that have been proposed in this country and abroad, about which there is considerable controversy."[24] As noted in Chapter 2, the committee was sponsored by the National Institute of Arthritis, Metabolism, and Digestive Diseases and the Division of Lung Diseases of the National Heart and Lung Institute, with input from the CF Foundation, the US Army, and the US Navy. The committee's 1976 report made several recommendations, including the assertion that "research to develop a reliable and safe neonatal screening test . . . for cystic fibrosis is essential."[25]

Drawing from three of the many examples of screening tests for CF that were proposed in the 1970s and implemented to varying degrees, this chapter documents the diversity of approaches to screening and examines how screening has both reduced and contributed to diagnostic uncertainty. Beginning with Kiss Your Baby campaigns that were implemented at least as early as 1973 by individual chapters of the Cystic Fibrosis Research Foundation (later renamed the Cystic Fibrosis Foundation), the first section reflects on how parents such as Jan Lowman were given the agency and responsibility to use their own sense of taste to screen for CF in their children.[26] The chapter then shifts to the "bucket test," proposed by a New Zealand physician in 1974 to detect rapid skin wrinkling following water exposure in people with CF; this test sheds light on the use of dermatological findings as a method to screen for systemic disease.[27] The chapter ends by examining the early years of the most widely adopted screening test for CF, first described in 1979 by physicians in New Zealand, which used blood spots from Guthrie cards that were developed for PKU screening to measure the level of a pancreas enzyme.[28] Even though this blood enzyme approach to newborn screening addressed concerns associated with the sweat test, such as failure to test in the first place, new challenges were introduced in the form of false positive and false negative screening results, which contributed to the persistence of uncertainty in the diagnosis of CF.

Urging Parents to Screen for Cystic Fibrosis with the Kiss Test

In 1978, a Cystic Fibrosis Foundation report pointed to a "well-known, old German proverb" that linked salty sweat to an early death and suggested it could be a possible reference to CF.[29] According to the report, the proverb "reads approximately, 'the baby who is kissed at birth and tastes salty will have a short life.' "[30] In fact, numerous German texts from the eighteenth and nineteenth centuries recount such a proverb, often referring to a salty forehead as a sign that the child would not survive long.[31] Following studies in the early 1950s documenting that people with CF had elevated electrolytes in their sweat, many parents of people with CF reflected on how a salty kiss was associated with the disease. For example, one mother who was involved in the Central Indiana branch of the National Cystic Fibrosis Research Foundation remarked in 1962, in reference to her daughter with CF, that "when you touch your lips to her temple, you get a strong taste of salt."[32] James Conniff, whose son Bobby was diagnosed with CF after he died in his crib at six weeks of age (as discussed in Chapter 2), noted in 1966 that "parents need not cringe before C/F's 90 percent mortality rate before the age of five . . . *if*, on noting that a kissed baby 'tastes salty' . . . , they insist on a sweat test."[33] Based on Conniff's extended account of his experience, it is clear that he believed that his son would have lived longer if he had been diagnosed with CF in a timely manner.

At least as early as 1973, in the midst of widespread concerns about negative health outcomes associated with delayed diagnoses, many individual chapters of the Cystic Fibrosis Research Foundation initiated Kiss Your Baby campaigns in which parents were urged to use their own sense of taste as a home screening test for the disease.[34] The campaigns both challenged and reinforced physician expertise, as parents who tasted excess salt on their baby's skin were instructed to ask their physicians to administer a diagnostic sweat test for CF, as Jan Lowman did. Similar to the "do not delay" campaigns initiated by the American Society for the Control of Cancer (which became the American Cancer Society) in the early twentieth century and its promotion of breast self-exams beginning in the mid-twentieth century, the Kiss Your Baby campaigns are an example of a disease-specific constituency placing responsibility on the public for more favorable health outcomes.[35] In the case of the Kiss Your Baby campaigns, the kiss test was presented to parents as both an affective interaction demonstrating love and as a technical interaction in which the parent played a key role as a partner in the diagnostic process by conducting a screening test for CF.[36] Furthermore, many descriptions of the kiss test included an image of a woman kissing a child, highlighting assumptions at the time about the gendered nature of caretaking.[37] However, despite the main focus on women as administers of the kiss test, it is important to note that the campaigns did not exclusively target women, as some Kiss Your Baby campaigns included images of men kissing children.[38]

In what appears to be the first such campaign, the Indiana chapter of the Cystic Fibrosis Research Foundation initiated Kiss Your Baby Week, May 6 to May 13, 1973.[39] As Indiana chapter president Leonard LeRoy explained, Kiss Your Baby Week "is one way we have to help parents become aware of the disease and insure [*sic*] an early diagnosis."[40] The Indiana campaign was widely advertised, with notice of Kiss Your Baby Week featured in newspapers from at least thirty-two states, and chapters in many other states initiated their own Kiss Your Baby Weeks following the Indiana campaign.[41] For example, as noted in *The Chicago Defender*, a Kiss Your Baby Week was held in Illinois in September 1973 to "help parents become aware of the disease" to ensure an "early diagnosis."[42] As the president of the Northern Illinois Chapter of the National Cystic Fibrosis Research Foundation noted, the campaign aimed to intervene in the professional diagnostic process because "too many children with C-F are misdiagnosed, or diagnosed only after the disease has progressed quite far."[43] Descriptions of Kiss Your Baby campaigns appeared in newspapers throughout the United States from at least 1973 to 1989, with articles typically highlighting parental responsibility and improved outcomes associated with early diagnosis.[44] As the executive director of the Iowa chapter noted in 1975, "many doctors as well as the general public are not familiar enough with the disease to be able to diagnose it immediately," and "cystic fibrosis can masquerade for years behind childhood colds and infections."[45] In other words, it was hoped that the kiss test would reduce uncertainty by prompting those who screened positive to receive a sweat test.

Some newspaper articles incorporated patient accounts to highlight the urgent need for Kiss Your Baby campaigns. For example, as noted in *The Atlanta Constitution* in 1977, Diane Rowland's concerns about her infant daughter's health were not taken seriously by the baby's physician, who said that she was simply "being an anxious mother" who was "overreacting."[46] However, after months of concerning symptoms, including several hospitalizations, Mrs. Rowland switched to a new physician, who "ran tests on Sonya, including the sweat test," and she was diagnosed with CF at five months of age, highlighting the role of physician error in delayed diagnosis.[47] After recounting the challenges associated with Sonya Rowland's diagnosis, the newspaper article highlighted that "the Georgia Chapter of the Cystic Fibrosis Foundation is kicking off 'Kiss Your Baby Week' today."[48] In another example from the mid-1970s, a North Carolina newspaper article featured two-and-a-half-year-old Robbie Boitnott, who was diagnosed with CF at nine months of age after his mother, who "had worked at a medical school," noticed that he tasted salty when she kissed him.[49] As Mrs. Boitnott explained, "I knew a little about the disease, so I told them that when I kissed Robbie, he tasted very salty."[50] Based on the results of his mother's kiss test, his physician ordered a sweat test and Robbie was diagnosed with CF.[51] After providing an account of Robbie's history and diagnosis, the news article promoted the upcoming Kiss Your Baby Week that was being held through the Winston-Salem Chapter of the CF Research Foundation.[52]

In addition to newspaper articles, the Kiss Your Baby campaigns were publicized by newspaper and magazine advertisements, bumper stickers, posters, dinner dances, and TV broadcasts.[53] For example, in 1975, the *Hartford Courant* ran a half-page advertisement that featured a young woman holding a baby in her arms; her lips were close to the baby's forehead while the baby lifted one hand to the woman's face.[54] On the top left side of the advertisement were the words KISS YOUR BABY in large font, with an extended message below about the importance of early detection and prompt treatment of CF. It began with, "You can't help but kiss your baby. He's so lovable. So wonderful. And, he needs you so much." The advertisement went on to say, "That's just why we ask you to 'kiss your baby.' If he should have cystic fibrosis, he needs you to do something about it. . . . Diagnosis and immediate treatment are vital to his life."[55] This image (or a slightly different one featuring the same woman and baby) was included in numerous advertisements and newspaper articles across the US between 1975 and 1980. Furthermore, a large version of this advertisement was framed and put on display during a CF Foundation dinner dance fundraiser held in New Rochelle, New York, in 1977 (Figure 3.3,

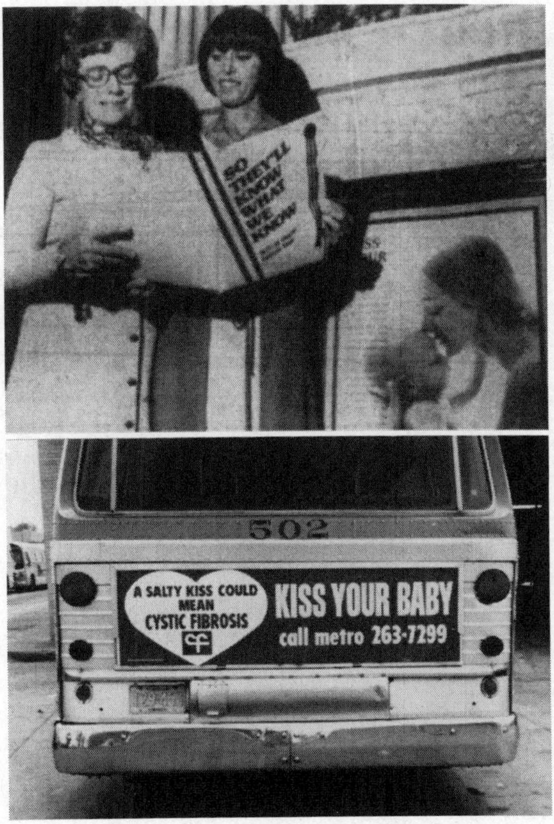

FIGURE 3.3. Cystic Fibrosis Foundation awareness and fundraising campaigns. *Top*: Photograph from A Kiss for Life fundraiser for cystic fibrosis held in New Rochelle, New York, in 1977. Pictured are event chair Gail Larocca and cochair Cathleen Nolan. Image appeared in "A Kiss for Life," *The Daily Item*, November 24, 1977. © Michael DeChillo–USA Today Network via Imagn Images. *Bottom*: KISS YOUR BABY advertisement on a city bus, undated. Photo courtesy of the Cystic Fibrosis Foundation.

top).[56] Reflecting on another approach to raising awareness about CF, a minister at a hospital recalled her early days on staff, explaining that "as I walked into work past the other staff cars, I noticed many of them had bumper stickers that read 'Kiss your baby' " and "I thought it was some kind of sweet reminder that new babies need kisses."[57] However, she "soon learned that . . . these bumper stickers were telling parents to literally kiss their baby and, if the baby tasted salty, to get him or her checked for cystic fibrosis."[58] Bumper stickers advertising the Kiss Your Baby campaigns also appeared on buses (Figure 3.3, bottom).

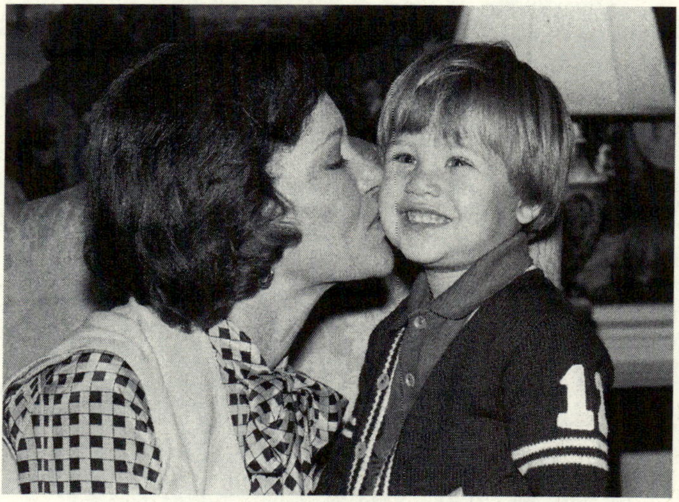

FIGURE 3.4. "This recent photo released by the White House shows First Lady Rosalynn Carter kissing her grandson Jason 'with very special attention' to assist the Cystic Fibrosis Foundation in its 'Kiss Your Baby' program." Image appeared in "Kiss Can Signal Cystic Fibrosis," *York Daily Record*, October 27, 1977. Courtesy Jimmy Carter Presidential Library.

As part of the CF Foundation's goal to "make the connection between salty skin and CF as widely known as the connection between a sharp pain on the right side and appendicitis," the Kiss Your Baby campaigns were associated with numerous well-known people, organizations, and events.[59] For example, Rosalynn Carter took part in the Kiss Your Baby campaign in 1977.[60] According to a *Newsday* report, the First Lady was approached by a sibling of someone with CF who worked in the White House mailroom, requesting that she be photographed performing a kiss test on her grandson Jason. The photo appeared in newspapers across the US, as well as at least one in Canada (Figure 3.4).[61] Also in 1977, the National Association of Insurance Women chose the "Kiss Your Baby public education program" as a service project and the organization later received the "Cystic Fibrosis Foundation award for the best first 'Kiss Your Baby' campaign."[62] The following year, two people from Pittsburgh broke the world record when they "continuously kissed for five days" to raise awareness for cystic fibrosis.[63] They began their kiss "beside a sign declaring the foundation's slogan: 'Kiss Your Baby,' a plea to parents to taste their children's skin for unusual saltiness."[64] As the Kiss Your Baby campaign continued into the 1980s, a number of prominent individuals, including comedian Joan Rivers, Speaker of the House of Representatives Thomas (Tip) O'Neill, and professional baseball player Bob Horner, were involved with outreach efforts on behalf of the CF Foundation.[65] Furthermore, while not mentioning the campaigns per se, the 1976 and 1985 editions of physician Benjamin Spock's widely circulated book *Baby and Child Care* highlighted the elevated level of salt in the sweat of individuals with CF, "which the parents may notice on kissing their baby."[66] In fact, Emily Kramer-Golinkoff was diagnosed with CF in 1985, at six weeks of age, after her mother "read about CF in the Dr. Spock book." As Kramer-Golinkoff explained, the book "said if you lick your baby's skin and it tastes like a salty pretzel then they may have CF, and so my mom licked my skin, I tasted like a salty pretzel and she asked the doctors to do a sweat test, which is how people with CF are diagnosed."[67]

It is unknown how many people directly benefited from the Kiss Your Baby campaigns. Reflecting on this topic in 2025, Robert Beall, former president and CEO of the CF Foundation, recalled that "there was never an assessment of the effectiveness of the campaign."[68] Furthermore, the false positive and false negative rates associated with this screening approach would have been nearly impossible to calculate, yet there exist numerous accounts of children who were diagnosed in response to an advertisement.[69] For example, in 1975, when Holly Sharp was about nine months old, "the CF Foundations 'Kiss Your Baby' public awareness campaign was being televised" and prompted her parents to get her tested for CF after they noticed that she tasted salty when kissed.[70] Just a few years later, around 1978, when Monica Durkin was about four years old, her mother noticed that she tasted salty after responding to a Kiss Your Baby Campaign advertisement. Despite the positive home test, "Monica's doctor didn't believe anything as serious as cystic fibrosis could be the problem, but at the Durkins' insistence, he ordered the salt test," and "the disease was confirmed."[71] As noted in the *Detroit Free Press* in 1980, Brian Webber "was born a very sick child," yet his parents, June and Jim Webber, were "glad the birth occurred during one of the Cystic Fibrosis Foundation's annual 'Kiss Your Baby Weeks.'"[72] The Webbers had "heard the ads, read the stories, kissed Brian and detected the taste."[73] Brian tested positive for cystic fibrosis soon after his parents performed the kiss test and began treatment for the disease, and he was reported to be "doing quite well" in 1980.[74] Similarly, Shelly McGee was diagnosed with CF in the mid-1980s, at seven months, as the result of an awareness campaign. As McGee explained while a senior at Mumford High School in Detroit, "Carmen Harlan (TV news anchor) advertised that if you kiss your baby and taste salt, you should have them tested for CF," and "that's how my parents discovered I had it."[75]

While many of the Kiss Your Baby advertisements appeared to be directed at parents, the CF Foundation did provide information about the campaign to physicians, some of whom performed the kiss test on their patients in the 1970s and 1980s as well.[76] For example, just days after Gayla Langford was born in Texas in 1975, "she started coughing," and by six months of age, she was hospitalized for bronchial pneumonia.[77] Because she was "not responding to any type of treatment," Gayla was transferred by ambulance to Children's Hospital in Dallas, where the physician "kissed her on the forehead and licked his lips."[78] Next, the physician "had the intern with him do the same thing," and "he asked the intern if his lips didn't taste salty."[79] After the positive kiss test, Gayla was given a sweat test and diagnosed with CF.[80] Something similar happened to Michael Griffin when he was about five months old and had a "chronic cough" and a tendency to "spit up his formula."[81] As noted in the *Dayton Daily News*, "after what seemed like a routine examination, the pediatrician did something peculiar . . . he picked up the baby and kissed him on his forehead."[82] While it is difficult to know whether these physicians were influenced by the Kiss Your Baby campaigns or simply drew from their awareness of the high salt content in the sweat of people with CF, it is clear that many children were diagnosed with CF following a positive kiss test. However, the Kiss Your Baby campaigns seem to have ended by the late 1980s, likely due to a range of factors. As Robert Beall recalled in 2025, CF "centers began to raise concern about the number of people" who "were sweat tested or evaluated after 'salty taste,'" but who then "often proved negative" for CF.[83] Furthermore, according to Beall, "in addition to burdening the centers, the anxiety it created with the parents as they waited for 'confirmation' created significant and sometimes unhealthful anxiety."[84] On a related note, the subjective nature of what constituted a salty kiss and the increasing availability of more quantitative screening methods for the disease may also have contributed to the decreasing prominence of the Kiss Your Baby campaigns in the late twentieth century.[85]

The Bucket Test as a Screen for Skin Manifestations of Cystic Fibrosis

As the Cystic Fibrosis Research Foundation was attempting to raise awareness of CF through the Kiss Your Baby campaigns, a New Zealand physician proposed a method that simply involved observing how quickly skin wrinkled following water exposure. Throughout the twentieth century, numerous texts were published that outlined the skin manifestations of systemic diseases to aid physicians in their use of cutaneous changes in the diagnostic process. For example, in 1906 New York dermatologist Lucius Duncan Bulkley published his lectures from the previous thirty years in a book titled *On the Relations of Diseases of the Skin to Internal Disorders*.[86] As Bulkley pointed out, "the occurrence of a cutaneous disorder may often be of the greatest service to a patient as a warning, a red signal flag of danger thrown out, which, if properly heeded and rightly cared for may save more serious consequences."[87] As physician and historian Justin Maxwell Rogoski explains, "clearly by the 1930s . . . skin had become a mirror of internal health . . . a key to deciphering what was on the *inside*."[88] The value of the skin in the diagnosis of systemic diseases was further reinforced in Wisconsin dermatologist Kurt Wiener's widely cited 1947 book *Skin Manifestations of Internal Disorders*.[89] In the text, Wiener acknowledged the value of modern laboratory technologies but also expressed concern that physicians of his day were no longer as skilled at incorporating observation into the diagnostic process. To address this concern and make it easier for physicians to consider skin changes in making diagnoses, Wiener coined the term *dermadrome*, "a synonym for true skin manifestations of internal disorders."[90] Wiener's book was reviewed by numerous physicians, including Paul di Sant'Agnese, whose work related to the sweat test for CF was discussed in Chapter 2.[91] While di Sant'Agnese thought that the topic was "well covered" in many respects, he did point to "some important deficiencies," including the omission of a discussion of cutaneous changes in "nutritional disturbances in infancy."[92] It is possible that Wiener's book may have influenced di Sant'Agnese's work on the changes in sweat electrolyte composition in people with CF, as the New York heat wave that preceded the sweat electrolyte observation occurred in the same year that di Sant'Agnese reviewed Wiener's book.[93] Almost two decades later, a Texas dermatologist pointed out that "the skin is often a window through which light may be shed on some underlying internal disease."[94] Physicians have continued to recognize skin changes as important signs that can help facilitate the diagnosis of systemic diseases such as lupus, Lyme disease, AIDS, and COVID-19, to name just a few.[95] In fact, as dermatologist Lisa Arkin explained in a 2021 oral history interview, "even when people are like, 'ah, it's just skin,' " she tells them, "you just wait for it because this is going to turn into more."[96]

It's unclear if physician Robert Elliott was aware of the broader work on the skin manifestations of systemic diseases when he was traveling from New Zealand to the United States by ship in the early 1960s, but he later recalled that he got the idea for a skin-based screening test for CF at that time. While on the ship, Elliott "noted that swimming in the onboard salt water pool for very long periods did not cause fingertip skin wrinkling unlike swimming in fresh water pools."[97] Aware of the altered salt content in the sweat of children with CF based on his experience as a CF physician, Elliott attempted to apply this observation about skin wrinkling to develop a possible screening test for CF. As Elliott explained years later, "I decided to try immersing the hands of CF children in fresh water and found their fingertips wrinkled much faster than normal children."[98] He went on to publish his findings in a short note in *The Lancet* in 1974, suggesting that "three minutes and a bowl of water might provide a cheap screening test for this condition."[99] Reflecting back on this publication more than four decades later, Elliott explained that "I claimed it was my discovery," yet "on questioning, mothers of CF children all knew this!"[100]

Less than a month after Elliott's publication, physician A. P. Norman and colleagues from London noted that Elliott's description of faster skin wrinkling in children with CF "may be an observation as important as that of di Sant'Agnese when he noted the high salt concentration of the sweat."[101] In their publication in *The Lancet*, the London physicians presented the results of a study in which six infants with CF exhibited "very marked wrinkling" within two to five minutes of exposure to water, a finding that they did not see in any but one control child "of similar nutritional state."[102] The control child whose fingers wrinkled more rapidly than the rest, with slight wrinkling by five minutes, was the twin sibling of a child diagnosed with CF. Other investigators would later postulate that this sibling was a carrier with one copy of a mutated CF gene.[103] As shown in Figure 3.5, the investigators highlighted the difference in skin wrinkling following exposure to water by providing photographs of the fingers of one child with CF and one "normal" child. A few months later, another physician published a note in *The Lancet* stating that Elliott had been "correct in attributing the rapid wrinkling of the skin in cystic fibrosis, which follows immersion in tap water, to the increased salt flux from the sweat glands," and provided a detailed hypothesis of the mechanism responsible for this phenomenon.[104]

Despite these early reports, not all physicians agreed with Elliott's claim that children with CF exhibited faster skin wrinkling upon exposure

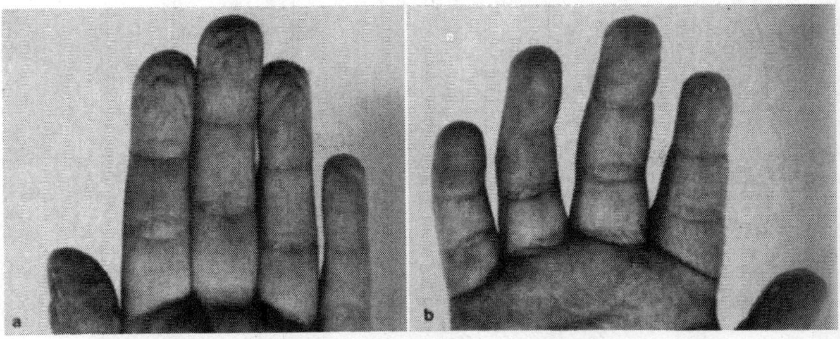

FIGURE 3.5. "(a) A cystic-fibrosis hand and (b) normal hand, after five minutes' immersion in hot water." Reprinted from A. P. Norman, M. L. Mall, and M. K. Johns, "Skin Wrinkling in Cystic Fibrosis," *Lancet* 304 (1974): 358–9. © 1974. Reproduced with permission from Elsevier.

to water than those without CF. For example, in the October 19, 1974, issue of *The Lancet*, physician C. Economou-Mavrou and colleagues from Athens, Greece, provided data that challenged the assertion that "excessive" skin wrinkling in children with CF "might provide an easy, cheap, and probably reliable screening test for cystic fibrosis."[105] To support their claim that rapid skin wrinkling was not "an abnormal phenomenon" specific to CF, the investigators included a table documenting that "immersion of the fingers in warm tap water for 5 minutes" resulted in "marked wrinkling" in a number of children with no apparent health problems and in those with a variety of diseases other than CF.[106] However, less than two months later in a note in *The Lancet*, Elliott reasserted his claim that skin wrinkling occurred faster in children with CF.[107] As Elliott explained, "the range of normality varies in different climatic conditions, and in Auckland wrinkling does not appear in cool tap-water (18–22°C) under 3 minutes in normals."[108] After noting the factors that could affect the time to skin wrinkling, such as age, recent exposure to sea water, and temperature, Elliott suggested "that 'normality' needs redefining in Athens if 6 of 17 'normals' were 'abnormal.'"[109] To reinforce his claim, Elliott included a table indicating the typical time for skin wrinkling to occur in the setting of different diseases and in healthy individuals, documenting that people with CF were the only ones whose hands wrinkled in 2.5 minutes or less.

The following year, Martin Johns of the Institute for Child Health and the Hospital for Sick Children in London weighed in on the topic of rapid skin wrinkling in people with cystic fibrosis and outlined methods for the photographic documentation of such changes in the journal *Medical and*

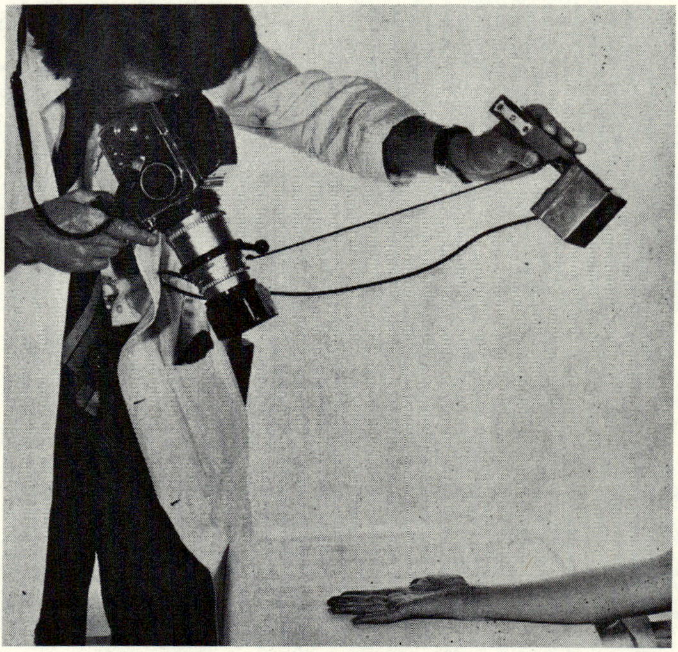

FIGURE 3.6. "The camera and lighting position. The length of the flash synchronising lead determines the position of the lighting within acceptable limits to give reasonably consistent results over a long series of patients in a number of different locations." Image from M. K. Johns, "Skin Wrinkling in Cystic Fibrosis," *Medical & Biological Illustration* 25, no. 4 (1975): 205–10. Copyright orphan.

Biological Illustration.[110] Using A. P. Norman's cases at the Hospital for Sick Children for the study, Johns stressed the importance of the proper placement of the camera and lighting source to document the extent of wrinkling present following water exposure (Figure 3.6). In other words, instead of simply visualizing the skin changes, Johns proposed that the screening technology expand to include a specific method of photographic documentation of skin wrinkling. In observing "a long series of children," Johns asserted that "almost without exception, the children with cystic fibrosis had noticeable wrinkling of the fingers within 2 min of immersion in hand-hot water, whereas normal children showed no (or minimal) wrinkling after 10 min."[111] Like Elliott had recalled, Johns also noted that many parents of children with CF had already been aware of this "rapid wrinkling at bath times," yet they "had either thought nothing of it or had not wanted to bother the doctors with such a trivial observation!"[112] Johns concluded that "this test would thus appear to provide a simple and cheap screening method for cystic fibrosis."[113] However, he stressed that the test "may not be absolutely reliable" because it was difficult to do accurately in newborns, one child with CF did not exhibit rapid wrinkling, and "one or two" control individuals did exhibit rapid wrinkling.[114]

Despite early interest in New Zealand and the United Kingdom, it appears that investigators did not continue to actively pursue skin wrinkling as a screening test for CF for the remainder of the twentieth century (although attention to the bucket test as a screen for CF would reemerge in the twenty-first century in many countries, including the United States, as noted in the epilogue).[115] In addition to concerns about the specificity of skin wrinkling to identify people with CF, it is also possible that physicians did not continue work on the bucket test in the final decades of the twentieth century because other screening tests were deemed more promising. Of particular note, New Zealand investigator Jeanette Crossley and colleagues, including Robert Elliott, provided evidence in 1979 that infants with CF had elevated levels of a digestive enzyme in the blood, a finding that was applied to newborn screening programs using Guthrie cards, a method that is still in use in many countries today.[116]

Newborn Screening for Cystic Fibrosis Using a Pancreas Enzyme in the Blood

As CF physicians were exploring various screening tests for the disease in the 1970s, E. Elias and colleagues of the Royal Free Hospital and Hoechst Pharmaceutical Research Laboratories in England described a new method to measure the level of a pancreas enzyme in the blood.[117] The investigators were not specifically focused on screening for CF, but rather on the early diagnosis of a range of pancreatic diseases. As Elias and colleagues explained, there were "no satisfactory blood-tests for screening" for pancreatic diseases at that time, and the "more invasive tests" were "not entirely reliable."[118] To address this issue, they developed a radioimmunoassay to measure the level of the pancreatic digestive enzyme trypsin in the blood, the same enzyme that was measured in the duodenal intubation test for CF discussed in Chapter 1.[119] As historian of science Angela Creager has documented, the radioimmunoassay was used by the 1970s for a range of applications and "the sensitivity and simplicity of the method led to its wide adoption in laboratory research and in medical diagnostics."[120] Consistent with this assessment, Elias and colleagues noted in 1977 that the "measurement of serum-trypsin at an early stage may simplify and shorten the sequence of tests undergone by many patients to obtain a definitive diagnosis in pancreatic disease."[121]

Drawing on the work of Elias and colleagues in developing the radioimmunoassay method to detect blood trypsin, investigators in New Zealand described a screening test for CF just two years later. As outlined in the March 2, 1979, issue of *The Lancet*, Jeanette Crossley and colleagues at the University of Auckland School of Medicine used the radioimmunoassay method to provide evidence that the digestive enzyme trypsin was elevated in the blood of young children with CF.[122] At that time, the investigators knew that digestive enzymes were produced by the pancreas and released into the intestine in healthy individuals, yet the enzymes were unable to leave the pancreas in many people with CF. As Robert Elliott, one of the 1979 coauthors (and the physician who proposed the bucket test in 1974), later explained, "the rationale was quite simple" because "we knew the ducts draining the pancreatic juices into the intestine are blocked in CF, so where were all the enzymes going?"[123] He postulated, "were the dammed up enzymes flowing back into the blood? The answer was YES."[124] After demonstrating that the pancreatic enzyme trypsin was elevated "in the first few months of life" in the serum of children with CF, Crossley and colleagues developed an assay for measuring the immunoreactive trypsin (IRT; later referred to as immunoreactive trypsinogen, the precursor to trypsin) present in dried blood spots.[125]

In particular, Crossley and colleagues used stored Guthrie cards from newborn screening that had been conducted for other conditions, such as PKU, including eleven from children who were later diagnosed with CF. There is an interesting parallel between the later reuse of stored Guthrie cards for CF testing and historian Joanna Radin's work documenting how scientists froze blood from indigenous peoples with the anticipation of future testing using technologies that had yet to be developed.[126] While the cost of the assay to screen for CF was a potential drawback, the New Zealand investigators argued that IRT screening using dried blood spots was preferred over existing screening methods because "the sample is already collected for other purposes in countries conducting Guthrie testing of the newborn" and "the test gives an abnormal result even for C.F. children with residual pancreatic function."[127] Since these children with at least some pancreatic enzymes available for food digestion would not be detected using screening tests targeting the pancreas that were already available (such as the stool trypsin or meconium albumin tests), the IRT bloodspot screening test would in theory be able to detect children with a wider range of disease manifestations.[128] Also in 1979, investigators in England addressed a key limitation of the IRT detection procedure outlined by Crossley and colleagues.[129] Of note, they used much smaller and more practical 4.25-mm-diameter dried blood spots, as compared to the 12-mm dried blood spots that Crossley and colleagues had used, to confirm that IRT was elevated in infants who were later diagnosed with CF and to document that IRT decreased in people with CF as they got older.[130]

Reflecting on her initial studies with colleagues from New Zealand, Crossley recalled in 2009 that "we were fortunate that our 1979 *Lancet* paper robustly established the potential of blood spot IRT for CF newborn screening, using the Hoechst-Behring Riagnost Trypsin Kit."[131] However, consistent with the critique by the investigators from England, Crossley acknowledged that the Hoechst–Behring "kitset as supplied required a relatively large sample size . . . , so our next step was modifying that method."[132] As Crossley explained, "for several reasons, economics being a main one, . . . we developed our own Auckland radioimmunoassay 'from scratch'" and found that it "was more sensitive . . . than our optimization of the Hoechst-Behring kitset assay."[133] In fact, using their newly developed "Auckland assay," Crossley and colleagues provided evidence in 1981 that this enhanced IRT method for newborn screening for CF (which used much smaller 3-mm-diameter discs from Guthrie cards) was highly sensitive in the context of both retrospective and prospective studies.[134] To conduct the retrospective study, Crossley and colleagues examined IRT levels from "the Guthrie cards of 24 confirmed cases of CF, and the two cards adjacent to each in the file (same hospital of birth, same date of birth)."[135] The results of their retrospective study demonstrated that the IRT levels from saved blood spots of those with CF were elevated compared to controls (Figure 3.7). Of particular importance, the elevated IRT levels occurred in infants with CF "whether or not they have residual exocrine pancreatic function," allowing for the detection of individuals with a broad range of clinical profiles.[136] Using the same assay, the New Zealand investigators then carried out a prospective study in which a second blood sample was collected from all infants with an elevated IRT at five days following birth.[137] The one infant who had a persistently elevated IRT subsequently had two positive sweat test results and "was under the continuing supervision of a paediatrician."[138]

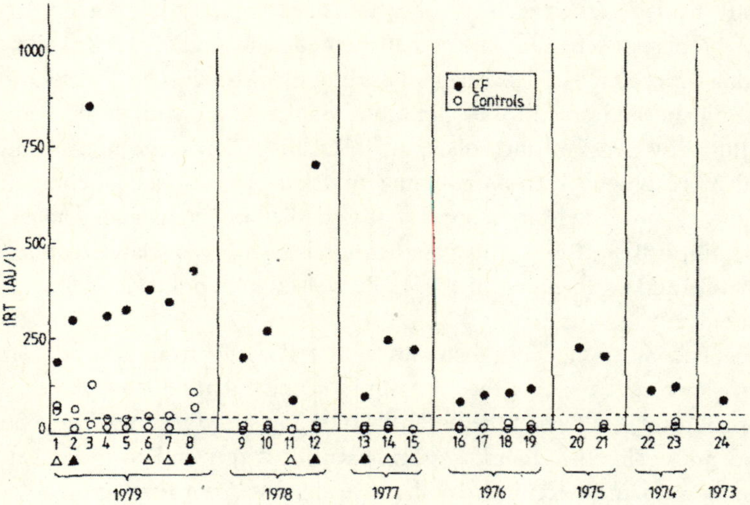

FIGURE 3.7. "A retrospective study of known cases of CF. IRT concentrations were measured in 3-mm diameter samples from the 5-day Guthrie cards, which had been stored at room temperature for up to 7 years. Stool trypsin levels on the 5th day were known for 10 of the babies studied: (▲) normal, (△) abnormally low." Reprinted from Jeanette R. Crossley, Patricia A. Smith, Brian W. Edgar, Peter D. Gluckman, and Robert B. Elliott, "Neonatal Screening for Cystic Fibrosis, Using Immunoreactive Trypsin Assay in Dried Blood Spots," *Clinica Chimica Acta* 113, no. 2 (1981): 111–21. © 1981. Reproduced with permission from Elsevier.

As part of their analysis of the new screening method, Crossley and colleagues also directed their attention in the early 1980s to the sensitivity and specificity of the IRT test for detecting cases of CF.[139] The use of the terms *sensitivity* and *specificity* in diagnostics can be traced to the early twentieth century, in the context of immunological concepts stemming from the development of serologic tests for syphilis.[140] As discussed earlier, the sensitivity of a test, such as IRT screening for CF, refers to the proportion of people who have the disease who test positive, and specificity indicates the proportion of people who don't have the disease who test negative.[141] Sensitivity and specificity will ideally be high, and, correspondingly, the false negative and false positive rates will be low. However, as Wilson and Jungner argued in their report to WHO in 1968, "a relatively high proportion of false positives can be accepted" in the context of a screening test, as a diagnostic test will follow.[142] In contrast, scholars have noted that a high false positive rate in a compulsory diagnostic test, such as for HIV or syphilis, is not acceptable because of the associated stigma that can result from such a finding.[143] When considering the appropriate level of specificity for the newborn IRT screening test for CF, Crossley and colleagues opted for lower specificity, and a correspondingly higher false positive rate, as they did not want to miss any infants with CF. Explaining their rationale for a lower IRT cutoff level and increased false positive rate, Crossley and colleagues noted that "a more extensive pilot programme may provide the justification for raising the cut-off value, . . . in the meantime, however, we prefer to err on the side of caution, and to accumulate information on those babies who are therefore designated 'false positives.'"[144] Based on the results of their initial studies, Crossley and colleagues noted that "no false negatives are yet known," although concerns about the sensitivity of the IRT test would eventually emerge.[145]

In addition to reflecting on the false positive and false negative rates associated with the IRT screening test for CF, Crossley and colleagues acknowledged in their 1981 report that "the justification for neonatal screening for CF is not universally accepted," as there were ongoing debates about the potential risks and benefits of an early diagnosis, including whether screening would translate to improved health outcomes in those with the disease.[146] However, several countries began implementing newborn screening for CF before widespread consensus about benefits were reached, and, as noted earlier, Colorado became the first US state to implement IRT-based newborn screening for CF in 1982.[147] Just a year later, in 1983, the US Cystic Fibrosis Foundation published a position paper on neonatal screening for cystic fibrosis, in which they pointed to a wide range of issues that needed to be addressed before screening should be implemented.[148] Even with earlier claims by the New Zealand investigators that people with some level of pancreatic sufficiency had elevated IRT as newborns, one of the CF Foundation's many concerns was that "to date, it has not been validated that newborns with CF who have normal pancreatic function will have an elevated IRT level."[149] Since about 10 percent of people with CF were thought to be pancreatic sufficient at that time, this translated to a "possible 10% obligatory false-negative rate for the IRT test."[150] Based on this and other potential drawbacks of screening, including the lack of clear evidence in support of improved health outcomes and the possible detrimental "effects on early parent-child interaction," the report emphasized in capital letters that "THE TASK FORCE STRONGLY RECOMMENDS THAT NO MASS POPULATION SCREENING FOR CYSTIC FIBROSIS BE IMPLEMENTED, EVEN IF A VALID AND RELIABLE TEST IS AVAILABLE."[151]

In subsequent years, numerous investigators would gather data to inform decisions about the possible implementation of IRT-based newborn screening for CF on a larger scale.[152] In addition to reflecting on the potential benefits and drawbacks of the early detection of infants with CF, investigators continued to contemplate how best to set up screening protocols to optimize for sensitivity and specificity and to correspondingly ensure that the false negative and false positive rates were as low as possible. For example, after screening 75,000 newborns in Australia and concluding that the "blood spot IRT assay . . . is an excellent screening test for detection of cystic fibrosis," Bridget Wilcken and colleagues acknowledged in 1983 that "sensitivity and specificity are satisfactory, but more experience is required before these can become optimal."[153] On a similar note, investigators at the Cystic Fibrosis Center at Johns Hopkins University described the IRT assay as "relatively simple, easily adaptable to automation, and inexpensive," yet they pointed out that "still to be determined are the sensitivity, specificity, and predictive value of the assay, optimum time for specimen collection, and the cut-off level at which retesting should be carried out."[154] Reflecting on newborn screening approaches more generally, the Johns Hopkins investigators stressed that while "the screening test itself may seem innocuous, . . . the potential for mislabeling is enormous . . . since every newborn is exposed to the procedure."[155] In fact, such concerns about mislabeling, in the form of false positive or false negative results following screening, would continue throughout the 1980s and beyond.

In the midst of widespread debates about the potential benefits and drawbacks of newborn screening for CF, as well as the reliability and validity of the IRT-based screening test itself, investigators in Wisconsin began a prospective study of CF newborn screening using dried blood spots on April 15, 1985 (Figure 3.8).[156] The trial was designed such that all infants whose parents did not opt out would be screened using IRT testing on blood spots already collected as part of newborn screening in that state, yet the results of only half of them would be shared at the newborn stage; the results of the other half would not be unblinded and shared until the child turned four. The study design allowed parents whose children were in the control group to ask for and receive the screening results, but "only 0.03% of parents ever asked for the results, including many residents who had babies during what turned out to be nine years of the study."[157] Despite extensive vetting by institutional review boards and funding agencies before the study began, associate investigator Norman Fost explained in an oral history interview that the study "has been controversial, to put it mildly."[158] Some expressed ethical concerns about the study design, suggesting that informed consent was inadequate, among other things, but as

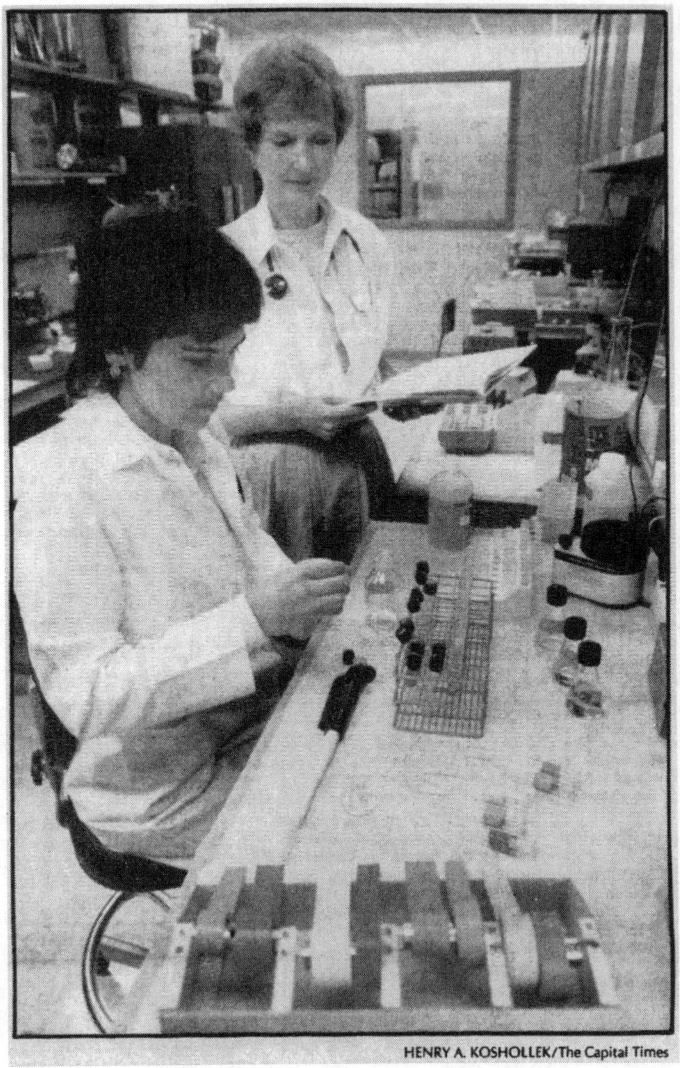

FIGURE 3.8. "Dr. Elaine Mischler (right), director of the University of Wisconsin Cystic Fibrosis Pulmonary Center, says research on the disease still has a long way to go. Anita Laxova (left) is research project manager for a newborn screening project." Reproduced with permission from Barbara Mulhern, "Cystic Fibrosis Study Raises Moral Issues," *Capital Times*, September 6, 1989. © *The Capital Times*.

principal investigator Philip Farrell explained years later, "clinical diagnosis was the standard in this country at that time," so the Wisconsin investigators justified having a control group that would not receive screening results at the infant stage.[159] When the Wisconsin study went forward, the hope was that it would allow investigators to determine the risks and benefits associated with IRT-based newborn screening for CF and provide needed information about the ideal test design as stakeholders decided whether to implement newborn screening on a larger scale in the US.

The debate about newborn screening for CF in the mid-1980s occurred within the context of deliberations about newborn screening more generally in the US and beyond.[160] For example, several months after the Wisconsin study began, at the Albany Birth Defects Symposium investigators from the US, Canada, and Japan discussed the advantages and disadvantages of newborn screening for a variety of diseases, including cystic fibrosis.[161] As a general note of caution, New York physicians pointed out that following the passage of the National Sickle Cell Anemia Control Act in 1972, "misguided but well-intended programs for screening for the disease" were implemented, resulting in a range of harms, including stigmatization.[162] Reflecting further on the sickle cell anemia case, they explained that the "results of screening programs were misused by industry, the military, insurance companies, etc., to exclude clients from positions or benefits."[163] In contrast, Robert Guthrie, who was honored at the symposium for his work on PKU newborn screening, pointed to the case of sickle cell anemia to support CF newborn screening, noting that CF "is a condition where we are screening primarily to start symptomatic treatment early and to permit genetic counseling" and "in these respects, it is like newborn screening for sickle cell disease, where it has been shown in New York State after ten years of screening, that it is significantly beneficial to have newborn screening carried out."[164] As Guthrie explained, "I think the controversy over screening for cystic fibrosis is definitely going to be resolved in favor of newborn screening."[165]

Several years after the Albany symposium, investigators continued to reiterate concerns about the sensitivity and specificity of IRT-based newborn screening for CF.[166] For example, an analysis of newborns who had been screened as part of the Wisconsin study between 1985 and 1988 revealed a 10.8 percent false negative rate.[167] The investigators noted that it would have been possible to detect CF in these newborns "if the neonatal cutoff value for the IRT assay is lowered" below 180 ng/mL, yet doing so would have "greatly increased . . . the number of false-positive results."[168] To illustrate their point with a specific example, the Wisconsin group explained that "if the neonatal cutoff point had been decreased to 160 ng/mL, only 1 of the 4 false-negative results in the newborn period would have been avoided, whereas there would have been 101 more false-positive results . . . almost twice as many."[169] In other words, the investigators were aware that there was a delicate balance between false positive and false negative results when considering screening test design. Data obtained from Wisconsin also documented that IRT levels in many individuals with CF fell in the weeks and months following birth, which the group predicted would further contribute to false negative results in newborn screening algorithms that involved taking a second blood sample for repeat IRT testing at a later date.[170]

In the early 1990s, investigators continued to point to challenges associated with IRT-based screening approaches. At the Fourth International Conference on Newborn Screening for Cystic Fibrosis in 1991, physician Beryl Rosenstein noted that "it is somewhat disappointing that 11 years after Dr. Crossley's initial report we are still encountering significant methodologic problems with IRT screening programs . . . attested to by the variety of assay kits and cut-off points in use and the plethora of proposed screening strategies."[171] Rosenstein also found it "disturbing that there are still many unresolved issues regarding reference standards and quality control" and encouraged conference attendees to take part in "an expanded international laboratory quality assurance program" led by UK clinical biochemist Mary Heeley and colleagues.[172] As investigators lamented the challenges associated with IRT-based newborn screening, there was still a lack of consensus about whether it was even appropriate to screen newborns for CF. For example, noting that the incidence of false positive results varied and could reach "as high as 80% on a single test," Wisconsin investigators felt in 1992 that the "potential adverse psychological and social effects of screening" were "particularly worrisome," especially since the "infant and family with erroneous results receive no medical benefits."[173] However, by 1994, the Wisconsin study would document improved nutritional outcomes for babies identified through CF newborn screening, a finding that contributed to the Centers for Disease Control and Prevention (CDC) recommendation of universal newborn screening for CF in 2004 and the eventual implementation of CF newborn screening in all US states by late 2009.[174] Furthermore, as Joëlle Vailly and others have noted, the Wisconsin study would play an important role in the adoption of CF newborn screening outside of the US as well.[175]

As investigators were weighing the possible risks and benefits of early diagnosis of CF in the late 1980s and early 1990s, many were also reflecting on the possible advantages and disadvantages of adding a DNA analysis step to IRT-based newborn screening. Following the identification of the gene associated with CF in 1989, which will be discussed in the next chapter, Wisconsin investigators suggested in 1990 that "the strategy for cystic fibrosis newborn screening will need to evolve into a true two-tier screening test," with the first tier being IRT analysis at the newborn bloodspot stage, followed by DNA analysis "performed on the same original blood spot" if the IRT value was above a certain cutoff level.[176] A year later, Wisconsin investigators further suggested that there would be "potentially great advantages with such an approach, including a much higher positive predictive value and reduced psychologic toxicity for the population at large."[177] Based on theoretical calculations, they estimated that the positive predictive value (the probability that someone with a positive screen actually has the disease) would increase from 13.7 percent with IRT alone to 48.6 percent with an IRT/DNA algorithm.[178] Excitement about a "drastically reduced" false positive rate with incorporation of DNA testing into IRT-based screening algorithms was also expressed in 1991 by Robert Elliott, the New Zealand physician who had proposed the bucket test in 1974 and was involved in the initial IRT study in 1979.[179] Many others also thought that an IRT-DNA screening strategy would significantly reduce the high false positive rate seen in IRT screening approaches, although physicians did acknowledge that incorporation of DNA testing into the algorithm would not reduce the false negative rate (for reasons that will be discussed in Chapter 4).[180] Focusing on the potential value of a two-tiered IRT-DNA algorithm, Wisconsin physicians Philip Farrell and Elaine Mischler asserted in 1992 that "great advantages will occur with such an approach . . . particularly with respect to false-positive families."[181] While researchers would eventually provide evidence that false positive test results were "greatly reduced" with the incorporation of DNA testing into IRT-based newborn screening algorithms, uncertainty following CF newborn screening remained a concern in the decades that followed, as Rachel Grob and Joëlle Vailly have documented.[182]

The next chapter will examine the incorporation of genetic testing into screening and diagnostic approaches for CF, highlighting how DNA-based strategies addressed some challenges while simultaneously introducing new forms of uncertainty, such that the quest for certainty in CF diagnostics remained elusive even in the context of DNA testing.

CHAPTER FOUR

Missing Mutations

Complexity and Uncertainty in Cystic Fibrosis Genetics

Soon after Rowland White was born in California in 2021, his blood was obtained through a heel prick and used to carry out routine newborn screening for a wide range of diseases, including cystic fibrosis. As a nurse explained to his mother, Cambrey White, "if there is something concerning on the newborn screen, don't worry, someone will call you."[1] Cambrey never received a call, but her son Rowland developed several symptoms consistent with CF in the months following his birth, including a cough and difficulty gaining weight, and he was eventually diagnosed with the disease at six months of age.[2] At the time of Rowland's diagnosis, CF had long been understood as a genetic disease that occurred when an individual received two disease-causing variants of the CF gene, one from each biological parent. As his mother recalled in 2022, the CF diagnosis came as a surprise for two reasons.[3] First, Cambrey had received a negative carrier screen result for CF when she was pregnant; as she recalled, her physician explained to her that the genetic test indicated that she did not carry a mutated version of the CF gene and therefore could not have a child with CF.[4] Second, Rowland had received a negative newborn screen result for CF shortly after he was born, a further indication that he did not have the disease.[5]

In a blog post just weeks after Rowland's diagnosis, Cambrey asked, "how in the heck could we be one of those rare cases that had two negative screenings yet a CF diagnosis (confirmed by something called a sweat test) for our son?"[6] While the answer to this question wasn't clear at the time, genetic testing completed several weeks later would provide some insight. White learned that she had received a false negative carrier test result, meaning that she actually was a carrier, but the carrier test came back as negative because her CF gene mutation was not included on the carrier screening panel, which "only tested for the 40 most common mutations."[7] At that time, more than two thousand variants in the CF gene had been described, yet only some of them had been characterized as disease causing, and many were not included on screening panels.[8] The complexity of CF genetics also contributed to Rowland's false negative newborn screening result, as Cambrey recalled that neither of his two CF gene mutations (identified after his CF diagnosis) were included on the panel of seventy-seven gene mutations that were evaluated when he was born in California in 2021.[9]

After Rowland's geneticist shared the specific mutations that he had inherited from each of his parents, Cambrey felt both "sad and fascinated at the same time."[10] As she explained, "during the time that we knew Rowland had CF but did not know his mutations, the geneticist suggested that my Ecuadorean ancestry could play a role in the mutation I carry." In fact, when Cambrey was told which CF gene mutation Rowland had inherited from her, she had already learned from the medical literature that it was the second most common mutation seen in Ecuador.[11] As Cambrey pointed out in 2022, "I have heard that CF is most common in people with European ancestry. However, more recently I have learned that isn't necessarily true—*rather CF has been well studied and documented in people with European ancestry compared to other races*."[12] In fact, the erroneous assumption that CF was a "white disease" or one seen primarily in people of "European ancestry" has played an important role in the composition of gene mutation panels for CF, contributing to significant disparities in diagnosis across racialized groups.[13]

The confusion surrounding Rowland's CF diagnosis following two negative screening tests can be understood within the broader context of the rise in genetic medicine over the last third of the twentieth century, coupled with the legalization of abortion following *Roe v. Wade* in 1973 that allowed for increased attention to carrier and prenatal testing.[14] As historians have documented, approaches to studying the genetic basis of disease have shifted over time as new technologies have been introduced into medical practice. Studies in the late 1950s and early 1960s focused on karyotyping, which allowed for the microscopic detection of changes in the total number of chromosomes (such as in the case of trisomy 21).[15] The advent of chromosomal staining techniques in the 1970s facilitated efforts to identify "discrete chromosomal abnormalities," as in the case of Prader–Willi

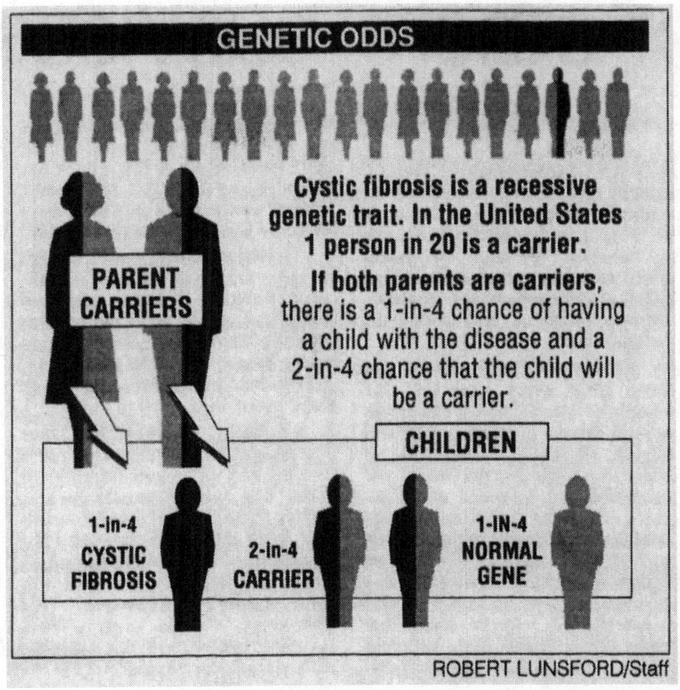

FIGURE 4.1. Illustration of the inheritance of CF included in a newspaper article on carrier screening for CF in 1990. Image from Charles Hite, "Unlocking the Genes: Genetic Screening Has the Potential to Raise More Questions Than It Answers," *Roanoke Times*, May 27, 1990, EXTRA4. © *The Roanoke Times*.

syndrome, which in the early 1980s was associated with a deletion in chromosome 15.[16] Also in the 1980s, scientists began mapping disease genes to particular chromosomes, and subsequent work focused on the identification and characterization of disease genes through positional cloning beginning in the mid-1980s. While many investigators hoped that localizing and subsequently identifying disease genes would lead to therapeutics, in most cases such information initially facilitated genetic testing approaches that were used in attempts to diagnose or reduce the incidence of the disease in question, often through reproductive interventions.

Consistent with broader trends in medical genetics, after the CF gene was characterized in 1989, scientists at academic institutions and biotechnology companies began work to develop a carrier test for preventive purposes (Figure 4.1).[17] In the decades that followed initial efforts to develop a CF carrier test in the late twentieth century, CF genetic testing was also applied to newborn screening protocols as well as diagnostic testing algorithms.[18] As the White case illustrates, CF genetic testing has been complicated by several factors, two of which will be explored in detail in this chapter. First, the inability of available genetic testing panels to definitively detect all disease-causing variants in the CF gene has resulted in false negative test results.[19] Second, even as scientists characterized additional CF gene mutations, expanded mutation panels were still unable to detect all disease-causing variants, with important differences in detection rates across racialized groups. Thus, diagnostic uncertainty in CF has persisted, albeit in different forms, following the availability of genetic testing. As such, the sweat test used to diagnose Rowland White, a variant of which was first developed in 1959 as discussed in Chapter 2, has remained the gold standard diagnostic to this day.[20]

Characterization of the "CF Gene" and Hopes for Treatment and Prevention

Early efforts to identify the gene associated with CF took place against a backdrop of widespread scientific interest in the localization of human genes, or what some scholars have referred to as the "cartography of the human genome."[21] Reflecting on the state of gene mapping efforts in 1983, a *Los Angeles Times* article explained that one scientist believed "that the new understanding of the organization of human chromosomes is bringing about a revolution in medicine comparable to that launched by the great 16th-Century scientist Vesalius, whose detailed study of human anatomy helped medical science out of the dark ages."[22] Many hoped that a human gene map would contribute to efforts to localize genes to particular regions on chromosomes, followed by the ability to treat and prevent genetic diseases. In fact, in 1983, scientists had mapped the Huntington's disease gene to a region on chromosome 4, and by 1985, the CF gene was localized to a region on chromosome 7.[23]

Despite narrowing the location of the CF gene to an individual chromosome in 1985, scientists still had to search through a region of over 1 million base pairs, or what a *Nature* editor would later refer to as a "vast genetic wilderness."[24] Almost four years later, by early summer 1989, Lap-Chee Tsui and John Riordan in Toronto, Francis Collins in Michigan, and "more than 30 collaborators" generated data that suggested they had identified the gene associated with CF.[25] While attending the Tenth International Workshop on Human Gene Mapping in Connecticut in June, Collins and Tsui "hovered over a fax machine in a freshman dorm room at Yale University."[26] As the fax came through, "reports from Tsui's lab brought the news they were waiting for," evidence that they had located the CF gene. However, they couldn't celebrate loudly because, as Collins recalled a few years later, "in the next room was one of our major competitors," and the "dorm walls were pretty thin, so we had to talk in whispers and not yell and scream."[27] According to an article in *The Boston Globe* later that summer, Tsui and Collins "kept the news quiet . . . because the hospital intends to patent the materials used in identifying the gene, as they are considered potentially commercially important for carrier and prenatal testing."[28] In fact, patents that would later be "jointly held by the University of Michigan and the Hospital for Sick Children in Toronto . . . have been nonexclusively licensed for diagnostic use, . . . making cystic fibrosis a model of collaborative and cooperative patenting and licensing practices," in contrast to the well-known controversy surrounding *BRCA1* and *BRCA2* patents.[29] By August 1989, a reporter who had heard about the discovery called Collins's lab to confirm that they had identified the CF gene, "and a graduate student, unprepared for the ambush, spilled the beans."[30] In response to the leak, press releases and news memos were issued by those involved in the research and joint news conferences were held in Toronto and Washington on August 24.[31] Just a few weeks later, on September 8, three articles describing the CF gene, as well as an editorial, were published in *Science*.[32]

Following the news of the CF gene discovery, many in the CF community expressed hope that new treatments for the disease, including gene therapy, would soon follow.[33] For example, Francis Collins, who would later go on to lead the Human Genome Project in the US and direct the NIH, described the identification of the CF gene as "a milestone of the highest order" and explained that "this advance *will* have an impact on treatment."[34] After the identification of the gene was announced at the Toronto news conference, Ashley Dyer, "a bubbly 4½-year-old patient," was the recipient of significant media attention.[35] Dyer "had become a sudden celebrity . . . not only because she is among the thousands of cystic fibrosis patients whose prospects may have taken an upward leap," but also because scientists had used DNA from Dyer and her family in their search for the CF gene (Figure 4.2).[36] For Sue Wallace, the parent of a child with CF, the gene discovery completely changed her expectations for her son's life expectancy. As Wallace explained, "When I found out my son

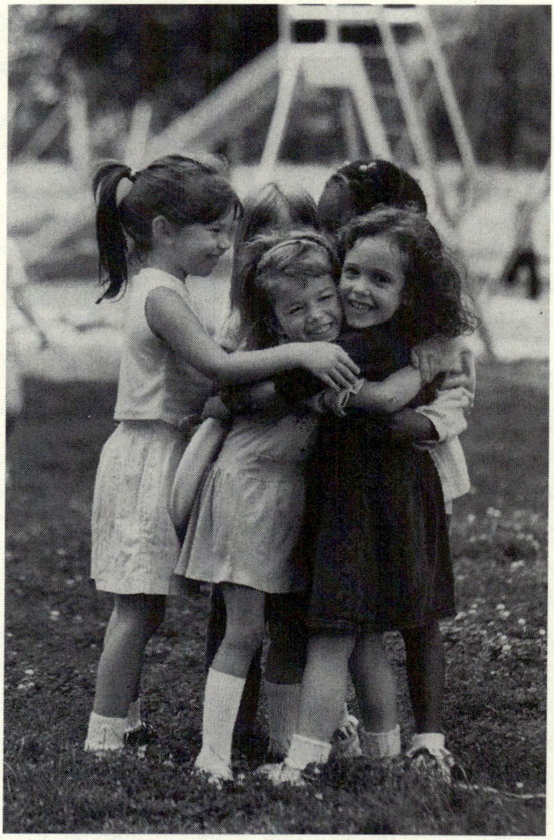

FIGURE 4.2. "Ashley Dyer, 4½ (right), who has cystic fibrosis, with playground friends." From Richard Saltus, "Race Is On to Apply Discovery: Cystic Fibrosis Gene's First Payoff Likely to Be in Prevention, Not Treatment," *Boston Globe* August 28, 1989. The photo, taken by Mike Slaughter, was originally published in the *Toronto Star*, August 24, 1989. Permission to reproduce granted by Getty Images.

had a fatal disease, I stopped worrying that he might run into the street and be hit by a car. It's illogical, I know. Yet somehow, it seemed, his fate was sealed."[37] She "never once thought there could be a cure. . . . Never, at least, until now."[38] In the days following the discovery of the gene, Wallace came "to believe that a miracle is hatching and cystic fibrosis will soon be an awful memory like polio. I guess I'd better start watching out for speeding cars again."[39] Similar sentiments of hope and excitement were expressed by children and adults with CF as well. In fact, just one day after the joint news conferences, an eight-year-old girl with cystic fibrosis described August 25 as "the most Best day ever in my Life" because of the gene discovery (Figure 4.3).[40] Enthusiasm in response to the CF gene discovery extended to the wider human genetics community as well. Reflecting years later on a talk that Tsui and Collins gave about the gene discovery at the American Society of Human Genetics (ASHG) conference in 1989, geneticist and physician Bob Nussbaum recalled that "the audience got to its feet as if it were a single organism and applauded—everyone was giddy with the realization that the vision of gene mapping had come to fruition."[41]

While many expected that a cure would soon follow the gene discovery, others were more cautious in response to the news.[42] For example, Denise Furtado, a thirteen-year-old girl with CF who was hospitalized at the time, said, "I think it's great. It gives me hope," but "it doesn't give me reason to celebrate. I'll celebrate when they come out with a cure."[43] And

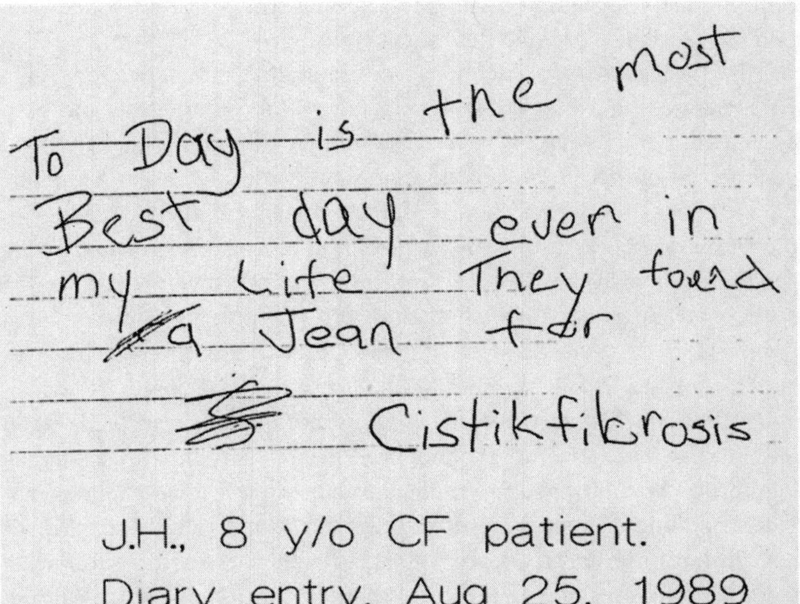

FIGURE 4.3. "Diary of Child with Cystic Fibrosis." From Francis S. Collins, "Realizing the Dream of Molecularly Targeted Therapies for Cystic Fibrosis." *New England Journal of Medicine* 381, no. 19 (2019): 1863–65. Reproduced with permission from Francis Collins, the National Human Genome Research Institute, and the Massachusetts Medical Society.

Barbara Palys, an adult with CF, felt that it would be many years before any therapeutic interventions would result from the discovery.[44] Consistent with these reactions, Francis Collins noted that "I wouldn't want to suggest that it will be 30 years before there is a cure for cystic fibrosis, but, yes, it is not an automatic progression once you find the gene."[45] In fact, as an article in the *Chicago Sun-Times* pointed out, "the difficulties of producing treatments and cures for a disease even after the genetic mutation is known is one reason for the lingering opposition to the proposed human gene-mapping project being organized by the National Institutes of Health and the Energy Department."[46] Despite opposition, both the NIH and the Department of Energy had budgets devoted to the Human Genome Project by 1990, some of which would eventually be used to focus attention on screening programs for genetic disease (including CF), genetic determinism, selective abortion and concerns about potential links to eugenics.[47] In particular, shortly after taking over the Office of Human Genome Research at the NIH, James Watson established a working group on the ethical, legal, and social implications (ELSI) of the Human Genome Project, which would fund these endeavors.[48]

As with DNA-based medicine more generally, characterization of the CF gene was followed by efforts to develop both genetic tests and therapeutics for the disease.[49] In the case of CF as in many other diseases, genetic testing became available much more quickly than therapeutic interventions.[50] Differing views about the use of CF genetic testing for preventive purposes can be placed within the broader context of more general debates at the time about the ethics of selective abortion based on genetic test results and whether such a practice constituted a form of eugenics.[51] Less than a year after the CF gene was characterized, genetic counselor Vickie Venne hinted at an additional challenge associated with the availability of genetic testing, noting that "counseling when a significant discovery is first announced means that you are challenged to interpret an unfinished story, which usually involves uncertainties that require additional time to resolve."[52] As this chapter illustrates, CF genetic testing has been associated with uncertainty in the decades following the gene discovery due to (1) the inability to detect all disease-causing variants in the gene, and (2) inequity in mutation detection rates across groups labeled by race or ethnicity. As the next section documents, these two factors jointly informed debates about whether it was appropriate to begin carrier screening with a single-mutation test that was unable to identify all carriers.

Debates About Whether to Begin CF Carrier Screening with a Single-Mutation Test

While scientists and medical professionals were aware that CF genetic testing could in theory be used for diagnostic or screening purposes, much of the emphasis following the gene discovery was placed on the development of tests to screen for carriers (individuals with a single CF gene mutation) to prevent the birth of children with CF. As investigators realized early on, the development of a genetic test to detect all carriers would prove challenging, in part due to the existence of more than one CF gene mutation. When the CF gene discovery was announced in 1989, approximately 68 percent of chromosomes in people with CF tested by the Toronto and Michigan groups had a single mutation, designated ΔF508.[53] (Pronounced "delta F508," the mutation consisted of a deletion of three base pairs in the DNA such that the corresponding protein was predicted to be missing a single amino acid, phenylalanine [F] at position 508.) At that time, many scientists predicted that an additional five or so mutations in the gene had yet to be discovered, and they expected that those mutations would account for the remaining 32 percent of chromosomes in people with CF.[54] As a CF Foundation newsletter pointed out, the different mutations could be understood "much as if a name was spelled wrong six different ways."[55] Yet it quickly became clear that the number of disease-causing mutations in the CF gene would be much higher than anyone initially predicted, complicating efforts to develop a genetic test.

As additional CF gene mutations remained to be discovered, debates ensued about whether to implement carrier testing. Some scientists felt that identification of additional mutations in the CF gene was necessary before it would be possible to offer carrier testing that was deemed "extremely accurate."[56] As Lap-Chee Tsui explained, "when those are identified, it will be possible to develop a screening test for the general population."[57] However, some researchers worried that there would be pressure to prematurely move forward with carrier screening from "companies wanting to market the tests."[58] In fact, by the end of October 1989, "at least half a dozen biotech companies [had] expressed interest in manufacturing the screening test for CF."[59] Many experts also predicted that physicians' fear of lawsuits would lead to quick adoption of carrier screening.[60] For example, as Arthur Beaudet at Baylor College of Medicine in Houston noted, "obstetricians might fear that if they don't offer the test, that a patient might have reason for litigation."[61] Beaudet went on to explain that litigation "is a legitimate fear, and that kind of reasoning could lead to rapid, premature implementation of testing."[62] While those expressing concerns about financial and legal pressure stressed that it was important to wait to implement testing until additional mutations could be detected, others thought it was imperative to move ahead right away to avoid the birth of children with CF. For example, as one London investigator argued shortly after the gene was identified, "the detection of carriers would make it possible to avoid the conception or birth of many currently unavoidable cases" of cystic fibrosis and should be carried out "now," before "all the mutations have been identified."[63]

In late October 1989, during this period of widespread deliberation about whether to implement carrier screening for CF before all of the mutations were identified, Robert Beall, executive vice president for medical affairs at the Cystic Fibrosis Foundation (and later CF Foundation president and CEO) asked both the NIH and the ASHG to take leadership roles in developing policy recommendations for CF carrier screening.[64] In a letter directed to Nancy Wexler in her role as chair of the ELSI working group on human genome research, Beall postulated that "CF carrier screening could become the largest genetic screening program in history" and suggested that Wexler's "committee of the Human Genome Project has the expertise to tackle this problem and perhaps use the [*sic*] CF as a model system in examining programs for the future."[65] It appears that Beall's letter circulated among those in leadership positions at the NIH, including Elke Jordan, deputy director of the National Center for Human Genome Research (NCHGR). As Jordan and one of her NIH colleagues pointed out in an internal letter in early November 1989, "the availability of a genetic test for cystic fibrosis raises the kind of questions that the human genome program is concerned about," and "the NCHGR is therefore interested in stimulating some discussion about these issues as they relate to cystic fibrosis before a test becomes generally available."[66]

However, a commercial genetic test would become available before the NIH had a chance to facilitate extensive discussions on the topic of CF carrier testing. By early November 1989, Integrated Genetics, which had been acquired by Genzyme Corporation, announced that it had developed a genetic test for CF that could detect a single mutation, ΔF508.[67] The test, at a cost of $185, was described as an effective means to "accurately identify 70 percent of all carriers of the defective gene" and diagnose people with CF "with a high degree of accuracy."[68] However, shortly after the single-mutation genetic test became available, a statement put out by the ASHG asserted that "carrier testing should be offered to couples in which either partner has a close relative affected with CF," yet they expressed "serious reservations" about more widespread use of the test, noting that "*routine* CF carrier testing of pregnant women and other individuals is NOT yet the standard of care in medical practice."[69] The ASHG was particularly concerned because "the current test detects only 70% of carriers, and there is little experience in the delivery of such complex information to large populations."[70] Many physicians supported this stance, noting that the single-mutation carrier screening test was associated with substantial diagnostic uncertainty due to its limited coverage and correspondingly high false negative rate. In other words, when an individual tested negative following the single-mutation carrier screening test, there was still uncertainty about whether they were truly *not* a carrier or simply had a mutation other than ΔF508.

Related to concerns about false negative results with a single-mutation test, an additional layer of uncertainty stemmed from the different frequencies of the ΔF508 mutation in various groups labeled by race or ethnicity.[71] As described in the February 1, 1990, issue of *The New England Journal of Medicine*, researchers in the United States and Canada used their own laboratory-based assay to determine that the ΔF508 mutation was present in 75.8 percent of CF chromosomes from what they defined as the "white population," 71 percent of CF chromosomes from the "Hispanic population," and 30.3 percent of CF chromosomes from "Ashkenazic families."[72] Of note, "North American black, Asian, and Middle Eastern families were excluded from the analysis."[73] While the investigators did not explain the exclusion, it may have been related to the relatively lower number of diagnosed cases of CF in individuals with those labels at that time.[74] In fact, inequity in the sensitivity of the ΔF508 single-mutation test across groups labeled by race or ethnicity can be partially traced to longstanding descriptions of CF as a "white disease," an assumption that had important implications for who was even tested for CF in the first place, as previous chapters documented.[75] Furthermore, the very definition of "white" has changed over time and in different contexts in the United States, where, as historians Keith Wailoo and Stephen Pemberton point out, "whiteness is an extremely flexible and potent concept."[76] Thus, as investigators had documented by early 1990, the frequency of the ΔF508 gene mutation varied across groups labeled by race or ethnicity, and data were not even available for some groups, which meant that a negative result for the ΔF508 carrier test would be associated with a very different level of certainty depending on the population in question.

Commentary in response to the *NEJM* article focused primarily on applications of the ΔF508 CF test for carrier and prenatal testing and included ongoing deliberation about who should have access to the test.[77] For example, with parallels to direct and indirect targeting of Black people for sickle cell testing in the early 1970s due to assumptions about race, reporter Gina Kolata pointed to the uncertainty about "whether health insurance companies will pay for the test . . . for anyone who wants it, including, for example, blacks and Asians, who face a far lower risk."[78] Such debates about who should have access to CF carrier testing were taking place long before scientists calculated the frequency of the ΔF508 mutation in different populations as outlined in the 1990 *NEJM* article. For example, in 1982, those in leadership roles at the Cystic Fibrosis Foundation recommended that future "carrier screening could be utilized by the entire U.S. population of childbearing age" because "unlike some other genetic disorders there is no ethnic or racial clustering of the gene."[79] In contrast, the President's Commission for the Study of Ethical Problems in Medicine and Biomedical and Behavioral Research took a different stance a year later, suggesting in 1983 that "just as individuals without eastern Jewish heritage are not screened for Tay-Sachs disease and Caucasians are not screened for sickle-cell anemia, CF screening of American blacks is probably inappropriate" because "CF is very rare in American blacks."[80] Thus, the long-standing debate about whether and to what extent CF was a "white disease" contributed to the uncertainty about which people to test.[81]

In ongoing discussions about who should have access to carrier and prenatal testing for CF aimed at the ΔF508 mutation, many commentators argued that such tests would move forward quickly because of financial incentives, an issue that had been raised shortly after the gene was identified, as discussed earlier in the chapter.[82] As one newspaper report noted following the *NEJM* article, "even before researchers have perfected a new test to detect adults who risk having children with cystic fibrosis, commercial laboratories are rushing to create the nation's first large-scale market for genetic screening services."[83] At the time, the president of Integrated Genetics, the company that developed a commercial ΔF508 CF test in November 1989, explained that "the genetic screening industry" had "nationwide gross sales of less than a million dollars a year."[84] However, many experts predicted that the market could expand dramatically. In fact, University of Wisconsin Medical School physician Norman Fost argued that "the potential market for this screening is at minimum a billion-dollar a year industry."[85] As Fost explained, "This is the gold rush. . . . This is the Klondike."[86] Yet as physician Michael M. Kaback, the American Society of Human Genetics president-elect, cautioned, "this is an example of moving technology ahead too fast."[87]

Although some stakeholders felt it was "probably too late to stem the rush for widespread testing in this country," many experts came together in early 1990 to discuss issues related to the availability of the single-mutation genetic test for CF.[88] At an NIH workshop on carrier screening for CF in March 1990, attendees concluded that the test was not ready for population-wide screening efforts because of "technical and ethical problems."[89] Not only was the single-mutation test "imperfect" because it could detect just 70–75 percent of carriers, but workshop participants expressed concern that mutation frequencies varied "according to racial and ethnic background, so that significant laboratory and counseling modifications would be required in different populations."[90] For example, experts felt that "the current test" targeting the single ΔF508 mutation "probably would miss mutations common in blacks and Jews of eastern European descent."[91] Given these concerns, workshop attendees argued that "widespread screening should be delayed until a test is developed that detects mutations in 95% of the gene carriers."[92] Yet according to Haig Kazazian from the Johns Hopkins School of Medicine, "with so many possible mutations, it may not be possible to develop a test (for 95% of the carriers) soon, or ever."[93] Amid concerns about widespread population testing, those on the panel "conceded that some adult Americans planning to have children already are being tested for the gene."[94] In fact, at that time, it was estimated that the "flawed" single-mutation ΔF508 test was "available from at least four genetic testing companies and many private hospital labs."[95] Despite words of caution from experts, Johns Hopkins physician Beryl Rosenstein pointed out that "you can't make believe (to patients) that a test doesn't exist when it does."[96]

The Search for Additional Mutations and Further Debates About Testing

While implementation of carrier and prenatal testing using the single ΔF508 CF mutation was being debated, scientists continued to work to characterize additional mutations in the gene not only to improve genetic tests, but also to develop therapeutics for the disease. One young scientist who hoped to identify novel CF mutations, Jeff Pinard, was a University of Michigan undergraduate working in the laboratory of Francis Collins in the summer of 1990.[97] Having played a key role in the CF gene discovery, Collins's lab continued to work in the field. As Collins explained, "it's really crucial to find the other mutations . . . every new mutation tells us something more about the gene: which regions of it are essential for its function, specific details we need in order to develop effective treatments."[98] Pinard joined Collins's lab because he had a special interest in the work: he had been diagnosed with CF as a child after "two serious bouts of pneumonia," multiple hospitalizations, and difficulty gaining weight.[99] According to Pinard, his doctor placed blame on his mother "for not feeding me properly," but he was eventually given a sweat test after his younger sister was diagnosed, as she "nearly died of dehydration at one and a half."[100] As Collins explained, Pinard "has had a fairly profound effect on my lab," since he was the first person with CF many of the scientists had "direct contact with."[101]

Pinard, who had a single copy of the ΔF508 mutation, felt that the identification of the additional CF mutation that he and his sister had would be helpful for carrier screening and future therapeutic options.[102] As Pinard explained, "one thing I hope is that the mutation we have will apply to a lot of other patients," because "that would cut down on the amount of tests that are needed to identify carriers."[103] Despite articulating his hope for improved carrier testing, Pinard explained to Barbara Walters during a 1990 interview that "even if it turned out that there was a 50/50 percent chance of my children having cystic fibrosis, I would still, I would still have children; I've never met another person with cystic fibrosis that has said, 'I regret the day I was born.' "[104] In the midst of widespread debates about the ethics of genetic testing for preventive purposes, Pinard spent forty to fifty hours a week working in the lab that summer and explained that "if there really are over 100 different CF mutations, it's going to be a bear!"[105] In fact, despite his analysis of "hundreds of DNA fragments," he was not able to identify his mutation nor "those of other atypical patients" (Figure 4.4).[106] Just when he thought he was getting close, he had to be hospitalized because of a "severe infection," during which time other researchers in his lab identified two new mutations "in the very batch of DNA he had been working with."[107] As Pinard recalled, "it was so frustrating . . . I was happy for them, but wished I could have reaped the fruit of all that labor!"[108]

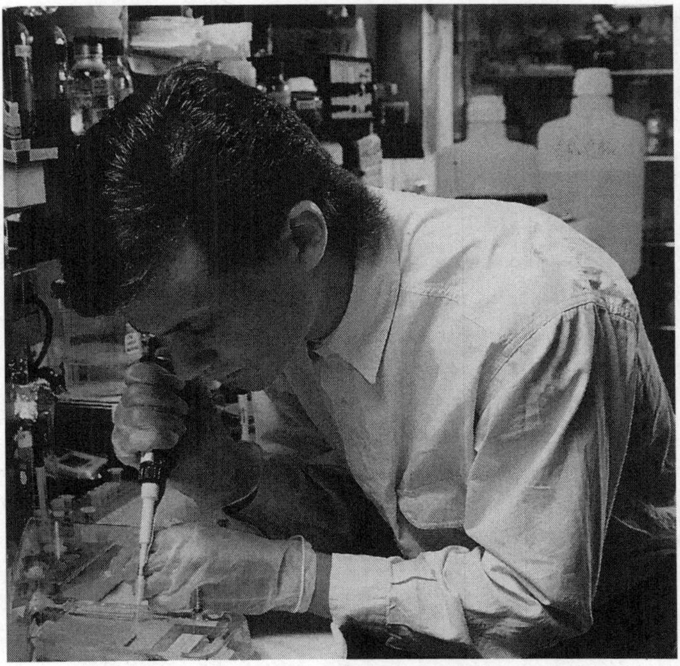

FIGURE 4.4. Image of University of Michigan undergraduate Jeff Pinard in the laboratory of Francis Collins. "He carefully inserts DNA mixed with dye into a well at the starting end of the gel. A different well is used for each patient." From Maya Pines, "Stalking a Lethal Gene," in *Blazing a Genetic Trail: A Report from the Howard Hughes Medical Institute*, 1991. Photograph by Kay Chernush.

At the time that Pinard was working in the lab in the summer of 1990, Cystic Fibrosis Genetic Analysis Consortium members had collectively identified over forty mutations in the gene.[109] The consortium had been organized by Lap-Chee Tsui and established with support from the Cystic Fibrosis Foundation shortly after the CF gene was described, with an emphasis on collaboration and open sharing of data as additional mutations in the gene were identified.[110] However, researchers continued to express concern that carrier screening would be challenging in light of the expanding number of mutations and the difficulty of testing for all of them, which was pointed to as a significant source of uncertainty.[111] These concerns about carrier screening for CF took place in the context of more general discussions about genetic testing in medicine. For example, in the summer of 1990, the ELSI working group was planning a workshop to discuss the "social and professional issues involved in the integration of genetic testing into mainstream medical practice, taking our unfolding experience with cystic fibrosis testing as a starting point."[112] During an ELSI workshop in September 1990, participants pointed to the need for pilot studies for CF genetic testing, while also discussing more general concerns about the integration of genetic testing into medicine, including issues of privacy, access to testing, laboratory quality control, and the lack of adequate resources and personnel.[113]

As stakeholders continued to debate best practices for the incorporation of genetic testing into medicine, both generally and in the context of CF, many expressed concern that CF testing was moving ahead before a sufficient number of mutations had been identified.[114] Furthermore, even as investigators characterized additional mutations in the CF gene, they weren't all included in mutation panels, and the sets of mutations tested varied across laboratories. By the summer of 1991, Arthur Beaudet estimated that "most DNA diagnostic laboratories test for anywhere from one to six or seven mutations," yet that was far fewer than the "98 probable CF mutations" that had been identified.[115] Despite concerns about false negative test results, one physician pointed out in 1991 that "the pressure is very powerful to test" because the "commercial molecular biology companies are pushing it hard."[116] Consistent with this claim, the company Collaborative Research was targeting genetic counselors and obstetricians with advertisements and brochures, and they hoped to "see a major, major market developed."[117] In fact, during the summer of 1991, the Office of Technology Assessment of the US Congress surveyed 431 genetic counselors and nurse geneticists because of "concern about the scientific, legal, economic, ethical, and social implications of the prospect that large numbers of people might be screened for their CF carrier status."[118] At a time when carrier screening was being offered more frequently for CF than for other diseases, genetic counselors and nurse geneticists varied widely in terms of their views about the suitability of CF carrier testing in the "general population," with one asserting "NO to widespread screening! Must be close to 100 percent detection for all CF mutations before it can even be considered," and another noting, "Let's go with screening! I can't believe we are not halfway through a pilot program by mid 1991."[119]

Debates about whether it was appropriate to offer widespread carrier screening for CF continued in the 1990s as additional CF gene mutations were discovered.[120] While the detection rate for carrier screening remained below the ideal of 95 percent in most stratified populations, there was one exception early on, in part due to the work of an Israeli scientist who had helped identify the CF gene in 1989. Knowing that the ΔF508 mutation was present in only about 30 percent of CF chromosomes from people in Israel, Batsheva Kerem and colleagues sought out and identified a novel mutation that was described as "the most common cystic fibrosis mutation in the Ashkenazi Jewish population in Israel."[121] Based on this and other research to lessen the uncertainty associated with carrier screening, the Genzyme panel had expanded to twelve mutations by November 1991, bringing the detection rate up "to 95% for Ashkenazi Jewish individuals and to 85% for Caucasians."[122] However, the detection rate remained much lower for other populations labeled by race or ethnicity.[123] In fact, an article published in *Newsday* in 1993 and widely reproduced in other newspapers visually depicted the notion that specific CF gene mutations were associated with certain groups, and labeled the mutation that Kerem and colleagues had identified (see position 1282, Figure 4.5).[124] Over the next several years, the number of identified mutations in the CF gene would grow, and the Genzyme CF panel expanded to thirty-two mutations by November 1993 and seventy by February 1997.[125] However, despite this expansion in the number of mutations on the Genzyme panel, the ability of the test to detect carriers still varied dramatically depending on how someone was labeled according to race or ethnicity, with most detection rates well below the target of 95 percent.

As investigators worked to improve carrier tests for CF, expanded genetic testing algorithms were often justified by the claim that the addition of mutations more prevalent in certain minoritized groups would increase the inclusivity of such tests. However, as numerous social scientists have documented, research that makes assumptions of difference to justify inclusion can reinforce problematic notions of the biological basis of difference. According to sociologist Steven Epstein, an "inclusion-and-difference paradigm" arose in medical research in the 1980s to try to shift from the standard white male as research subject to a more diverse group of subjects, including women and minoritized groups (and later the elderly and children), yet such efforts to reduce discrimination have focused on defining and then including groups based on the assumption of biological difference.[126] Furthermore, reflecting on efforts in the field of pharmacogenomics to reduce health disparities, anthropologist Duana Fullwiley points out that "one cannot but wonder if genomics' new emphasis on human difference . . . will perhaps irrationally exacerbate social notions

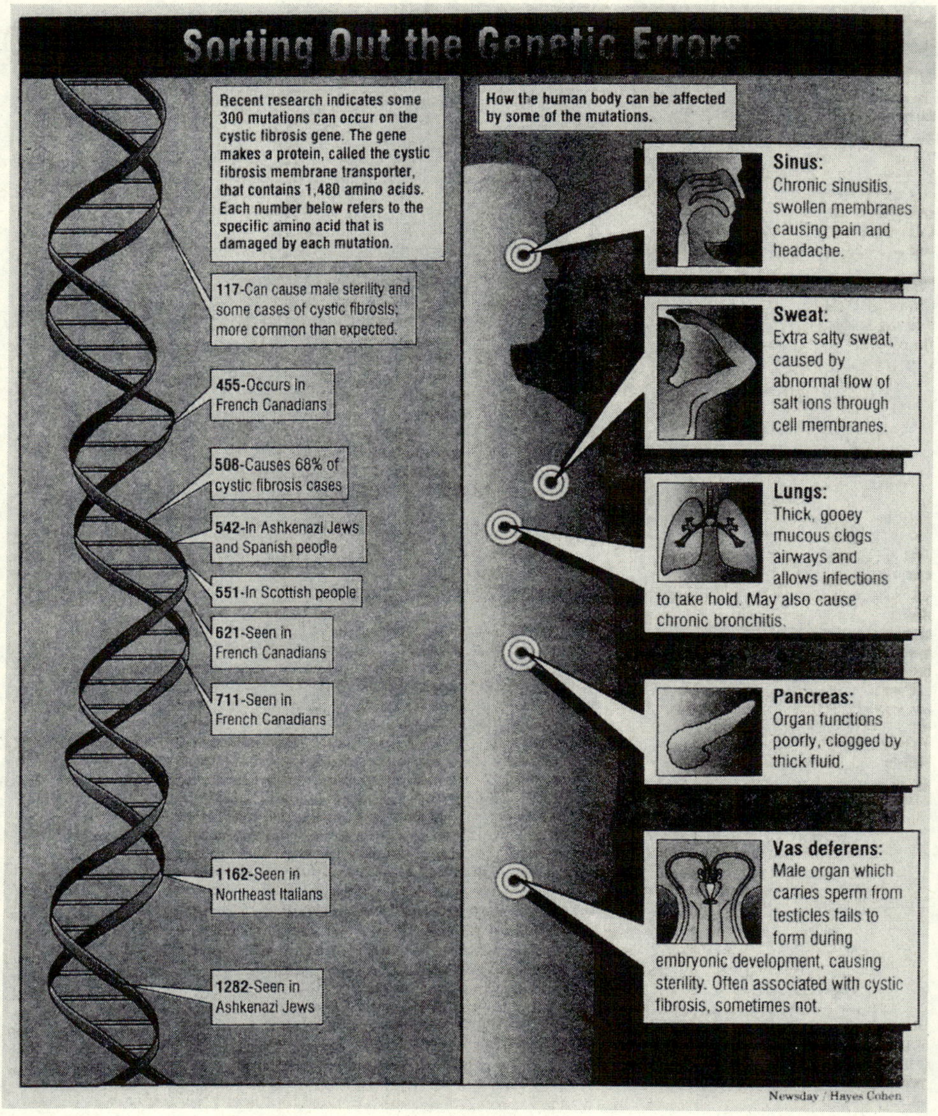

FIGURE 4.5. Diagram highlighting select mutations and their location on the CF gene, as well as regions of the body that can be affected in the setting of CF. From Robert Cooke, "A Deadly Gene's Surprise," *Newsday (Suffolk Edition)*, August 17, 1993. © 1993 Newsday. All rights reserved. Used under license.

of difference and the inequalities that these have traditionally borne," an issue of particular relevance as stakeholders contemplated the ideal makeup of a CF mutation panel, as will be discussed in the next section.[127]

Efforts to Standardize a CF Mutation Panel for Carrier Detection

As the number of identified mutations in the CF gene continued to increase in the late 1990s, many stakeholders felt there was a need for guidelines indicating the ideal makeup of a carrier panel. To gain insight into the range of CF mutation screening panels in use in 1997, the Biochemical and Molecular Genetics Resource Committee of the American College of Medical Genetics (ACMG) and the College of American Pathologists surveyed laboratories that were already involved in their proficiency challenge program. Survey results from forty-three laboratories documented "a wide range in the number of mutations tested, from just 1 to 70," indicating a lack of standardization reminiscent of challenges with previous tests described earlier in the book (Figure 4.6).[128] To provide a forum for discussions about CF mutation panel standardization and related issues, the NIH held the Consensus Development Conference on Genetic Testing for Cystic Fibrosis in Bethesda, Maryland, in April 1997.[129] Although participants did not end up making a recommendation on a specific number or set of mutations to test, they did suggest that "laboratories providing molecular diagnostic capability should utilize tests that achieve a mutation detection rate of approximately 90 percent or better for Caucasians or a detection rate for African-Americans, Asian-Americans, Hispanics, Ashkenazi Jews, Native Americans, and others comparable to that available at present."[130] However, despite efforts to increase the inclusivity of genetic tests for CF, drawbacks of the "inclusion-and-difference paradigm" remain when using such labels.[131] Furthermore, following the

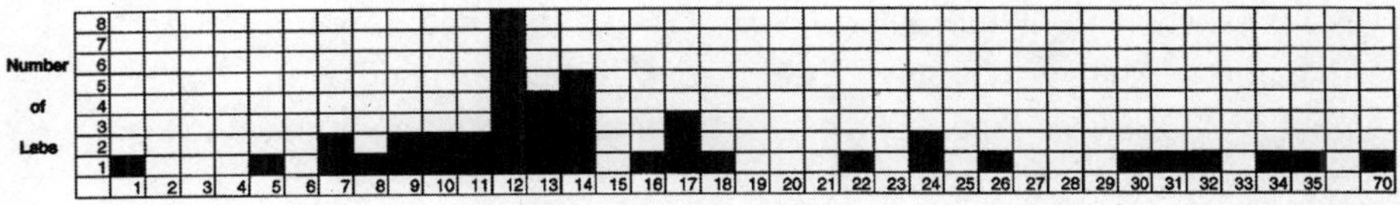

FIGURE 4.6. "Number of CFTR mutations screened by participating laboratories." Reprinted from Wayne W. Grody, Robert J. Desnick, Nancy J. Carpenter, and Walter W. Noll, "Diversity of Cystic Fibrosis Mutation-Screening Practices," *American Journal of Human Genetics* 62, no. 5 (1998): 1252–54. © 1998. Reproduced with permission from Elsevier.

NIH consensus conference, investigators who had surveyed laboratories in 1997 lamented that "the choice of number and type of mutations in CF test panels has been left to the discretion of the individual laboratories" and argued that it "would be prudent and helpful" to provide "more explicit guidelines specifying particular mutations and minimal test panel sensitivities for each ethnic population being screened."[132] As deliberations about the ideal makeup of a carrier screening panel were taking place in 1997, "more than 600 mutations and DNA sequence variations" had been described, further complicating matters.[133]

Guidance regarding a standard carrier screening panel would come several years later, in April 2001, when the CF Carrier Screening Working Group of the ACMG recommended a "pan-ethnic" panel of twenty-five mutations. The group formulated the carrier screening panel by including "all CF-causing mutations with an allele frequency of ≥ 0.1% in a general U.S. population."[134] In reflecting on the recommendations that were published in the March/April 2001 issue of *Genetics in Medicine*, Wayne Grody and colleagues noted that "implementing the delivery of mass population screening for CF carriers raised many issues and concerns including . . . the differing prevalence of individual *CFTR* mutations among various ethnic, demographic, and racial groups."[135] The ACMG recommendations were "incorporated into a joint ACMG/ACOG/NIH Steering Committee document" that was expected to be "widely distributed."[136] The steering committee recommended that carrier screening "be *offered* to non-Jewish Caucasians and Ashkenazi Jews, and *made available* to other ethnic and racial groups."[137] Acknowledging that test sensitivity was low in some groups, the committee recommended "that an extended panel should not be offered routinely . . . to couples testing positive/negative with the standard panel" because it "would provide very low additional yield."[138] Also in 2001, the year that "prenatal and preconception carrier screening for CF was introduced into routine obstetric practice," a CF carrier testing brochure was put out by the American College of Obstetricians and Gynecologists (ACOG) and included a figure indicating that one's "chance of being a CF carrier" varied "depending on race/ethnicity."[139] At that time, "CF became the first target of pan-ethnic universal carrier screening by molecular methods."[140]

While some physicians and scientists were supportive of the ACMG's recommendation of a twenty-five-mutation "pan-ethnic" carrier screening panel, others expressed concerns.[141] For example, Cornell University physician Fred Gilbert argued that the twenty-five-mutation panel "is not optimal as a screening standard for the United States because it excludes mutations that are important in population groups that are significant components of the American mosaic."[142] Genzyme scientists expressed similar sentiments in the May/June 2001 issue of *Genetics in Medicine*, where they presented data suggesting that a "pan-ethnic" panel of fifty to seventy mutations "may provide a practical test that maximizes sensitivity" compared to the twenty-five-mutation panel recommended by the ACMG.[143] Several years later, in 2004, Genzyme scientists reiterated this sentiment and argued that an expanded "panel that reflects diversity is necessary."[144] As they pointed out, "with 14% of our carrier screening referrals being from Hispanic and African American individuals, and another 12% from individuals with ethnicities other than the ACMG/ACOG recommended Caucasian or Ashkenazi Jewish, it is evident that clinicians are offering or making CF carrier screening available to a diverse population, many of whom choose testing."[145] Also in 2004, investigators in Maine and Maryland provided evidence that the clinical sensitivity of the twenty-five-mutation panel, a measure of how well a carrier couple or fetus with CF can be detected, varied dramatically based on how the carrier couples were labeled according to race or ethnicity.[146] As shown in Figure 4.7, the clinical sensitivity of each group labeled by race or ethnicity increased to varying degrees as the number of mutations analyzed increased, yet sensitivity plateaued very quickly for most groups even as additional mutations were added. Consistent with concerns about the "inclusion-and-difference paradigm" in clinical research noted earlier, the investigators acknowledged that their use of the five "racial/ethnic categories" included in the study was "less than ideal."[147] The investigators also noted that the study was limited in that "all of the results . . . assume that each individual belongs to a single racial/ethnic group and that both of the partners belong to the same racial/ethnic group."[148] Despite these limitations, the study data illustrated the extent to which false negative results were associated with the twenty-five-mutation panel. By that time, experts had already estimated that hundreds of thousands of people were being tested annually, indicating that many individuals were directly affected by decisions about the makeup of carrier screening panels.[149]

As limitations to the twenty-five-mutation panel were being discussed, guidelines for who should be tested were also being reconsidered. For example, in 2005, ACOG put out an update on carrier screening for CF.[150] As they noted, although the 2001 guidelines "recommended that cystic fibrosis carrier screening be *offered* to Caucasian couples (including Ash-

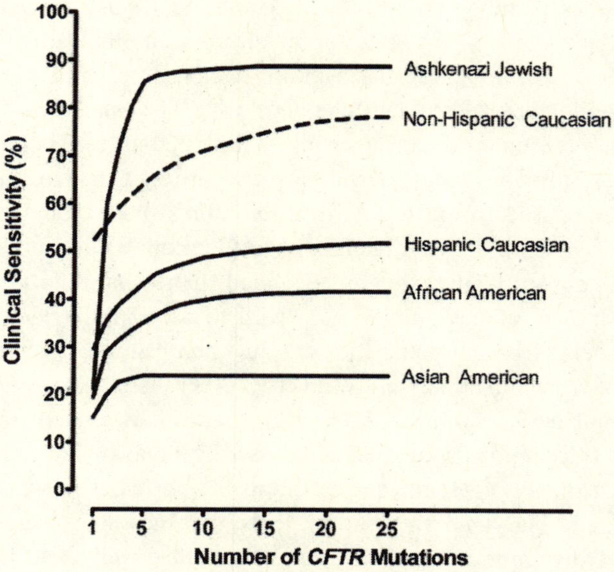

FIGURE 4.7. "Clinical sensitivity for detecting cystic fibrosis, using a panel of 25 *CFTR* mutations in five racial/ethnic groups. Clinical sensitivity (the square of the proportion of detected disease-causing mutations) is the proportion of carrier couples or affected fetuses that can be identified and is shown on the vertical axis. Horizontal axis shows the American College of Medical Genetics recommended panel of 25 mutations. For each group, the mutations are added in order from most to least common within that group. The clinical sensitivity reported is considered a maximum, as analytic sensitivity is assumed to be 100%." This figure appeared in Glenn E. Palomaki, Stacey C. FitzSimmons, and James E. Haddow, "Clinical Sensitivity of Prenatal Screening for Cystic Fibrosis via *CFTR* Carrier Testing in a United States Panethnic Population," *Genetics in Medicine* 6 (2004): 411. Reproduced with permission from Springer Nature.

kenazi Jews) . . . and be *made available to* all patients, . . . in practice, two thirds of obstetricians offer cystic fibrosis carrier screening to all pregnant patients rather than using the selective criteria."[151] Reasoning that it was "becoming increasingly difficult to assign a single ethnicity," ACOG determined that it was "reasonable to offer cystic fibrosis carrier screening to all pregnant patients, provided that women are aware of their carrier risk and of the test limitations."[152] However, ACOG still provided distinct guidance for specific groups, noting that "cystic fibrosis carrier screening *should* be offered before conception or early in pregnancy when both partners are of Caucasian, European, or Ashkenazi Jewish ethnicity."[153]

Amid ongoing discussions about who should be offered testing, debates about the ideal number of mutations on CF genetic testing panels continued as well. By 2005, Genzyme was offering a panel of ninety-seven mutations, which it argued was better at detecting CF mutations in "Caucasian," "African American," and "Hispanic" populations than the recently updated ACMG/ACOG-recommended panel (which had been reduced from twenty-five to twenty-three mutations in 2004 because one of the mutations did not meet the 0.1 percent frequency threshold and the other was reclassified as one that did not cause CF).[154] However, UCLA School of Medicine physician and geneticist Wayne Grody and colleagues critiqued the expanded mutation panels as lacking "scientific rigor," arguing that they "appear to render low additional yield" and were designed "based on arbitrary or spurious criteria."[155] They also expressed concern that "CF carrier screening has now become a commodity, and a highly competitive one at that," alluding to concerns about financial conflicts of interest in testing approaches that had been voiced since the CF gene was first identified.[156] Of particular relevance to the issue of diagnostic uncertainty, they argued that expanded mutation panels offer a "false sense of security" because even if one hundred mutations were included, "the individual could still carry any of the other 1400 *CFTR* variants that had not yet been tested."[157] The geneticists also critiqued the focus on the increased sensitivity of expanded mutation panels, noting that a "more useful parameter is . . . positive predictive value," defined as "the proportion of individuals with a positive test result who in fact have the diagnosis (or in this case, carrier state) in question."[158] As they explained, with rare mutations included in expanded carrier screening panels, "the probability that a positive result is due to a technical error (false-positive) begins to exceed the probability that the tested person is in fact a carrier," something that "one can choose to ignore . . . only at one's peril," highlighting that as one source of uncertainty was addressed, new sources of uncertainty arose, contributing to the persistence of uncertainty.[159]

In addition to critiquing the use of expanded mutation panels for CF carrier screening, Grody and colleagues reflected in 2007 on the question, "Why not just go to complete gene scanning/sequencing?"[160] At that time, CF gene sequencing was "being used almost exclusively for diagnostic testing," in large part because it was too expensive to be incorporated into routine screening programs.[161] In fact, Genzyme had already begun offering CF gene sequencing in 2006, while also continuing to offer the ninety-seven-mutation test.[162] In addition to concerns about cost, Grody and colleagues argued that gene sequencing was not a solution to the issue of false negative test results in carrier screening because of the difficulty of interpreting variants of "unknown clinical significance."[163] In other words, if sequencing were employed in the setting of carrier screening, additional uncertainty would be introduced "because interpretation of the disease-causing potential of the vast majority of rare *CFTR* mutations is not possible."[164] In an effort to determine whether uncharacterized variants in the CF gene were disease causing, the Clinical and Functional Translation of CFTR (CFTR2) project was established in 2010.[165] By 2011, 126 of the more than 1,800 variants in the CF gene had been characterized as disease causing, but the vast majority of the variants remained of uncertain clinical significance.[166] Reflecting on the challenges associated with gene sequencing for CF and other diseases in 2014, physician and geneticist Garry Cutting noted that as the application of gene sequencing approaches expanded over time, the detection of variants of uncertain significance grew at a higher rate than the annotation of such variants (to determine whether they were disease causing), resulting in an ever-increasing "interpretive gap."[167]

Over the last decade, clinicians and scientists have continued to reflect on the advantages and disadvantages of different CF genetic testing approaches. For example, in 2019, Kyle Beauchamp and colleagues from Myriad Genetics and Myriad Women's Health argued that next-generation sequencing with pathogenic variant reporting was favorable over the twenty-three-mutation panel based on their analysis of carrier screening done on approximately 100,000 individuals.[168] In contrast, the ACMG continued to recommend the twenty-three-mutation panel "as the minimum list of *CFTR* variants that should be included" for carrier screening in 2020, the same year that Cambrey White had a forty-mutation carrier test in Hawaii.[169] At that time, the ACMG did acknowledge that "laboratories may want to consider adding additional variants to their panel depending on the ethnic composition of their expected test population."[170] Just a few years later, in 2023, the ACMG updated its recommendations for CF carrier screening, noting that "improved equity in variant detection is both necessary and desirable" because "CF has been reported across all races, ethnicities, and ancestries."[171] Drawing from the prior twenty-three-mutation panel as well as the CFTR2 database (which included 401 annotated, disease-causing variants at the time of their study), the workgroup recommended expanding the minimum panel to one hundred mutations, having "set a minimum 95% carrier detection rate for all biogeographic ancestries."[172] Even with this recommendation to increase the minimum number of mutations on carrier screening panels, additional CF-causing *CFTR* variants continue to be characterized, resulting in the persistence of false negative results and continued uncertainty in CF carrier testing.[173]

As investigators have debated various approaches to carrier testing in the decades following the 1989 gene discovery, similar concerns about equity and uncertainty have been expressed about CF newborn screening algorithms with a genetic testing component.[174] Recall from Chapter 3 that early CF screening protocols for newborns examined the level of a pancreas enzyme, immunoreactive trypsinogen (IRT), in the blood; following the gene discovery in 1989, many states updated their algorithms to include a DNA testing component if the initial IRT level was elevated, and newborn screening protocols would vary across states in terms of IRT cutoff level and DNA testing method in the following decades.[175] When Rowland White was born in California in 2021, the state was employing a three-tier screening protocol, in which an elevated IRT was followed by a seventy-five- or seventy-seven-mutation DNA test, and if at least one mutation was identified, *CFTR* gene sequencing was carried out.[176] Although Rowland's IRT level was elevated, prompting DNA testing, neither of his CF gene mutations were included on the California panel, which meant that DNA sequencing was not done, and he received a negative newborn screen for CF. Around the time that Rowland underwent newborn screening, states varied widely in how many *CFTR* variants they tested for, from a low of 1 to a high of 365, further contributing to uncertainty depending on where in the US someone was born (Figure 4.8).[177] Given the increasing awareness of false negative newborn screening results such as Rowland's, the Cystic Fibrosis Foundation put out updated consensus guidelines on newborn screening in 2025.[178] Drawing insight from a multidisciplinary committee, which included Cambrey White as a community representative, the foundation recommended that "CF newborn screening algorithms should not limit *CFTR* variant detection to the F508del variant or variants included in the ACMG-23 panel."[179] Instead, the committee recommended screening "for all CF-causing *CFTR* variants as identified by CFTR2," which had reached 1,085 disease-causing variants by that time.[180] The CF Foundation also recommended that newborn screening algorithms include a "*CFTR* sequencing tier . . . to improve the specificity and positive predictive value of CF newborn screening."[181] In fact, by the time that the 2025 CF Foundation consensus guidelines were published, some states were already taking such an approach.[182]

While the 2025 CFF recommendations were based on evidence that such approaches would improve the detection of CF in newborns, the committee did acknowledge that a "byproduct" of CF newborn screening is the detection of CF carriers and those with indeterminate diagnoses who do not meet the diagnostic criteria for CF but who also do not clearly

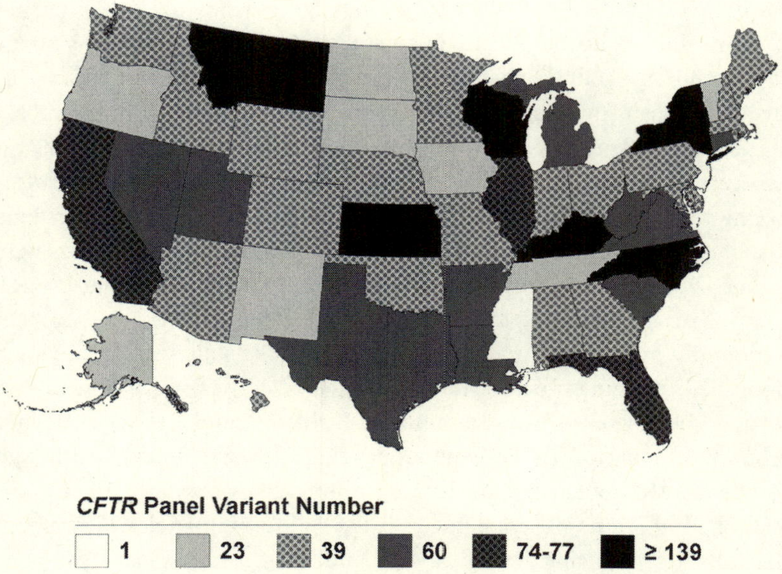

FIGURE 4.8. "Geographic distribution of CFTR variant analysis by state." Reproduced from M. R. Rehani, M. S. Marcus, A. B. Harris, P. M. Farrell, and C. L. Ren, "Variation in Cystic Fibrosis Newborn Screening Algorithms in the United States," *Pediatric Pulmonology* 58, no. 3 (2023): 927–33. Permission for use granted by John Wiley & Sons.

fit into the "normal" category.[183] In other words, as investigators have worked to reduce diagnostic uncertainty by expanding the DNA testing component of CF newborn screening algorithms over the past several decades, new uncertainties have continued to arise in the process, with "considerable implications for families and the support and resources required for follow-up," as will be discussed in the epilogue.[184]

* * *

In 2019, thirty years after the CF gene was discovered, and thirty years after genetic testing for the ΔF508 CF gene mutation first became available, the FDA approved Trikafta, a three-drug combination (elexacaftor/tezacaftor/ivacaftor) developed by Vertex Pharmaceuticals that targeted the root cause of cystic fibrosis.[185] This therapeutic intervention was the result of the venture philanthropy model pioneered by Robert Beall, in which the CF Foundation invested in Aurora Biosciences (now Vertex Pharmaceuticals) "to discover compounds that might correct the malfunctioning protein in people with CF."[186] Trikafta was the very type of intervention that many hoped would be available soon after the identification of the CF gene. Recall the statement that Francis Collins made in 1989, in which he clarified that the availability of therapeutics following the gene discovery "is not an automatic progression" yet emphasized that "I wouldn't want to suggest that it will be 30 years before there is a cure for cystic fibrosis."[187] And while Trikafta isn't a cure, many people with CF have expressed great optimism following FDA approval.[188] In fact, Jenny McGlincy, who wrote the diary entry included in Figure 4.3 when she was eight, cried when she learned of the news thirty years later.[189] As McGlincy explained in 2019, "To think of my lung function improving or my digestion increasing, or even adding a few years to my life that I could spend with my daughter. . . . Now that it's available, I'm a little like, 'Is this really happening?' "[190] Julie Desch, a retired physician and adult with CF, described Trikafta as "life changing" and noted that her cough "literally disappeared" within days of starting the drug.[191] As Desch explained in 2020, with Trikafta, CF "feels like it's more of . . . a chronic health condition that I live with . . . I don't have . . . the same feeling of, this is killing me slowly, that I used to have."[192]

Yet even as the prospects for many with CF have improved following the availability of Trikafta, not all people with the disease are able to benefit from the drug. In addition to issues related to access and side effects, one key limitation of Trikafta is that it works only in people with certain mutations in the CF gene.[193] As alluded to in previous chapters, the CF gene (*CFTR*) codes for the CFTR protein, which serves as a chloride channel located in the outer membrane of certain cells in the body. Some mutations in the CF gene result in proteins that are altered such that they don't fold into the proper shape, resulting in problems with the function and/or cellular localization of the protein. As explained in an article in *The Boston Globe* in 2019, "the new Vertex medications—called modulators—aim to restore normal CFTR activity by tweaking errors in the location and shape of the protein that are introduced by the genetic mutation."[194] However, the modulators are effective only if there is CFTR protein present to "modulate" in the first place, leaving about 10 percent of people with CF unable to benefit from the drugs because of their specific mutations. As CF Foundation president and CEO Michael Boyle explained in 2020, "that last 10% will require other approaches, because a significant portion of that group has mutations that do not make protein."[195]

Individuals with CF who are not able to take Trikafta because of their specific mutations, an inability to tolerate the drug, or lack of access have expressed feelings of being "left behind" as the improved prospects for the majority of those with the disease do not apply to them.[196] In fact, shortly after Cambrey White's son Rowland was diagnosed with CF, she found out that he was part of "the final 10%" who were ineligible for Trikafta or other modulators.[197] As Cambrey explained in 2023, "learning that my son, Rowland, has two rare cystic fibrosis variants and is currently unable to access highly effective modulator therapies was emotionally challenging and isolating for me."[198] According to Cambrey, "what I want more than anything is for Rowland to have access to a modulator when he is older (preferably sooner rather than later) because it will increase his life expectancy and help keep him healthy."[199] Many other parents and people with CF who do not currently qualify for modulators have expressed similar concerns about how the lack of availability of treatments such as Trikafta will have profound effects on health outcomes.

Furthermore, in part due to earlier, erroneous views that CF was a "white disease" coupled with the corresponding design of genetic testing algorithms for CF going back decades, those in certain minoritized groups are less likely to qualify for a modulator. According to physician Meghan McGarry of the University of California, San Francisco and her colleagues, "over 90% of non-Hispanic White people with CF in the U.S. have *CFTR* mutations that qualify for a CFTR modulator," yet "only 70% of American Black, 75% of Hispanic, and 80% of other racial minorities with CF have qualifying mutations."[200] Thus, "medical stereotyping" not only has influenced which patients are recommended for genetic testing and the composition of those genetic testing panels for screening and diagnostic algorithms, but such assumptions also have carried over into the development of therapeutics for the disease, further exacerbating health disparities.[201] In the setting of these challenges, many scientists and physicians have placed great emphasis on addressing these disparities.

As this chapter has documented, the introduction of genetic testing into screening and diagnostic algorithms for CF has addressed some forms of uncertainty while concomitantly introducing others, a theme that has persisted in efforts to diagnose CF from the late 1930s to today. In the next chapter, we will see how diagnostic uncertainty has extended to secondary diagnoses in people with CF in the setting of efforts to identify microbial infections.

CHAPTER FIVE

Elusive Microbes

Uncertainty in the Context of Secondary Diagnoses

Less than a month after WHO characterized COVID-19 as a pandemic, Michelle Patrovani, mother of two young adults with cystic fibrosis, remarked that "everyone else on earth must understand now what it is like to live with Cystic Fibrosis."[1] Patrovani was not unique in making this connection, as many others in the CF community reinforced the similarities between CF and COVID-19 in the spring of 2020. For example, Paul Quinton, an adult with CF and a scientist who studied the physiological basis of the disease for many decades, observed in May 2020 that "everybody's behaving like they have cystic fibrosis."[2] Furthermore, CF Foundation president and CEO Michael Boyle pointed out that "social distancing is the norm" for those with CF and suggested that "people who are struggling with current distancing recommendations" in the face of COVID-19 might "learn from the CF community's experience."[3] As Boyle explained, as early as 2013 people with CF had been asked to stay six feet away from others with the disease, following the release of infection control guidelines that "bear a striking similarity to what the CDC is asking of us now."[4]

Yet, how is it that the experience of CF, long defined by medical professionals as a chronic genetic disease affecting primarily the respiratory and gastrointestinal systems, could be likened to an infectious disease such as COVID-19? New York physician Dorothy Andersen, who is often credited with the first comprehensive description of CF in 1938, as discussed in Chapter 1, initially acknowledged that "a fetal infection of unknown origin" was a "possible explanation" for the etiology of the disease, yet she and others soon came to believe that CF was genetic.[5] As a 1957 newspaper article stressed, "cystic fibrosis is not contagious; it is transmitted to children by means of a recessive gene inherited from both parents."[6] Throughout the subsequent decades and up to the present time, CF has been understood as a genetic disease. In fact, during the last third of the twentieth century, as the median life expectancy for people with CF increased into the teens and beyond, many communities of people with CF thrived in North America and Europe.[7] Anthropologist Paul Rabinow has used the term *biosociality* to describe communities formed around a shared genetic makeup or marker, and the earlier CF communities (before the identification of the *CFTR* gene in 1989) functioned in much the same way.[8] Furthermore, numerous scholars have documented the important role that community formation can play in the lives of those with disabilities, noting that such groups can provide social support systems, advocate for access to resources, and work to reduce stigma.[9] However, the CF case stands out in disability history because by the late twentieth century, most in-person communities had been disbanded due to fears of patient-to-patient transmission of a pathogenic microorganism referred to at the time as *Pseudomonas cepacia* (later renamed *Burkholderia cepacia*). Reflecting on these changes in 2007, Isabel Stenzel Byrnes, an adult with CF, remarked that "CF had evolved into an infectious disease."[10]

By examining the history of attempts to identify *P. cepacia* in those with an established CF diagnosis, it is possible to see how diagnostic uncertainty has persisted not just in the context of the diagnosis of CF itself (as outlined in Chapters 1–4), but also in the setting of secondary diagnoses. In diseases such as CF, an initial CF diagnosis often raises follow-up questions about the disease state—for example, is this particular case of CF complicated by a *P. cepacia* diagnosis? The presence of a *P. cepacia* infection, which could not be eradicated with available antibiotics, had important implications for treatment, prognosis, and the risk of transmission of infection to others with CF. However, as this chapter illustrates, physicians came to realize that it was difficult to determine with certainty whether an individual with a primary CF diagnosis had a secondary *P. cepacia* diagnosis. I argue that this diagnostic uncertainty, or the inability to consistently determine whether someone with CF was infected with *P. cepacia* despite testing for it, contributed to the reframing of CF as a type of genetic/infectious hybrid disease. Still considered a genetic disease that could not be transmitted through exposure to others, CF nevertheless became associated with contagion among individuals with CF, challenging the traditional dichotomy of infectious versus inherited disease.[11]

The chapter begins by documenting physicians' initial concerns in the late 1970s about the rapid and often fatal decline in health associated with a *P. cepacia* diagnosis and subsequent efforts to prevent the spread of the microorganism. Amid debate about the source of *P. cepacia*—ranging from contaminated hospital surfaces to the natural environment to patients themselves—some physicians began to exclude *P. cepacia*–infected people from CF summer camps and other settings beginning in the 1980s in an effort to curtail the spread of the microorganism. By the 1990s, however, many physicians had come to believe that people with CF did not always test positive for *P. cepacia* when infected, in large part because of difficulties isolating and identifying the microorganism.[12] I argue that these sources of diagnostic uncertainty, coupled with the severe health decline linked to the infection, prompted those in leadership positions in the CF community to eventually consider each person with CF as a potential source of the microorganism, thereby limiting all in-person contact between those with CF by the early twenty-first century. This shift in the framing of CF, prompted by the diagnostic uncertainty associated with a microbe, had an immense impact on the lives of those living with the disease and those who cared for them.

The Segregation of People with CF by Microbial Status

Bacterial infections of the respiratory tract have long been observed in people with CF, yet the specific microorganisms described have changed somewhat over the last eighty years. In the period before widespread antibiotic use, doctors pointed to the microorganism *Staphylococcus aureus* as the main respiratory infection and the leading cause of death in people with CF.[13] With the advent of antibiotic treatment for *S. aureus*, the incidence of other microorganisms increased.[14] Of particular note, *Pseudomonas aeruginosa* "emerged as the most important bacterial pathogen in lung disease of CF patients" in the time after the advent of antistaphylococcal antibiotics.[15] While *P. aeruginosa* remains a common pathogen, many physicians have suggested that antibiotics directed against *P. aeruginosa* in turn selected for the growth of *P. cepacia* in people with CF.[16] Although *P. cepacia* was first described as a plant pathogen in 1950, reports of infection in humans began to appear in the 1970s.[17] Initially, such reports involved contaminated medical equipment or chemical solutions, and infections were typically noted in "hospitalized persons with serious underlying disease."[18] For example, a Minnesota study published in 1972 described forty-one cases of *P. cepacia* infection among outpatients or hospitalized individuals, one of whom had CF.[19] While additional details concerning this individual with CF are not available, it may represent the first documented case linking *P. cepacia* to CF.

Around the time that isolated cases of *P. cepacia* were first described in people with CF, summer camps for those with the disease were just beginning to form in North America and Europe (Figure 5.1).[20] Many children with CF reported feeling "normal" during summer camp, where they could complete hours of medical treatment aimed at staving off lung disease and take pills to aid in their digestion without feeling self-conscious.[21] Writing in her diary in 1986, fourteen-year-old Isabel Stenzel (quoted above describing CF as an infectious disease) noted that the California CF camp she attended "is the best place in the world where you meet new friends, no one stares, and you get all the food you want."[22] At CF camp, kids talked openly about their shorter life expectancy, adult counselors with CF served as role models, and participants developed lifelong friendships and support systems. Many parents, patients, and health care workers believed that CF summer camps functioned effectively to reduce patient isolation and increase therapeutic adherence, an observation that has important parallels to the community formation that occurred in polio rehabilitation wards in the 1940s and 1950s.[23] Reflecting back on the CF camps years later, one physician noted that "they were certainly good for morale," yet he also remarked that "I am sure they all infected each other."[24]

In fact, in the decade after the isolated case of *P. cepacia* was reported in 1972, several additional isolated cases of *P. cepacia* infection in people with CF were documented in Canada and the United States, followed by reports of larger clusters of infected individuals.[25] For example, in what would later be described as a "seminal report," physicians at the Hospital for Sick Children in Toronto provided evidence that the prevalence of *P. cepacia* in people with CF increased from 9.6 percent in 1970 to 18.1 percent in 1981.[26] The clinical course of such patients was quite variable, with physicians describing three possible outcomes. One group had no change in lung function, a second group experienced a slow decline over an extended period, and a third group faced rapid deterioration resulting in death within weeks to months of the *P. cepacia* diagnosis.[27] While CF had long been associated with increased mortality due to lung disease, this third group was particularly concerning because of the rapid

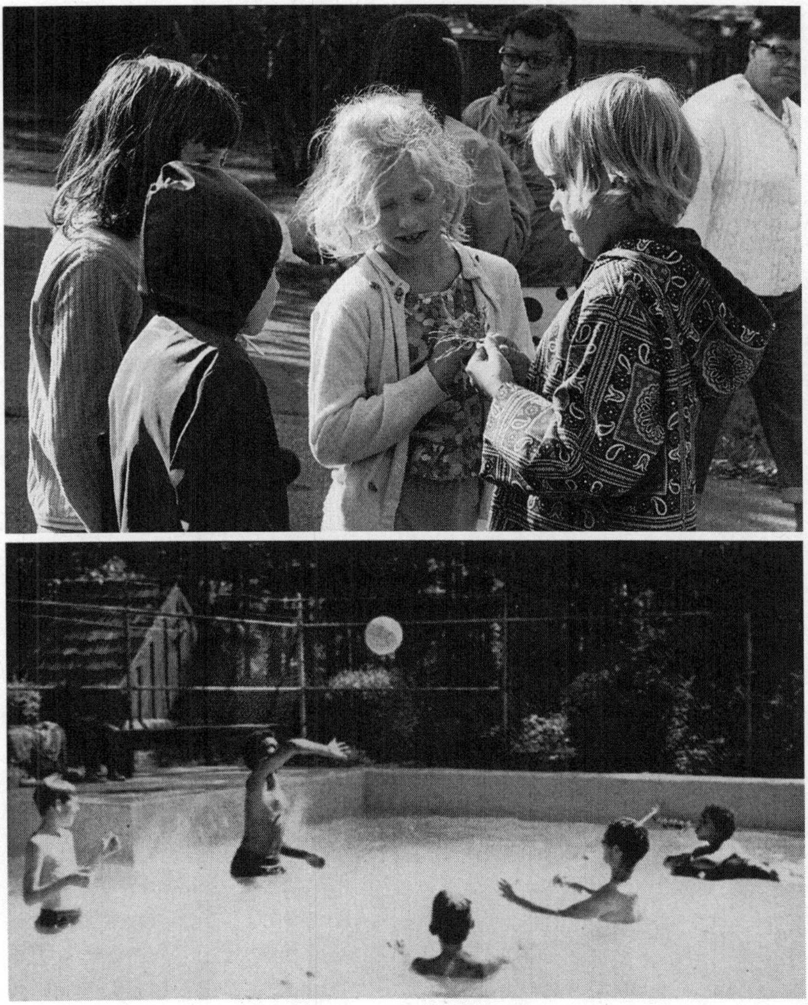

FIGURE 5.1. Camp Ho Mita Koda, Ohio, 1970. *Top*: "C/F Camp Makes Out of Doors a Reality for 50 Children," *The Archway*, October 1970, 4–5. Located in the Cystic Fibrosis Loose Folder, Stanley A. Ferguson Archives, University Hospitals of Cleveland. Photograph from *The Archway* courtesy of the Stanley A. Ferguson Archives of University Hospitals of Cleveland. *Bottom*: S. Stadnyk and N. Bindschadler, "A Camp for Children with Cystic Fibrosis," *American Journal of Nursing* 70, no. 8 (1970): 1691–3. Located in the Cystic Fibrosis Loose Folder, Stanley A. Ferguson Archives, University Hospitals of Cleveland. Reproduced with permission from Wolters Kluwer Health.

and unexpected decline often referred to as "cepacia syndrome."[28] As the Toronto investigators noted, *P. cepacia* was a "major threat to patients with CF" because it was "resistant to most commonly used antimicrobial agents."[29] While acknowledging that the "origin of the outbreak has not been determined," the Toronto group did have some evidence that the *P. cepacia* cases were the result of nosocomial (hospital-acquired) infection and stressed that thorough cleaning of medical equipment was key for prevention.[30]

P. cepacia was a growing concern at several hospitals in the US at this time. At St. Christopher's Hospital for Children (SCHC) in Philadelphia, *P. cepacia* was identified in fifty-four people with CF between July 1973 and December 1976, and 26 percent of the patients had "died from respiratory failure" by 1977.[31] In response to the growing number of cases of *P. cepacia* at SCHC, physician Daniel Schidlow "called the CDC and got them involved" in the mid-1980s.[32] Based on a retrospective analysis of SCHC patient samples from January 1979 to December 1983, the CDC and Philadelphia colleagues noted that 45 percent of thirty-eight people with CF died following *P. cepacia* infection.[33] In contrast to the Toronto study in which an "outbreak" was deemed responsible for the *P. cepacia* cases, investigators in Philadelphia concluded that "*P. cepacia* colonization of patients with CF was endemic in the hospital."[34] *P. cepacia* infection in people with CF was also a significant concern at Rainbow Babies and Childrens Hospital in Cleveland by the early 1980s.[35] Not only did the prevalence of the microorganism among patients receiving care at the Cleveland hospital increase from 7 percent to 15 percent between 1978 and 1983, but death associated with *P. cepacia* infection increased from 9 percent to 55 percent over the same period.[36] Furthermore, in an epidemiologic study done in 1984, investigators at Rainbow Babies and Childrens Hospital and the CDC documented that *P. cepacia*–infected people with moderate to severe CF had significantly worse outcomes than noninfected controls with the disease (Figure 5.2).[37]

Although the Cleveland hospital responded to *P. cepacia* infection with increased attention to cleaning, as in Toronto and Philadelphia, additional, unique measures were implemented in Cleveland to reduce the incidence of *P. cepacia* in people with CF. Faced with significant morbidity and mortality in the CF patient population, but without clear evidence in support of nosocomial spread, Cleveland area physicians implemented a comprehensive policy that included the "physical separation" of people with CF based on *P. cepacia* status in hospital and summer camp settings begin-

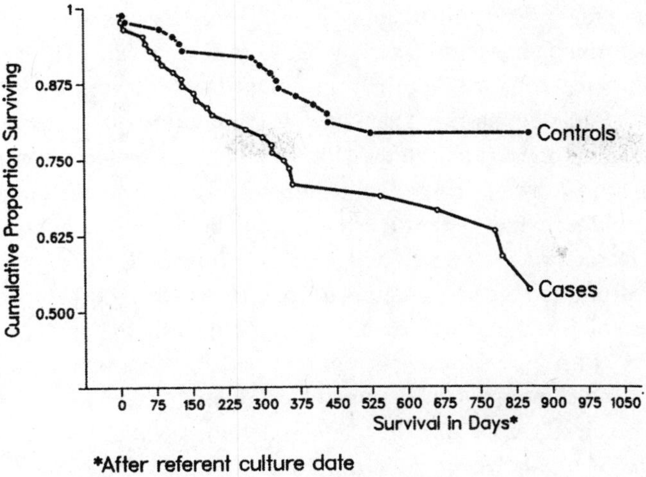

FIGURE 5.2. "Survival of patients colonized with *P cepacia* who had cystic fibrosis and matched control patients with cystic fibrosis at Rainbow Babies and Childrens Hospital, Cleveland, from January 1981 to June 1984." Reprinted from O. C. Tablan, W. J. Martone, C. F. Doershuk, R. C. Stern, M. J. Thomassen, J. D. Klinger, J. W. White, L. A. Carson, and W. R. Jarvis, "Colonization of the Respiratory Tract with *Pseudomonas cepacia* in Cystic Fibrosis. Risk Factors and Outcomes," *Chest* 91 (1987): 527–32, 529. Reproduced with permission from Elsevier.

ning in August 1983.[38] Although the changes in Cleveland were associated with a marked decrease in new cases of *P. cepacia*, the patient separation component of the policy received some criticism due to the lack of controls in the study and the negative impact on patients.[39] Responding to the Cleveland study, Epidemic Intelligence Service officer Ofelia Tablan and colleagues at the CDC pointed out that it was difficult to know whether the "resulting decrease in acquisition rate of *P. cepacia* was due to dividing patients into cohorts or other changes in practices."[40] For instance, in addition to segregating Cleveland patients by *P. cepacia* status in the 1980s, changes included sterilizing respiratory equipment, discontinuation of a breathing test that required people with CF to share equipment, a focus on handwashing, and patient education efforts.[41] In 1987, CDC investigators acknowledged that patient-to-patient transmission of *P. cepacia* was theoretically possible, but stressed that this mode of transmission had "not been demonstrated."[42]

In an attempt to determine with certainty how *P. cepacia* was spread among people with CF, physicians developed and employed new technologies to identify different versions, or strains, of the microorganism.[43]

For example, in 1988 Philadelphia investigators described a method to type bacterial subspecies, including those of *P. cepacia*.[44] The "ribotyping" technique compared the chromosomal DNA of various *P. cepacia* isolates.[45] Philadelphia physician John LiPuma and colleagues used the ribotyping method to analyze the DNA of *P. cepacia* isolates from people with CF who took part in an educational program over the summer of 1989, providing evidence that *P. cepacia* could be transmitted between patients.[46] Described as a "watershed moment" for the CF community, these findings prompted the investigators to conclude that "unnecessary contact between colonised and non-colonised cystic fibrosis patients should be avoided."[47] Further evidence in support of patient-to-patient transmission of *P. cepacia* came out of CF summer camp studies conducted through joint efforts by the CDC and the CF Foundation. As described in the *Morbidity and Mortality Weekly Report* published by the CDC in 1993, studies in the late 1980s and early 1990s of four North American summer camps provided evidence that *P. cepacia* was transmitted between campers.[48] In the same year, the CF Foundation recommended that summer camps be suspended. Many of the summer camps that remained open after 1993 excluded individuals who tested positive for the microorganism.[49]

By the early 1990s, segregation or exclusion of those with *P. cepacia* had become increasingly widespread because of concerns about patient-to-patient transmission of the microorganism.[50] As recounted by Daniel Schidlow during a 2016 interview, one of his *P. cepacia*–infected patients with CF felt "incarcerated" following the adoption of a segregation policy at St. Christopher's (Figure 5.3).[51] As seen in a drawing done by this individual, the hospital room contains bars, as if it were a prison cell, and the patient is depicted as an onion. The image operated on several levels: not only was the onion connected to the tears of the isolated patient, but the microorganism *P. cepacia* was first isolated from a rotten onion by Cornell University plant pathologist Walter Burkholder in 1947.[52] As Schidlow recalled, the isolation experienced by this patient "didn't sit very well; isolation never sat very well with the patients because all social contact was negated, they couldn't leave their rooms, it became a real problem for the patients. On the other hand, . . . as much as it was a problem, it had to be done."[53] Another person with CF, Jacquie Romano, became infected with *P. cepacia* in 1992 at age twenty-two. As a result, she was eventually forced to discontinue her active in-person involvement with the Canadian Cystic Fibrosis Foundation (later renamed Cystic Fibrosis Canada) because of the fear that she would infect others.[54] Being asked to restrict her work

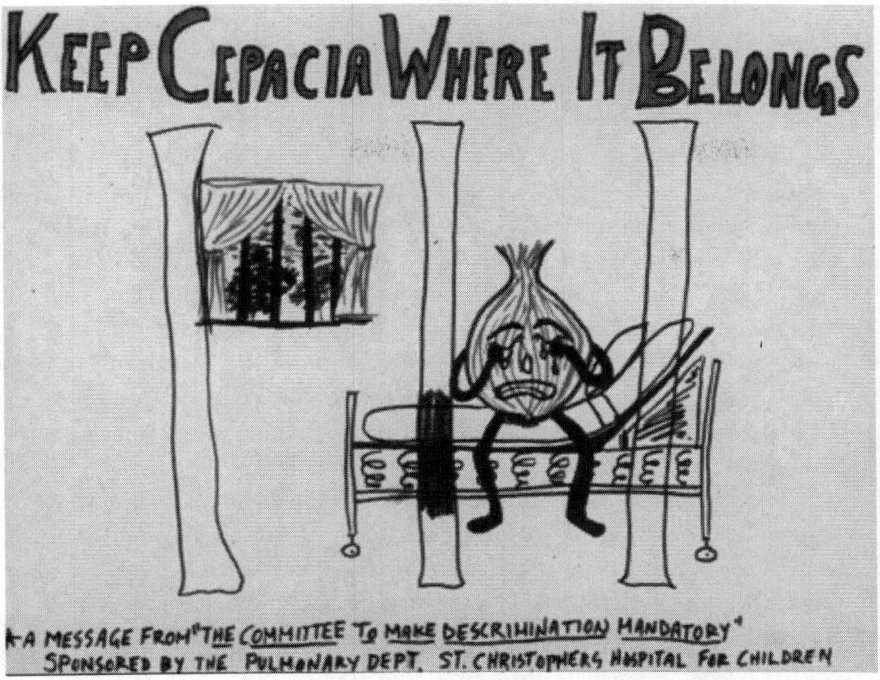
KEEP CEPACIA WHERE IT BELONGS
A MESSAGE FROM "THE COMMITTEE TO MAKE DESCRIMINATION MANDATORY"
SPONSORED BY THE PULMONARY DEPT. ST. CHRISTOPHERS HOSPITAL FOR CHILDREN

FIGURE 5.3. Drawing by a *P. cepacia*–infected person with cystic fibrosis at St. Christopher's Hospital for Children in Philadelphia, circa 1980s, after the isolation of *P. cepacia*–infected patients was implemented. The drawing was given by the patient to Dr. Daniel Schidlow, who was the patient's physician at St. Christopher's. Permission to reproduce the drawing granted by Dr. Daniel Schidlow.

with the foundation to email and telephone interaction was "incredibly isolating" and she would at times "feel like a leper."[55] As Canadian physician David Speert reflected, "Nobody wanted to create a group of lepers within the CF community. But it's an issue of balancing risk against humanity."[56]

Although strict segregation of patients according to microbial status was not recommended according to guidelines put out by the US CF Foundation in 1994, segregation policies in many locations continued to involve separating hospitalized patients with *P. cepacia* or excluding *P. cepacia*–infected patients from other social activities.[57] For example, when young siblings Lauren and Paul Chrest tested positive for *P. cepacia* in the mid-1990s, "it wreaked havoc for their family."[58] Lauren first found out that she was positive while hospitalized and sharing a room with her friend Jessica, who also had CF. When St. Christopher's realized that she was positive, Lauren's mother "didn't know how to tell her that she couldn't stay with Jessica" anymore and would need to be "quarantined."[59] Furthermore, many of the Chrests' close family friends no longer wanted to get together socially due to the fear that their own children (who had CF) would become infected by Lauren and Paul, and the family expected that they would not be invited to the Christmas party at St. Christopher's that year.[60] Reflecting on these experiences, Lauren's and Paul's mother recalled that "it was hard being told they had the pseudomonas cepacia and that they wouldn't be allowed to be around other kids who had cystic fibrosis. . . . I wouldn't want them to be treated like lepers."[61] In fact, around the same time, several physicians pointed to the "logistic and social consequences of draconian infection control measures reminiscent of mediaeval approaches to leprosy."[62]

As controversial as such practices were, an important part of making segregation policies work to prevent cross-infection was having diagnostic clarity about who was infected. However, as the next two sections will document, it was not always possible for physicians to determine with certainty if someone was infected with *P. cepacia*. In the final section, I argue that *P. cepacia*–associated diagnostic uncertainty contributed to a change in policy such that all people with CF were treated as potential reservoirs of infection and asked to refrain from in-person contact with others with CF.

Diagnostic Uncertainty and Challenges with Microbial Growth

When physicians began segregating people with CF by *P. cepacia* status, there was an assumption that those who tested negative were not infected with the microorganism. Since people with CF were regularly tested for respiratory infections, regardless of symptoms, this public health measure appeared sound from an infection control standpoint.[63] However, microbiologists began to express concerns in the mid-1980s that *P. cepacia* could "present a challenge in the laboratory" because it was so difficult to detect in CF sputum samples.[64] If one could not accurately determine whether someone was infected with *P. cepacia*, then methods such as segregation would not effectively curtail patient-to-patient spread of the microorganism. This inability to reliably detect infected patients, and corresponding challenges to public health measures, has parallels to the phenomenon of the healthy carrier in diseases such as typhoid fever and diphtheria.[65]

In both situations, it can be difficult to know who is infected with the microorganism in question.[66] In the case of the healthy carrier, the failure to detect a microbe is often attributed to the lack of testing due to the individual's asymptomatic nature. However, the history of *P. cepacia* diagnosis sheds light on a different challenge, which is that despite testing, the microbe can remain undetected. This latter example of difficulty detecting a microbe in the context of performing a laboratory test is an important, yet less well studied, source of diagnostic uncertainty.[67]

P. cepacia was first identified as the causative agent of a type of onion rot by Walter Burkholder in 1947.[68] After suspecting that the plant disease was of bacterial origin based on his observation of the affected onion bulb tissue and noting "an abundance of bacteria" using microscopy, Burkholder proceeded to determine which specific "type" of bacteria was the cause of the "sour skin."[69] Using standard microbiology techniques, Burkholder placed the affected onion tissue on nutrient agar plates, spreading it in such a way as to dilute any bacteria present. Once the bacteria had sufficient time to reproduce on the plates, Burkholder noted three main types of colonies, or visible clumps of bacteria each originating from a single bacterial cell. Consistent with Koch's postulates, Burkholder "severed and smeared" onion bulb tops with each type of isolated bacteria and observed infection "within a few days" following inoculation with the "true pathogen," a novel species he designated *Pseudomonas cepacia*.[70] As additional confirmation that *P. cepacia* caused onion rot, he isolated bacteria from the newly infected onion bulbs, exposed healthy onion bulbs to the bacteria, and again observed onion rot consistent with the original disease pathology.

In the course of his work, Burkholder noted that the *P. cepacia* colonies appeared "in rather limited numbers, at times only three or four to a plate and frequently scattered among" the other types of bacteria isolated from diseased plant tissue.[71] This relative scarcity of *P. cepacia* colonies on nutrient agar plates was also noted when specimens from people with CF were studied. For instance, *P. cepacia* grew very slowly under standard microbiology laboratory conditions, requiring seventy-two hours or more before bacterial colonies could be seen on agar plates containing growth medium.[72] Complicating matters, the microorganism *P. aeruginosa*, often present in sputum samples derived from people with CF, could grow much faster on the standard laboratory media and thus mask the presence of *P. cepacia*.[73] As investigators in Philadelphia suggested in 1984, *P. cepacia* may have been underdiagnosed in earlier studies because of limitations in "techniques used to isolate and identify this organism."[74]

In an attempt to remedy the inconsistencies in the ability of laboratories to isolate *P. cepacia*, investigators at St. Christopher's Hospital for Children in Philadelphia and several other institutions developed a new growth medium for isolating the microorganism.[75] Their goal was to formulate a medium (which they would call PC medium) that would allow for growth of a wide range of isolates of *P. cepacia* while inhibiting growth of other organisms. As described in 1985, the investigators began with fifty strains of *P. cepacia* derived from patients with CF at SCHC and further confirmed by the CDC Hospital Infection Program. Highlighting the importance of effective media in reducing instances of diagnostic uncertainty, the investigators noted that 40 percent of the tested strains could be isolated only on their new PC media.[76] Furthermore, the PC media effectively inhibited growth of the vast majority of other microorganisms, such as *P. aeruginosa*, typically isolated from people with CF. Two years later, another group described a second *P. cepacia* medium, termed OFPBL, which was also superior to the standard laboratory media in selectively promoting *P. cepacia* growth.[77] An additional group confirmed that PC and OFPBL media were able to grow *P. cepacia* from patient samples and noted that PC agar was better at inhibiting non-*cepacia* microorganisms.[78]

Aware of concerns related to *P. cepacia* detection, the CDC and the CF Foundation carried out a laboratory proficiency test from December 1985 to February 1986.[79] They found that most laboratories could identify a pure sample of *P. cepacia*, yet only 32 percent of 115 US CF centers could identify *P. cepacia* when it was provided as part of a simulated CF sputum sample containing more than one microorganism. The type of isolation medium used was a significant factor in the ability of laboratories to detect *P. cepacia*. In fact, 95 percent of labs using either PC or OFPBL selective isolation media were able to detect *P. cepacia*, whereas only 22 percent of those not using a selective medium were able to detect *P. cepacia*. Once these labs that had initially failed to detect *P. cepacia* were allowed to try again using a selective medium, 97 percent could then identify *P. cepacia*.[80] This study highlighted how challenging it was to determine the incidence and prevalence of *P. cepacia* at various CF clinics because of the variety of laboratory methods employed in practice. According to CDC epidemiologists, most laboratories were using selective media after 1986.[81]

In a follow-up study, epidemiologists from the CDC compared selective media for isolating *P. cepacia* from patients with CF, from patients without CF, and from the environment.[82] They tested three media types and found that the PC medium was most effective at promoting *P. cepacia* growth from all samples.[83] While selective media certainly increased the detection of *P. cepacia*, the CDC investigators did point out that other factors could affect recovery, such as how and whether the sputum is prepared before plating and whether the sputum is refrigerated. Even though they identified a medium that was relatively effective at isolating *P. cepacia* from patient samples, they did conclude by saying that "there is probably a need for an improved medium for detecting *P. cepacia* in environmental specimens."[84] At that time, in the late 1980s, *P. cepacia* had been described not just as a plant and human pathogen, but also as a microbe capable of carrying out bioremediation, or the degradation of environmental pollutants.[85] In fact, Rebecca Mueller has documented how the CF community worked with the Environmental Protection Agency to reduce the environmental use of the microbe given the significant health concerns for people with CF.[86] By 1994, the CF Foundation recommended both PC medium and OFPBL medium for the microorganism, which had been renamed *Burkholderia cepacia*, and stressed the importance of letting plates incubate for longer periods to allow sufficient bacterial growth for detection.[87]

Despite the availability of selective media for *B. cepacia* complex species, investigators in Vancouver and Philadelphia noted that misidentification remained an issue in 1997.[88] Of the 819 isolates sent to the reference laboratory in Vancouver, 3.4 percent had been misidentified. To address the problem of misidentification, the group developed the BCSA isolation medium, which was "more enriched for the growth of *B. cepacia*" and "more selective against other organisms than currently available selective agars."[89] However, several years later, investigators in the US and Europe noted that there was still "poor laboratory proficiency" in identifying *B. cepacia* complex and related species.[90] Pointing to a 1999 study of US CF centers, they stressed that "less than half . . . surveyed employ '*B. cepacia*'-specific selective media or incubate cultures for extended periods, both of which improve the yield of this organism."[91] Thus, even in the setting of improved media and laboratory methods to promote the selective growth of *B. cepacia* complex microorganisms, not all laboratories took advantage of these resources in practice.

Years later, Cleveland physician Robert Stern reflected on the challenges that some laboratories had in identifying *B. cepacia* and related microorganisms and the impact this had on people with CF. As Stern recalled, "we saw a couple of new patients from [location X] who had never had *cepacia*, and they had it here on the original culture. Turned out that the lab in [location X] was just not culturing it."[92] Even more striking, Stern recalled a "couple of patients from here who moved to [location Y] and they had *cepacia* when they left here, they never had it in [location Y], had it when they moved back." As Stern concluded, "obviously, they missed it down there."[93] Physicians in the UK noted a similar situation, highlighting the differences in the ability of individual laboratories to detect *P. cepacia*.[94] In addition, they provided evidence of transmission of *P. cepacia* between people with CF before an individual was positive by sputum sample, and suggested that it might be necessary to isolate all patients from each other.[95] Differences in the ability of laboratories to culture *B. cepacia* complex microorganisms was an important source of diagnostic uncertainty, though taxonomic complexity further contributed to diagnostic challenges.

Diagnostic Uncertainty and Taxonomic Complexity

Just as segregation by *P. cepacia* status only worked if one could reliably culture or identify the microorganism in the setting of infection, such public health practices required that *P. cepacia* have a stable definition across locations and over time. However, the medical relevance of *P. cepacia* in the CF community, coupled with efforts to trace the mechanism of *P. cepacia* spread, prompted scientists to generate "an unusually large amount of taxonomic data" beginning in the 1990s.[96] Reflecting on this work years later, John LiPuma recalled that "as we started taking a hard look at these bacteria that we were recovering from people with CF and noticing that they had different characteristics, that sort of promoted our interest in sorting out the taxonomy."[97] As a result of this attention to *P. cepacia*, extensive changes in microbial taxonomy followed, making it increasingly difficult to determine whether a person with CF was infected with *P. cepacia* or a different, related microbe.[98] As John LiPuma explained in a 2016 interview, "initially this was considered one species and what we've learned . . . [from] analyzing these strains from people with CF is there are really now 20 distinct species," only some of which were associated with a poorer prognosis in CF.[99] Furthermore, not all laboratories used these new species designations as they were established, as such changes required knowledge and resources that were not universally available. In addition, many people with CF, and even some physicians, continued to use the generic term "*cepacia*" long after the original species had been redefined, leading to confusion about the significance of a particular diagnosis. Although many scholars have examined the transformation of classification systems, including the reevaluation of the species concept itself in microbiology, this section will provide insight into how taxonomic change has contributed to diagnostic uncertainty in medicine.[100]

Examining Burkholder's published account of *P. cepacia* in 1950, it is not surprising that this "new species" would eventually be reclassified and moved out of the *Pseudomonas* genus many decades later.[101] While this newly described Gram-negative aerobic bacterial species had characteristics that aligned with the features of the *Pseudomonas* genus, including the placement and presence of flagella for movement, Burkholder pointed out in 1950 that "certain characters . . . show that it does not fit in too well with the majority of the plant pathogens of this genus."[102] For example, *P. cepacia* contained a "yellowish, water-soluble pigment" that Burkholder argued was "probably not the same as the green pigment" seen in other *Pseudomonas* species.[103] In addition, the microorganism was able to grow at a higher temperature range than other members of the *Pseudomonas* genus.[104] In the decades that followed Burkholder's 1950 report on *P. cepacia* and onion rot, scientists and clinicians reworked the classification of this and other microbes. Of particular relevance, two independently named microorganisms linked to bioremediation (*Pseudomonas multivorans*) and human disease (*Pseudomonas kingii*) were described and determined by 1973 to be synonymous with *P. cepacia*.[105] Since Burkholder's *P. cepacia* had been published first, that name was given priority, and all three species names were merged into one. An image of the microbe and its flagella can be seen in Figure 5.4.[106]

By the early 1970s, taxonomists were using molecular techniques to revise the "classification and nomenclature of many established genera."[107] In fact, investigators from the University of California, Berkeley, examined the similarity of nucleic acids to reexamine the relationship between species in the *Pseudomonas* genus. At that time, the region of the bacterial genome that coded for ribosomal RNA (rRNA, involved in protein synthesis) was understood to be "more conserved in the course of evolution than the bulk of the genome" and therefore an ideal target for such studies.[108] To determine how closely related the various *Pseudomonas* species were to each other, the Berkeley group examined the rRNA of each species and subdivided the genus into five groups.[109] They noted that the five groups "seem to be very distantly related to each other phylogenetically" and suggested that they "deserve at least independent genus (and possibly

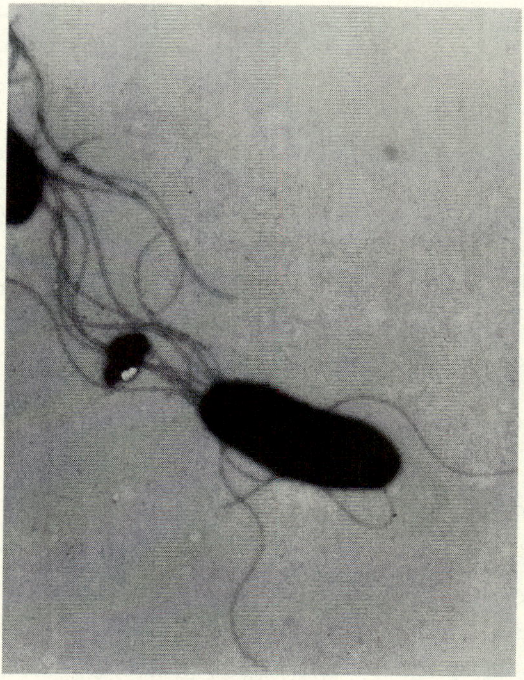

FIGURE 5.4. "Electron photomicrograph of field strain no. A32/69 [*P. cepacia*], showing 11 to 12 polar flagella and a few flagella apparently winding back upon the cell and appearing to emerge laterally." Image magnified 30,000 times. Republished with permission of Microbiology Society, from J. J. S. Snell, L. R. Hill, S. P. Lapage, and M. A. Curtis, "Identification of *Pseudomonas cepacia* Burkholder and Its Synonymy with *Pseudomonas kingii* Jonsson," *International Journal of Systematic Bacteriology* 22 (1972): 127–38, 133. Permission conveyed through Copyright Clearance Center.

family or order) assignment."[110] As illustrated in Figure 5.5, *P. cepacia* was placed in the rRNA homology group II.[111]

Almost two decades later, scientists from Japan reevaluated the composition of the genus *Pseudomonas* and moved all seven members of rRNA homology group II, including *P. cepacia*, to a new genus.[112] The genus was "named after W.H. Burkholder, the American bacteriologist who first discovered the etiologic agent of rotten onion," and *P. cepacia* was correspondingly renamed *Burkholderia cepacia*.[113] Also in the early 1990s, investigators noticed a great deal of variation among *B. cepacia* strains, making "correct identification problematic."[114] By the mid-1990s, many investigators had provided evidence that techniques to identify *B. cepacia*

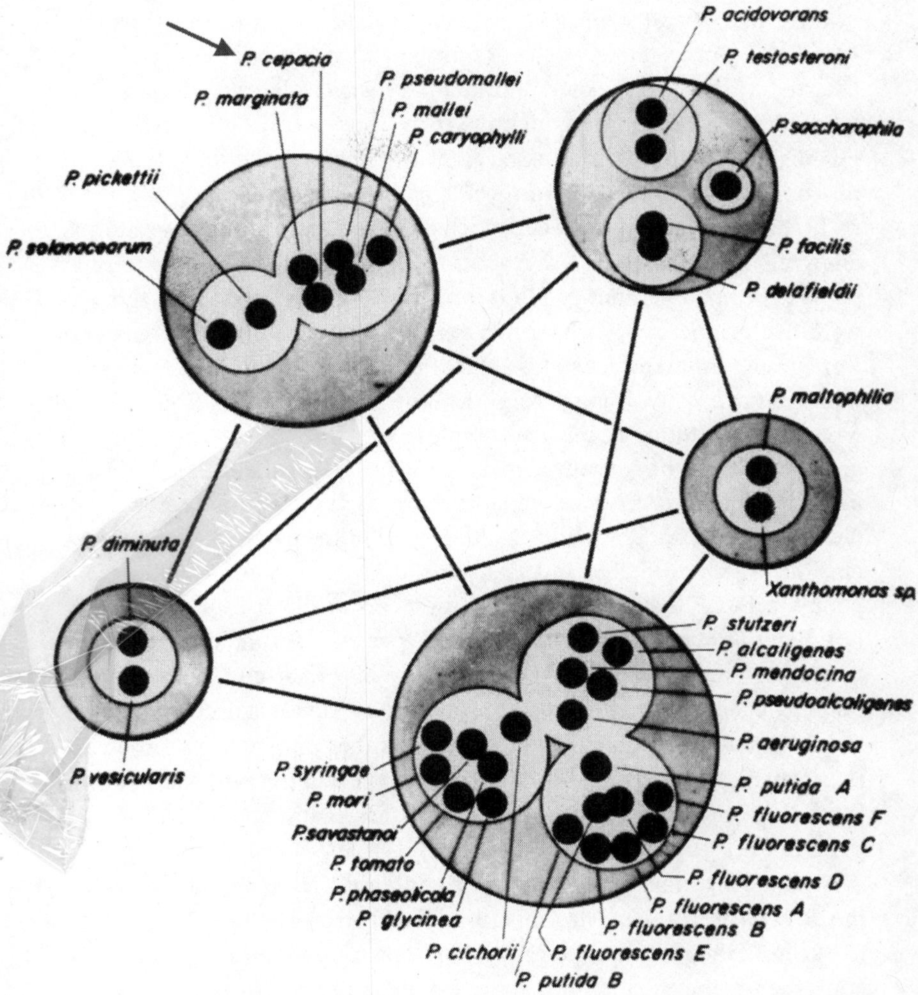

FIGURE 5.5. "Pseudomonas species and biotypes arranged according to rRNA and DNA homologies. The shaded circles represent rRNA homology groups." Arrow added to indicate *P. cepacia*. The authors note that "The relative distances of the five homology groups from each other are shown in the figure as well as we could achieve in a simple two- dimensional graph." Republished with permission of Microbiology Society, from N. J. Palleroni, R. Kunisawa, R. Contropoulou, and M. Doudoroff, "Nucleic Acid Homologies in the Genus *Pseudomonas*," *International Journal of Systematic Bacteriology* 23 (1973): 333–39, 338. Permission conveyed through Copyright Clearance Center.

"were either not very sensitive, not very specific, or neither sensitive nor specific."[115] For example, as North Carolina microbiologist Peter Gilligan asserted in 1996, "only 60–80% of the *B. cepacia* isolates recovered from CF patients are accurately identified" by commercial typing systems.[116] Highlighting the challenges associated with defining and identifying this microorganism, some asked in 1996, "what is a true *B. cepacia*?"[117]

In the context of these diagnostic challenges, investigators from Europe analyzed numerous *B. cepacia* isolates derived from plants, soil, water, and people with and without cystic fibrosis and identified what they thought were five distinct species based on genomic analysis (although only two were given formal species status at that time).[118] At the International *Burkholderia cepacia* Working Group meeting held in British Columbia in May 1997, the term "*B. cepacia* complex" was "proposed to refer to this group of five phenotypically similar species."[119] Over the next several decades, additional *B. cepacia* complex species were defined and reclassified, making diagnostics especially challenging.[120] In the early 2000s, researchers in the United States and Canada identified eighteen isolates from people with CF that appeared to be members of the *B. cepacia* complex but didn't fit into one of the established species.[121] Along those lines, the "unsurpassed taxonomic complexity" of the *B. cepacia* complex served to "rapidly challenge newly developed molecular identification approaches by the discovery of novel 'atypical' isolates that do not fit into the current classification system."[122] As John LiPuma pointed out, "what we've learned about taxonomy in *Burkholderia* has really been driven by its place in CF."[123]

And the taxonomy only got more complicated. By 2007, a decade after the *B. cepacia* complex was initially defined with what appeared to be five species, the complex had grown to ten such species.[124] Just three years later, the number had jumped to seventeen, and by 2016, twenty species within the *B. cepacia* complex had been defined, as John LiPuma pointed out.[125] By 2018, investigators had characterized twenty-four *B. cepacia* complex species, only some of which were associated with severe medical consequences in people with CF.[126] John LiPuma noted that when people discuss "this group scientifically," they typically use the term *B. cepacia* complex to refer to the group of species "or they'll specifically talk about [individual species such as] *B. multivorans* or *B. dolosa* or *B. cenocepacia*, etc."[127] However, "the more sort of jargony popular term that's used is *B. cepacia* and that does cause confusion." Indeed, while there is a single species called *B. cepacia* within the larger *B. cepacia* complex, many people with CF have also pointed out that the term *B. cepacia* or simply *cepacia* is used to refer to all species within the *B. cepacia* complex, which serves as a source of confusion about whether one is talking about the single species or the collective group of microbes. Furthermore, as LiPuma noted in 2016, "*B. cepacia* per se, that species is one of the ones that's not as regularly found in CF . . . we don't see much *B. cepacia* in CF as it turns out."[128] This taxonomic complexity, coupled with the challenges in isolating *B. cepacia* complex microorganisms in the laboratory, made the diagnostic process especially challenging. As the next section will demonstrate, this diagnostic uncertainty contributed to a change in infection control measures that profoundly impacted the daily life of many with CF.

The Isolation of All People with Cystic Fibrosis

While the initial restrictions placed on patient contact typically involved separating those infected with *P. cepacia* from those without the microorganism, many clinicians eventually decided that all people with CF posed a safety risk to each other, in part because laboratory methods were not robust enough to detect *B. cepacia* complex species in everyone who was infected. In response to these and other concerns related to infection control, the CF Foundation sponsored a consensus conference in 2001 to make policy recommendations.[129] As outlined in the updated infection control guidelines put out by the CF Foundation in 2003, "practices that contain respiratory secretions and prevent transmission of respiratory tract pathogens . . . must be followed with all CF patients."[130] Justifying this move away from segregation practices, investigators pointed out that infection control "cannot be implemented according to the specific microbiology results of individual CF patients because microbiology methods are not 100% sensitive for the detection of CF pathogens."[131] Since "respiratory secretions of all CF patients potentially could be infected with epidemiologically and clinically important microorganisms," the guidelines recommended that "contact between CF patients should be limited."[132]

Reflecting back on the 2003 guidelines years later, physician John LiPuma recalled that the restrictions placed on patients "were harsh and at the time extremely controversial."[133] According to LiPuma, people with CF and their families had many questions about the specifics of the new policy, such as how far patients needed to be from each other, how long they could stay in the same room, the size of the room, and whether attendance at the same school as another person with CF was advisable, "for which we often didn't have good answers." As LiPuma noted, the "very draconian . . . measures that were put into place" were "really hard on caregivers and on patients."[134] By 2013, in the setting of continued concerns about patient-to-patient transmission of microorganisms in the *B. cepacia* complex, as well as other pathogens such as *P. aeruginosa* and methicillin-resistant *S. aureus* (MRSA), the CF Foundation put out updated infection control guidelines.[135] The recommendations, developed by "an interdisciplinary committee of healthcare personnel with expertise in CF, 3 parents of children with CF, and an adult with CF," stressed the need to "separate all people with CF from others with CF, regardless of their respiratory tract culture results, at least 6 feet (2 meters) in all settings, to reduce the risk of droplet transmission of CF pathogens."[136] In addition, the guidelines noted that "only 1 person with CF may attend a CF Foundation-sponsored indoor event."[137] The efficacy of this approach was emphasized in the CF Foundation's 2013 patient education manual, which noted that "the infection prevention and control policy includes practices and activities to promote safety and reduce the risk of cross-infection among people with CF."[138]

Parallel to some of the debates that have arisen during the COVID-19 pandemic about mask use, social distancing, and lockdown mandates, parents and people with CF varied greatly in their response to the 2013 guidelines. Some welcomed the recommendations, whereas others felt that they were overly paternalistic. For example, Julie Desch, the adult with CF and retired physician mentioned in the last chapter, acknowledged that the CF Foundation "does an amazing job raising money and awareness in the fight to cure CF," yet stressed that "I don't take kindly to being excluded from an event sponsored by the very organization that is supposed to be my advocate."[139] As Desch argued in her 2013 blog post, "the CFF is attempting to control our behavior, at least when it comes to this 'one person' rule," and she stressed that she had the right to make her own decisions as someone living "in a free country where we are free to decide what risks we want to take."[140] Many who responded to the blog agreed with Desch and noted that the CF Foundation guidelines made those with CF feel even more isolated and excluded. In fact, it is possible to see how the infection control guidelines, which limited the ability of people with CF to form in-person communities, were at odds with the diversity model of disability, which "encourages self-acceptance and the deliberate rejection of shame and internalized ableism."[141] For example, one adult with CF remarked that "I hate feeling like a leper," and another was "furious when the notice came out" and stopped donating money to the foundation. However, others, in particular parents of children with CF, favored the CF Foundation's guidelines.[142]

The following year, in light of the continued debate about the 2013 guidelines, the journal *CHEST* published a set of point/counterpoint editorials that addressed their most controversial recommendation, namely the decision to restrict attendance at indoor CF Foundation–sponsored events to only one person with CF. Arguing in the affirmative, Chicago physician Manu Jain and colleagues, including John LiPuma, stressed that the mandate was necessary because (1) it was possible for people with CF to transmit pathogenic microorganisms to each other, (2) the acquisition of pathogenic microorganisms could "lead to clinical deterioration and possibly death" in people with CF, and (3) limiting contact between people with CF reduced transmission of *B. cepacia* complex and other microorganisms.[143] Those in support of the guidelines did acknowledge how "unfortunate" the recommendation was, as it added "to the burden of disease as the value of the psychosocial support provided by participation in CF community activities cannot be overstated."[144]

Arguing against the recommendation to limit attendance at indoor events, Steven Shepherd and three other people with CF, including Julie Desch, pointed out that the policy was "unfounded, misguided, unnecessary, and harmful."[145] In addition to contending that the recommendation was not grounded in scientific evidence, they stressed that "the ban damages what for many patients is an already fragile sense of self-worth" because it conveys to those with CF "that they are unfit to be around other people like themselves, that they are a source of contagion, and that they are a danger to others."[146] Reminiscent of debates about paternalism in medical and disability history more generally, they noted that for adults "the ban carries the additional message that they are incompetent to make their own decisions."[147] In the rebuttal from Jain and colleagues, they pointed out that the one-person rule had also been implemented by organizations in the UK and Canada and cautioned that people with CF were "variably informed about infection risk."[148] Shepherd and colleagues, however, reiterated their view that "the ban is causing more harm than good and should be revoked."[149] The one-person policy was further debated in an April 2014 podcast, in which the two lead authors of the point-counterpoint *CHEST* articles expressed differing views about whether the guideline committee (which included one adult with CF and three parents of children with CF) was representative of all people with CF, whether and to what extent the views of other people with CF were considered before implementing the policy, and whether it was possible to allow more than one person with CF to attend meetings from a safety standpoint.[150]

While acknowledging the range of views held by individuals, the recommended isolation of those with CF from others with the disease has had a profound impact on the CF community.[151] Paul Quinton, the adult with CF quoted at the start of this article and coauthor of the 2013 counterpoint editorial in *CHEST*, was impacted on a professional as well as a personal level. As a scientist involved in CF research, Quinton "was usually on a committee or doing a talk or organizing group sessions or something pretty active" at the annual North American CF Foundation conference for years before the 2013 policy was implemented. However, as he recalled in a 2020 interview, the guidelines restricting attendance to one person with CF left "a number of us feeling really, really shut out, kind of like pariahs for the CF Foundation."[152] Another adult with CF, Erin Evans, stated that "I understand why . . . you're not supposed to be around other people with CF," yet she pointed out that "it's a choice that everybody with CF has to make."[153] As Evans explained, she is friends with a married couple, both of whom have CF, and she also knows others "who would never go in a room with somebody with CF." Evans described her own stance as "kind of in the middle of it," in that she does at times choose to see others with CF in person, yet she is "very careful," being "mindful of what we're touching," keeping a distance, and avoiding close contact such as hugging.

Many parents of people with CF, even those in support of the guidelines, expressed a sense of loss following the recommendation that those with CF avoid contact with each other. For example, Peter Evans, father of Erin Evans mentioned above, recalled that the contact they had with another family after Erin was diagnosed was "extremely helpful." However, as he recalled in a 2020 interview, "when it was instituted that we couldn't get together anymore, I felt like we lost a lot." He went on to note, "I was really sad about that but . . . I think the benefits of not interacting far outweigh what we lost but we lost quite a bit I think."[154] Another parent, Virginia S., recalled that "it progressively got to be worse and worse of a problem" following the implementation of infection control guidelines when her daughter Erica was in grade school.[155] For example, when Erica and twins with CF were invited to a birthday party, Virginia reached out to the other mother to see if they might coordinate so the twins could go for half of the time and Erica could go the other half. However, the other mother "would not hear of it" and made it clear that her daughters would be "staying the whole party," leaving Erica's family to decide whether to follow the infection control guidelines or allow her to go to her friend's birthday party. As these accounts highlight, the reframing of CF as a type of genetic/infectious hybrid disease has had widespread implications for people with CF, their loved ones, and the medical community.[156]

* * *

In 1994, several years after *P. cepacia* was reclassified as one species within the *B. cepacia* complex, the CF Foundation pointed to concerns related to diagnostic uncertainty and noted that "if the techniques used to detect the presence of *B. cepacia* are too insensitive, or the isolates are erroneously identified as *B. cepacia* when they are not, then the patient may be misclassified."[157] The foundation cautioned that "such misclassification may have significant medical and psychosocial implications."[158] In fact, as I have argued, diagnostic uncertainty associated with *B. cepacia* complex microorganisms contributed to the reframing of CF. Reflecting on this change in a 2019 interview, Atlanta physician Eric Sorscher explained that CF "is a disease you can't 'catch,' but that needs to be qualified in some important ways if you are a person with CF because there are infections you can acquire from someone else with the disease."[159] In other words, CF is now understood to be not only a genetic disease, but also one associated with contagion, challenging the strict dichotomy of inherited versus infectious diseases.

The very fact that people have been able to choose whether or not to follow the infection control guidelines in situations outside the purview of the CF Foundation or CF care centers has at times led to increased stigma and blame when an unfavorable health outcome follows an in-person encounter. For example, in 2009, eighteen-year-old Katie Donovan and seventeen-year-old Dalton Prager connected on Facebook given their shared experiences living with CF.[160] When Dalton began making plans to travel almost four hundred miles to see Katie in person, his mother "flat-out opposed the meeting" in light of the infection control guidelines in place at that time.[161] However, Katie justified taking the risk, and possibly acquiring the *B. cepacia* complex microorganism that Dalton harbored, stressing that she'd "rather be happy—like really, really happy—for five years of my life and die sooner than be mediocre happy and live for 20 years."[162]

In fact, Katie did become infected soon after meeting Dalton at a Dairy Queen in Kentucky, but they remained "relatively healthy" for the several years before and after their marriage in 2011.[163] However, the two died in 2016, shortly after their fifth wedding anniversary.

In response to what became a very public relationship between Katie and Dalton Prager, many in the CF community debated whether people with CF should have in-person contact.[164] Some adults with CF, such as Gunnar Esiason, were strongly opposed to such meetings. As Esiason stressed in a 2016 blog post, "I'm not one to say that what Katie and Dalton did was wrong," but "I wholeheartedly believe that people with CF should not be near each other, nor should patients follow in Katie and Dalton's example."[165] Esiason described such person-to-person transmission of antibiotic resistant microorganisms as "a public health concern" because "interaction between people with CF creates a breeding ground for infection to spread."[166] In other words, Esiason argued that people who chose to meet in person put not just themselves but others at risk as well.[167] The responses to Esiason's post varied widely, with some in strong support of his stance and others defending those with CF who chose to interact in person. For example, as Paul Quinton explained, "it saddens me to read that some think and imply (carefully) that Katie and Dalton should have been more fearful, had better sense, and never exposed themselves to loving and living together."[168]

Some have also changed their views about the infection control guidelines. In a 2020 interview, Julie Desch recalled that at first, the restrictions on patient contact "really infuriated me because . . . I was not really thinking about it from the perspective of somebody who might actually be afraid, because I wasn't afraid."[169] She went on to explain, "I knew how to take precautions around other people with CF and so I didn't experience fear." She continued to explain that "during this COVID thing, I experienced, really for the first time, the fear of a mother for her children's health and now I'm kind of looking back at how those parents of kids with CF must have felt when they were made aware of the risk that their kids were exposed to from other kids or other people with CF." Desch explained that "now I totally, I grok that fear, I understand that fear now because I've felt a similar fear for my own kids." Despite this newfound understanding, Desch stressed that "it's not like I suddenly agree with the CF Foundation's policy . . . but I understand the intention behind it in a way that I don't think I did when I wrote that post" in 2013. Nevertheless, Desch pointed out that in the setting of such a policy "people end up feeling excluded . . . like a walking, talking pathogen as opposed to a human being," encapsulating the significant effect that diagnostic uncertainty, and the subsequent reframing of the disease, has had on the CF community.

Thus, as this chapter has illustrated, diagnostic uncertainty has persisted not just in the setting of the diagnosis of CF itself, but also in the context of secondary diagnoses. Given the possibility of person-to-person transmission of *B. cepacia* complex and other microorganisms among people with CF, and the difficulty of knowing whether someone is infected with a particular pathogen, uncertainty regarding a CF diagnosis affects not just the person in question but extends to those who might come in contact with them as well.

Epilogue

In 2020, about a month into the COVID-19 pandemic, twenty-five-year-old Michelle Mastrianni noticed that her hands began to "wrinkle up really, really badly" after brief exposure to water.[1] Despite spending much of her childhood swimming, Michelle had never before experienced "this extreme level of wrinkling."[2] She eventually saw a dermatologist and was diagnosed with aquagenic wrinkling of the palms in 2021.[3] Her dermatologist told her that this rare skin condition had a "strong link to cystic fibrosis" and suggested that she get tested, postulating that Michelle might be a carrier for CF since she didn't have the lung or gastrointestinal symptoms characteristic of the disease.[4] Instead of being a carrier, however, Michelle was unexpectedly diagnosed with CF after further testing and much uncertainty, and she was asked to be seen every three to four months at a CF clinic so she could be monitored for the development of additional symptoms. Reflecting on her experience in 2021, Michelle explained that "at the beginning of all of this I kind of thought that my hands had betrayed me by suddenly developing this symptom and being essentially allergic to water, but now I feel like they saved me in a sense . . . because I was able to find out about this [CF] diagnosis as a result of this [skin] condition."[5]

Recall from Chapter 3 that in the 1970s some CF physicians suggested using the "bucket test" to detect rapid skin wrinkling following exposure to water as a way to screen for CF and reduce diagnostic uncertainty. However, other physicians critiqued the use of the bucket test at that time because they felt that early skin wrinkling following water exposure was not specific to CF. In the decades after the screening tool was first proposed in 1974, the bucket test was not widely adopted, yet more recent scientific reports list early skin wrinkling, or aquagenic wrinkling, as one of the many features of CF.[6] Furthermore, in the twenty-first century, the medical literature has increasingly urged dermatologists who diagnose aquagenic wrinkling with the bucket test to refer patients for CF testing (with a sweat test or a genetic test), just as Michelle's dermatologist did. After Michelle was diagnosed with aquagenic wrinkling, she went through months of diagnostic uncertainty about whether she had cystic fibrosis. According to the "gold standard" diagnostic sweat test for CF, Michelle's sweat chloride concentration fell in the intermediate range (30–59 mmol/L), meaning that it wasn't high enough to be diagnostic for CF, but it wasn't low enough to be considered "normal."[7] When Michelle's genetic counselor later told her that she had two CF gene mutations, Michelle initially assumed that meant that she had CF, because she "thought the definition of having CF was having two mutations."[8] However, Michelle soon learned that the medical professionals involved in her care were unsure whether she should be diagnosed with cystic fibrosis or CFTR-related disorder (CFTR-RD).[9]

At the time that Michelle's diagnosis was up in the air, the CFTR-RD label was reserved for individuals who did not meet the diagnostic criteria for CF but who had evidence of CF gene dysfunction and symptoms in a single organ system.[10] In 2020, when Michelle initially noticed that her skin wrinkled rapidly following exposure to water, numerous CFTR-related disorders had been identified in the medical literature, including not only aquagenic wrinkling, but also pancreatitis, bronchiectasis, and a form of male infertility caused by congenital bilateral absence of the vas deferens.[11] CFTR-RD is not the only diagnostic category that involves possible CFTR dysfunction in the absence of a CF diagnosis. Recall from Chapter 4 that as newborn screening for CF has expanded, an increasing number of individuals have been identified who do not meet the diagnostic criteria for CF but who also do not clearly fit into the "normal" category. For example, in 2005, Richard Parad and Anne Marie Comeau of the New England Newborn Screening Program documented these diagnostic dilemmas in detail, and many investigators have weighed in on how to define and respond to this type of uncertainty over the past few decades.[12] These newborns are now given the label CFTR-related metabolic syndrome (CRMS) or CF screen positive, inconclusive diagnosis (CFSPID), as their results are inconclusive for CF based on genetic and sweat testing carried out in response to a positive newborn screen.[13] Since some people with CFTR-RD and CRMS/CFSPID diagnoses ultimately convert to a CF diagnosis, individuals with these labels are typically followed by

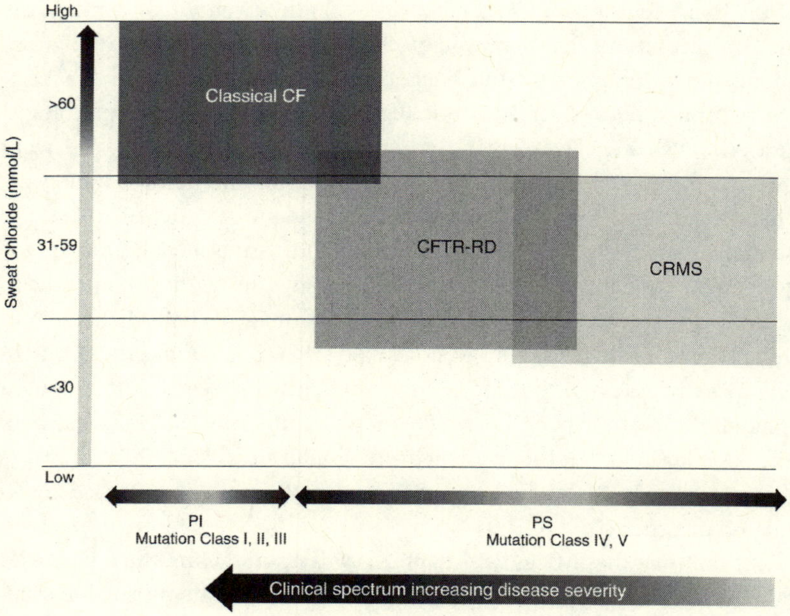

FIGURE E.1. Characteristics of patients in a Wisconsin study spanning 1994–2012. "Clinical descriptors of our cohort capture the overlaps and distinctions among CF, CFTR-RD, and CRMS. Sweat chloride measurements are from the time point closest to diagnosis. CF, cystic fibrosis; CFTR-RD, cystic fibrosis transmembrane conductance regulator-related disorder; CRMS, CFTR-related metabolic syndrome." Reproduced from H. Levy et al., "Refining the Continuum of CFTR-Associated Disorders in the Era of Newborn Screening," *Clinical Genetics* 89, no. 5 (2016), with permission from John Wiley and Sons.

CF centers for the development of symptoms and signs consistent with CF.[14] In fact, some investigators have suggested that CF, CFTR-RD, and CRMS/CFSPID constitute a spectrum, as illustrated in Figure E.1.[15]

Reflecting on her experience with the confusion about whether she should be given a CF or CFTR-RD diagnosis, Michelle explained that "it feels like it's somewhat arbitrary . . . whether you have CF or not," but once her physicians did further genetic testing of her parents, "they were more comfortable saying, 'okay, you have CF.' "[16] Even after Michelle was ultimately diagnosed with CF, she continued to experience uncertainty about what the diagnosis would mean for her long term. As she explained, "I don't know when my symptoms might worsen. I mean, I don't really have any lung symptoms at the moment, but I don't know when I might . . . develop them. It's possible that I will never develop them."[17] Michelle's experience with the diagnosis of CF in the absence of respiratory or gastrointestinal symptoms is reminiscent of numbers-based diagnoses of diseases such as hypertension or the conflation of risk and disease in the case of breast cancer.[18] However, unlike these cases, in which treatment is sometimes initiated to reduce risk, Michelle's physicians recommended against the modulator therapy Trikafta, which may have functioned to treat the hand wrinkling, because they felt that any potential benefits did not outweigh the risk of side effects from the drug.

Thus, while Michelle was not subjected to the potential harms of a therapeutic intervention in the absence of respiratory or gastrointestinal symptoms, she was still faced with the challenges associated with being a "patient-in-waiting" who was living in a "limbo state" between health and disease.[19] As Michelle explained, "I have this chronic illness but I don't currently feel chronically ill so it feels like . . . just a weird juxtaposition of things."[20] Similar accounts of the "patient-in-waiting" have been documented for those with CFTR-RD and CRMS/CFSPID diagnoses. For example, as Álvaro La Parra-Pérez, parent of a child with CRMS, explained in 2023, "our annual check-ups at Children's Hospital are always a brutal reminder of the threat that looms . . . yet, we know we are fortunate," because "our daughter is growing up without any symptoms that would make us think that the CRMS potential threat is manifesting in any way."[21] Similarly, Anna, parent of a child with CFSPID, explained that "we do know that he's got a faulty gene that does affect, it doesn't work as well as ours does at getting the salt and the chloride around the body, we do know that he's not completely healthy even though he looks it."[22] As Russell, parent of a five-year-old child with CFSPID, noted, "It was a massive shock to us . . . I mean obviously I'm glad she doesn't have full CF . . . but we have to live with the possibility of it every day . . . we factor it in to decisions we make in life . . . like where we live: are we near a decent CF centre . . . ? Is there anyone else with CF in her school that could infect her? So we prepare for the worst, but hope for the best."[23] Such reflections by parents of children with CRMS/CFSPID are particularly striking because the uncertainties they face are a direct result of prior efforts to reduce diagnostic uncertainty through newborn screening for CF, highlighting how uncertainty persists in medicine despite, and because of, the introduction of new technologies.[24]

* * *

In October 2020, around the time that Michelle Mastrianni developed aquagenic wrinkling of the palms, I was learning more about the range of health conditions associated with *CFTR* gene variants while virtually attending the North American Cystic Fibrosis Conference. Providing introductory remarks for the session titled "Beyond CF: A Spectrum of CFTR Variation & CFTR-opathies," genetic counselor Karen Raraigh explained that "as we learn more about variation with the *CFTR* gene, our understanding of the phenotypic spectrum of conditions related to CFTR dysfunction grows."[25] Particularly relevant to my own clinical history, University of Iowa physician Douglas Hornick presented a talk titled "Are CF Carriers at Increased Risk for a Broad Range of CF-Related Conditions?"[26] Hornick began by pointing to the "pretty widely held opinion" that CF carriers do not have associated health problems by providing evidence from a number of sources, and his assertion was consistent with descriptions of the "healthy carrier" or "healthy heterozygote" that have been widespread throughout the twentieth and much of the twenty-first centuries.[27] However, as Hornick's talk documented, this view of CF carriers as completely healthy has become increasingly untenable. Referring to work that he had recently published with Aaron Miller and colleagues, Hornick argued that "our analyses showed evidence for multi-organ morbidity within the CF carrier population."[28]

While the possibility of disease manifestations in those with a single *CFTR* gene variant had been noted for many decades, Hornick's presentation of the University of Iowa data was particularly striking to me because it was the first large-scale case-control retrospective study documenting the increased risk of fifty-seven health conditions in CF carriers.[29] After listening to the conference presentation, I immediately read the corresponding *Proceedings of the National Academy of Sciences* article and supplementary material. As I went through the list of CF-related conditions that were more prevalent in carriers such as myself, I noted that I had seven of them, including pancreatic steatorrhea (another name for pancreatic insufficiency). As I contemplated this link between certain health conditions and CF carrier status, I recalled that I was tested for CF with the eighty-seven-mutation Genzyme panel and the gold standard sweat test shortly after I was diagnosed with pancreatic insufficiency. At that time, more than two decades ago, none of my physicians suggested to me that my carrier status might explain my pancreatic insufficiency; instead, my gastroenterologist had suspected that the pancreatic insufficiency was due to two *CFTR* gene mutations, only one of which had been identified.[30]

As I continued to learn about the University of Iowa study, I initially suspected that the "CF carriers" with CF-associated health conditions were *not* in fact carriers, but instead people with undiagnosed CF due to the failure to detect a second mutation. Yet the investigators anticipated

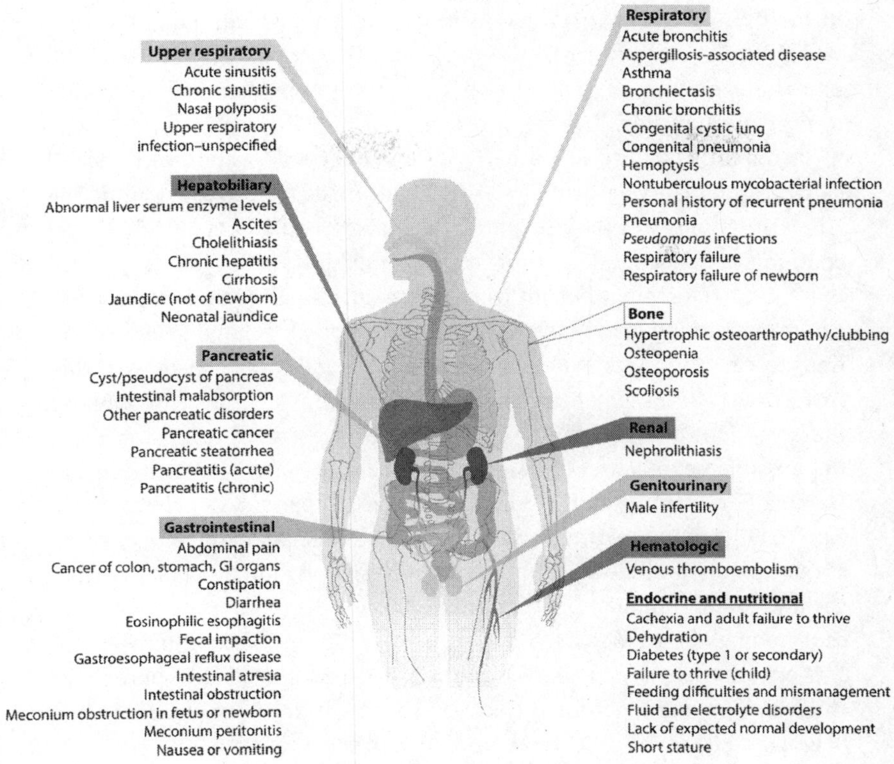

FIGURE E.2. "CF-related conditions for which CF carriers may be at increased risk." Reprinted with permission from P. M. Polgreen and A. P. Comellas, "Clinical Phenotypes of Cystic Fibrosis Carriers," *Annual Review of Medicine*, 73 (2022): 563–74, 568.

this critique and specifically noted that "our findings cannot be explained by misclassification bias, that is, people with CF misclassified as CF carriers due to undetectable *CFTR* mutations on 1 allele."[31] The University of Iowa investigators went on to assert that even though the *absolute risk* of CF-related health conditions was relatively low in carriers, the increased *relative risk* compared to controls, coupled with the existence of more than ten million CF carriers in the US, meant that the "disease burden attributable to the CF carrier status is likely substantial."[32] Several years later, two of the University of Iowa investigators further reflected on the CF-related health conditions seen more frequently in CF carriers in an *Annual Review of Medicine* article and provided a visual depiction of the organ systems involved (Figure E.2).[33] When I read the article, I realized that I had developed several additional CF-related health conditions, including an intestinal obstruction, in the years after I learned of the University of Iowa study. However, even with these connections, I was still uncertain about whether and to what extent my own carrier status related to my clinical profile.

Given the high disease burden presumed to be associated with the CF carrier status, University of Iowa investigators suggested that "identifying CF carriers may aid the prevention, diagnosis, and treatment of several common and uncommon disorders."[34] Other physicians also suggested that CF carriers might benefit from treatment using CF therapeutics. For example, pointing to the increased prevalence of CF-related health conditions in carriers, investigators in both the US and France suggested that carriers with disease manifestations might benefit from CFTR modulator therapy.[35] However, some individuals have expressed apprehension about the possible negative repercussions of this change in how CF carriers are framed. For example, in the editorial that accompanied the *PNAS* publication, University of Toronto physician David Fisman expressed concern about the possibility of "pathologizing widespread and important genetic variation within human populations."[36] In fact, even before the more recent findings of an increased risk of CF-related health conditions in CF carriers, physicians and social scientists had recognized that parents of children who were identified as carriers through newborn screening had heightened levels of concern about the child's health.[37]

Considering the evidence that CF carrier status confers an increased risk of CF-related health conditions, physician Philip Farrell and colleagues noted in 2021 that "in place of the traditional discrete model of *gene-to-disease*, we suggest a more advanced and realistic model of *genotype-to-risk*."[38] Pointing to the role of risk calculations in treatment decisions for the prevention of such conditions as cardiovascular disease and bone fractures, the authors suggested that the genotype-to-risk paradigm for *CFTR* gene variants could allow physicians to provide patients with their relative risk of developing certain health conditions.[39] In other words, this challenge to the "dogma of the healthy heterozygote" meant that genetic test results for CF would not only provide information used for the possible diagnosis of cystic fibrosis, but such test results might also alert individuals to their increased risk for a host of CF-related health conditions. Given the difficulties associated with risk-based medicine and the expansive number of *CFTR* gene variants that are not well characterized, diagnostic uncertainty associated with *CFTR* genotype is likely to become even more pronounced over time.[40] In addition to debates about whether someone should be diagnosed with cystic fibrosis, we may soon be faced with an expanded number of people who are told that they are at increased risk of CF-related health conditions because of their CF carrier status. In fact, some have suggested that CF carriers should be screened at an earlier age for certain conditions such as colon cancer.[41]

As we can see, documentation of the increased risk of CF-related health conditions in carriers has served to further challenge the strict dichotomy of simple Mendelian genetic diseases versus complex diseases such as cancer, diabetes, and heart disease.[42] On the one hand, there is great value in identifying people with an elevated risk of disease if interventions can mitigate that risk, but at the same time, new kinds of harms can emerge in the process. Furthermore, the type of reframing that has been taking place regarding CF carrier status has extended to other Mendelian diseases as well, especially as genetic testing expands and as large-scale studies of the clinical profile of those with common genetic variants become increasingly feasible.[43] To further complicate matters, a study published in 2025 using data from the *All of Us* Research Program found that only four CF-related health conditions had "moderate evidence of increased risk" in carriers, in contrast to the fifty-seven conditions identified by the Iowa group.[44] Also in 2025, investigators at Vanderbilt University provided evidence from prenatal carrier testing that female CF carriers were at increased risk of pancreatitis, a finding consistent with the Iowa study but not the *All of Us* study, pointing to continued uncertainty about the nature of the risks associated with CF carrier status.[45] This shift in the definition of a carrier, from that of a "healthy" person to one who may be at risk of disease, and the continued uncertainty about the nature and extent of risk associated with carrier status, is likely to make it even more challenging to determine whether an individual should be given a disease label, further highlighting the elusive nature of attempts to achieve diagnostic certainty in medicine.

* * *

While we have witnessed uncertainty in the setting of expanded diagnostic labels associated with possible *CFTR* gene dysfunction, ranging from the CF carrier state to CFTR-RD and CRMS/CFSPID, uncertainty related to the diagnosis of CF itself has continued as well. As *Challenging Diagnosis* has illustrated, diagnostic uncertainty associated with CF has persisted for more than eighty years despite numerous developments in screening approaches and diagnostic technologies. To be fair, many people have been diagnosed with CF early in their disease course ever since the first detailed characterization of the disease in 1938, yet efforts to reduce diagnostic uncertainty related to CF from the late 1930s to today have been fraught with challenges. One difficulty in reaching the goal of widespread timely diagnosis of people with CF is that the very definition of the disease has changed dramatically over time. In the late 1930s, CF was often described as a disease of the pancreas with an average life expectancy of less than a year and diagnosis occurred through an invasive duodenal intubation test that revealed the absence of pancreatic enzymes in digestive juices. Today, while some people are still diagnosed with CF in the setting of pancreatic insufficiency, others, such as Michelle Mastrianni, have received a CF label in the absence of the gastrointestinal or respiratory symptoms characteristic of the disease. Over the last eight decades, as certain sources of diagnostic uncertainty were addressed by the introduction of the sweat test in the 1950s, screening tests in the 1970s, and genetic testing in the late 1980s, new uncertainties have arisen in their place, such that uncertainty in CF diagnostics has been a constant.

Reflecting on the persistence of diagnostic ambiguity, we can see how technical solutions have consistently fallen short in the elusive quest for certainty. In conducting the research for this book, I was particularly struck by how often I came across accounts of people with CF who were overlooked by medical professionals for years and even decades despite having symptoms consistent with the disease. From accounts of "neurotic mothers" concerned about the health of their infants to adults whose diagnoses were delayed due to assumptions that CF was a "white disease" or that their symptoms were psychogenic, the diagnostic odyssey that many with CF have gone through is remarkable. Even after someone receives a CF diagnosis, many kinds of uncertainty remain. For example, people diagnosed with CF are faced with uncertainty about whether they will receive a secondary diagnosis, such as a *B. cepacia* complex infection, with important implications for their prognosis. Furthermore, in the setting of CRMS/CFSPID, or what we might refer to as a formalized label of uncertainty, individuals face regular healthcare encounters because they may convert to a CF diagnosis in the future. And of course, uncertainty remains about whether and to what extent a CF carrier is at risk of developing a range of CF-related health conditions. Many have suggested that the incorporation of artificial intelligence (AI) into the diagnostic process could effectively address the problem of uncertainty, not only for CF but for other diseases as well.[46] However, if the history of efforts to reduce CF-related diagnostic uncertainty through the introduction of new diagnostic and screening technologies is a predictor of future outcomes, it is more likely that AI in diagnostics will address some sources of uncertainty while concomitantly introducing new ones.

Acknowledging that uncertainty is inherent in medicine more generally, many physicians have suggested that diagnostic uncertainty should be tolerated or even embraced.[47] For example, medical professionals have worked in recent years to develop frameworks and tools to help physicians and patients address uncertainty.[48] Reflecting on one such approach to address diagnostic uncertainty in 2024, Boston physician Sonja Solomon explained that "the conversation can't just stop with 'I don't know' "; instead, "even where there is a high degree of uncertainty, there's always a way forward."[49] Consistent with this assertion, when a patient has debilitating symptoms in the absence of a diagnostic label, medical professionals can play a critical role in that patient's experience of illness by first acknowledging the legitimacy of their suffering and then working with the patient to address their symptoms while also seeking a diagnosis. At the same time, medical professionals could benefit from a culture in which discussions about diagnostic uncertainty among colleagues are the norm.[50] Such attention to providing resources for those facing uncertainty also applies to situations in which patients have a diagnosis in the absence of symptoms or an elevated risk of disease in the future. Given the persistence of diagnostic uncertainty in the case of CF and in the setting of more complex and contested diseases, *Challenging Diagnosis* supports a revised medical framework that places greater emphasis on supporting patients and physicians in the face of uncertainty.

Acknowledgments

In 2012, my father-in-law sent me an article about eleven-year-old Colman Chadam, who had been transferred out of his Palo Alto junior high school because administrators believed that Colman had CF and therefore posed a health hazard to the two siblings with CF who attended the same school. At the time, medical professionals advised people with CF to avoid in-person contact due to the possibility of person-to-person transmission of a particularly pathogenic microorganism among individuals with CF, yet school administrators and Colman's own physician disagreed about whether Colman even had cystic fibrosis. When I read the article, I was on the faculty in the Department of Biological Sciences at Wellesley College, and my colleagues and I often used CF as a case study when teaching key concepts in cell biology, molecular biology, and genetics. I also had a personal connection to the disease, as one of my relatives was diagnosed with CF when I was a kid. However, I lacked the tools at that time to fully examine the many layers of diagnostic uncertainty that the Chadam case illuminated. Prompted in part by a desire to better understand what happened to Colman Chadam, as well as my growing interest in the history of biology and medicine more generally, I decided to go back to school to obtain formal training in the history of science. I would like to acknowledge the many people who helped me along the way, and who made this book possible.

The Department of the History of Science at Harvard University provided a welcoming and intellectually engaging home during my time working on the book. I would like to begin by thanking David Jones, who has been instrumental in my ability to write this book. David has consistently gone above and beyond expectations to support me in my pursuit of this new career path, and I continue to feel incredibly fortunate to have found such a brilliant and selfless mentor who has always made time to provide me with detailed, thoughtful, and prompt feedback on my scholarship and career decisions. Allan Brandt has been such a joy to work with, and I am particularly grateful for his exceptional support, warmth, and encouragement over the years. Allan has an amazing ability to celebrate strengths while also being honest in his assessment of areas for growth, and I always leave our conversations feeling valued and hopeful. Hannah Marcus has been a wonderful mentor, providing kindness, enthusiasm, and insightful engagement with my scholarship while also offering thoughtful advice about my professional development. I benefited greatly from being part of a community of Hannah's students through her weekly writing group, Historians of Hope, which I found extremely inspiring, in large part because of Hannah's great skill in building community and trust. Sophia Roosth has provided me with invaluable guidance as I navigated the transition into this new field, and I continue to be amazed by her vast knowledge of the social study of the life sciences. I have especially appreciated Sophia's ability to provide an engaging environment in which to discuss key concepts and sources in the field while also being demanding in her expectations and thoughtful with her feedback. I am so appreciative of David, Allan, Hannah, and Sophia for providing extremely helpful suggestions on multiple drafts of individual chapters, the full manuscript, and presentations.

Also at Harvard, I am grateful for the advice, mentorship, support, and guidance at various stages of the book project provided by Elizabeth Lunbeck, Gabriela Soto Laveaga, Evelynn Hammonds, Rebecca Lemov, Eram Alam, Charles Rosenberg, Anne Harrington, Sarah Richardson, Alex Csiszar, Linda Schneider, and Allie Belser. My time as a student at Harvard and beyond has been greatly enriched by Alyssa Botelho and Jacob Moses, who have both been such wonderful friends and colleagues, providing insightful and thoughtful feedback on the book project, drafts of written work, and presentations. I am also grateful for the valuable advice, feedback, and encouragement provided by Emily Harrison, Lisa Haushofer, Kiran Kumbhar, Yvan Prkachin, Colleen Lanier-Christensen, Gili Vidan, Angélica Márquez-Osuna, Miriam Rich, and Shireen Hamza, as well as Juanis Becerra, Frank Blibo, Brad Bolman, Rory Brinkmann, Emma Broder, Cara Kiernan Fallon, Anna Christensen, Hannah Conway, Iman Darwish, Max Ehrenfreund, Erin Freedman, Maud Jansen, Juhee Kang, Gustave Lester, Ben Maldonado, Wythe Marschall, Jamie Marsella, Eli Nelson, Tiffany Nichols, Udodiri Okwandu, Meg Perret, Kat Poje, Ángel Rodriguez, Christopher Rudeen, Tasha Schoenstein, Alexis Turner,

Aaron van Neste, Molly Walker, Jiemin Tina Wei, Che Yeun, and Jongsik Christian Yi. I also appreciate the helpful suggestions and community provided by attendees of Harvard's History of Medicine Working Group and Modern Sciences Working Group.

I have benefited tremendously from being part of the Department of History at Purdue University during the final stages of writing this book, and I am particularly grateful for the insightful feedback, guidance, and support provided by Frederick Davis, Wendy Kline, and Kathryn Cramer Brownell, as well as David Atkinson, Ekaterina Babintseva, Huiying Chen, Christopher Ewing, Debbie Fleetham, O. T. Ford, Ariel de la Fuente, Tina Irvine, Kathryn Maxson Jones, Jonathan Lande, Zachary Loeb, Angie Teel, Subodhana Wijeyeratne, and Melinda Zook. I am also grateful to the graduate students who provided feedback on a chapter draft, including Keri Blair, Zach Logsdon, Secret Permenter, Nathan Halder, and Abby Riehl, and I especially appreciate Alicia Venchuk for so carefully proofreading the entire manuscript. In addition, I am grateful to the students I have mentored at Purdue and Harvard for their enthusiasm and insight when engaging with various components of the book project.

I would also like to express my sincere gratitude to those mentors and colleagues who read and provided invaluable insight and advice on an earlier version of the full manuscript. The book is significantly improved because of their insights, and any errors that remain are mine alone. Robert Aronowitz, Joel Howell, and Susan Lindee took part in a manuscript workshop made possible by a grant from Purdue University, and they each provided me with incredibly thoughtful and detailed feedback that greatly strengthened the book. In addition, I am grateful to Philip Farrell for providing me with excellent suggestions for how to improve the book based on his experience as a CF physician, Stephen Pemberton for generously offering to read the full manuscript and providing me with such insightful and thoughtful feedback, and the anonymous reviewers at the University of Chicago Press for so carefully engaging with my work and offering such helpful suggestions. I am especially grateful to Karen Darling for her enthusiastic support of this book project and insightful feedback on the manuscript; Fabiola Enríquez Flores for her invaluable assistance as I worked to prepare the manuscript; Jon Dertien, Susan Fleshman, Tamara Ghattas, Anne Strother, and Theresa Wolner for their insights and guidance during the final stages of the publication process; and the University of Chicago Press for publishing this book.

I have also benefited from many additional mentors, colleagues, and friends who provided important insight about the book in the form of feedback, advice, support, and encouragement. I am especially grateful to Diane Paul, Meredith Krevosky, Diana Horrigan, Sara Press, Andrew Lea, and Katherine Warren, as well as Sari Altschuler, Itamar Avneri, Andy Baker, Simon Brausch, Mary Carpenter, Christina Goeltz Clarke, Rachel Derr, Deborah Doroshow, Hughes Evans, Alfred Freeborn, Brigette Freeman, Elise Frketich, Scott Gilbert, Corinna Gilley, Dave Gilley, Lori Green, Amy Heim, Stefan Helmreich, Wei Hong, Rebecca Jackson, Henry Kalter, Richard Keller, Lara Keuck, Yang Li, Maren Linett, Ilana Löwy, Michele Luchetti, Kate MacCord, Jane Maienschein, Robert Meunier, Sam McLaughlin, Alex Miller, Sandra Moose, Amy Moran-Thomas, Gregory Morgan, Rebecca Mueller, Molly Nebiolo, Maureen Nunes, Luísa Reis-Castro, Whitney Barlow Robles, Lila Rosenthal, Leigh Rudikoff, Robin Scheffler, Klara Schwalbe, Carolyn Shapiro-Shapin, Annabelle Slingerland, Yui Suzuki, Cecilia Tenorio, and Hanna Worliczek. I would also like to thank Angela Creager and Katharine Park for their generosity in providing advice as I considered making a career change.

For much-needed support and camaraderie during the writing process, I would like to thank Andrea Bohlman, Marielle Debos, Rosanna Dent, Amy Hay, Elena Jackson Albarrán, Elaine LaFay, Alison Lefkovitz, Ann Reynolds, Elizabeth Saleh, and Elvira Vilches, as well as Caroline Murphy, Sarah Koval, Madeline McMahon, Kelly Minot McCay, Maryam Patton, Ashley Gonik, Hannah Kaemmer, Etha Williams, Alexandria Brown-Hedjazi, and Megan Baumhammer. I am also grateful for suggestions provided by attendees of talks I have given at the Max Planck Institute for the History of Science, the Indiana University School of Medicine, Harvard University, the History of Science Society annual conference, the American Association for the History of Medicine annual conference, and the Rocky Mountain Interdisciplinary History Conference.

I am so grateful to the people who allowed me to interview them for this project, including Lisa Arkin, Jim Bolek, Anne Marie Comeau, Julie Desch, Gunnar Esiason, Erin Evans, Peter Evans, Debra Maloney-Evans, Philip Farrell, Cyrus Hopkins, Lucy Lester, John LiPuma, Marvin Lough, Michelle Mastrianni, Maryanne O'Hara, Michelle Patrovani, Robyn Petras, Paul Quinton, Charles Rabkin, Erica S., John S., Virginia S., Danieli Salinas, Thomas Sandora, Daniel Schidlow, Eric Sorscher, Robert Stern, and Cambrey White. The oral history interviews for this project were either deemed exempt (IRB19–0251 and IRB20–0580) or approved (IRB16–0460) by the Harvard University Institutional Review Board. In addition, I appreciate the helpful advice and insight provided by Scott Granter and Richard Mitchell.

I would also like to express my gratitude for assistance with archival documents and suggestions for resources provided by Scott Podolsky, Jessica Murphy, Carolyn Hayes, and Dominic Hall (Center for the History of Medicine, Francis A. Countway Library of Medicine, Harvard Medical School), Keith Pierce (Countway Library, Harvard Medical School), Fred Burchsted (Widener Library, Harvard University), Emily Bell (Lamont Library, Harvard University), Nicholas Webb and Barbara Niss (Icahn School of Medicine at Mount Sinai), Michele Lyons (Office of NIH History and Stetten Museum, National Institutes of Health), Zach Utz, Kris Wetterstrand, and Christopher Donohue (National Human Genome Research Institute, National Institutes of Health), Rebecca Fullerton, Alina Morris, and Teri Hedgpeth (Boston Children's Hospital), Stephen Novak and Katherine Satriano (Augustus C. Long Health Sciences Library, Columbia University Irving Medical Center), Jeffrey Mifflin (Massachusetts General Hospital), Jodi Aoki (Trent University Archives), Margaret Burzynski-Bays (University Hospitals of Cleveland), Dalia Zemaityte (University Hospitals and Rainbow Babies & Children's Hospital), Heather J. Robinson-Mooney and Ann K. Sindelar (Cleveland History Center of the Western Reserve Historical Society Library, Archives & Genealogy Center), Russell Knapp (Ball State University), Kevin Blowers (Bethel University), Youlanda Logan (Jimmy Carter Presidential Library & Museum), Jocelyn Wilk (Columbia University Libraries), Carlee Kessler and Frankie Piker (Wisconsin Historical Society), Joseph DiLullo (American Philosophical Society), and Allison Gibbs (Wright State University). I would also like to thank Francis Collins for providing permission to reproduce the diary entry in Figure 4.3, Lee Rosner for granting permission to reproduce the photo taken by Kay Chernush in Figure 4.4, Daniel Schidlow for allowing me to reproduce the drawing in Figure 5.3, and Dianna Poissant of Bruker Biomedical Systems for providing me with the image of the sweat collection device that appears on the cover of the book. I am also grateful to the Cystic Fibrosis Foundation for access to their archival materials, and I especially appreciate the generous assistance of Marybeth McMahon and Christina Pietrasanta, as well as Quynh Tu Tran, Sarah Hempstead, Paula Lomas, Suzie Conway, Azi Kaider, and Tricia Hopkins. I am also grateful for the invaluable insight about the Kiss Your Baby campaigns provided by Robert Beall.

I appreciate the financial support provided by Harvard University, including the Harvard University Graduate School of Arts and Sciences Dissertation Completion Fellowship and the Strominger Prize Dissertation Research Fellowship through the Department of the History of Science, the Sandra Ohrn Family Graduate Student Dissertation Fellowship, an ENGAGE grant and numerous ASPIRE grants through the College of Liberal Arts at Purdue University, the Purdue Books Initiative, and generous start-up and research funding through the History Department and College of Liberal Arts at Purdue.

I would also like to thank the *Journal of the History of Medicine and Allied Sciences* and *OBM Genetics* for allowing me to reproduce material originally published in the following two articles: Michelle Lynne LaBonte, "Diagnostic Uncertainty, Microbes, and the Isolation of People with Cystic Fibrosis," *Journal of the History of Medicine and Allied Sciences* 72, no. 3 (2022): 186–216, https://doi.org/10.1093/jhmas/jrab056; and Michelle Lynne LaBonte, "Addressing Uncertainty: The Emergence of the CRMS/CFSPID Diagnostic Category Following Newborn Screening for Cystic Fibrosis," *OBM Genetics* 5, no. 3 (2021): 1–20, https://doi.org/10.21926/obm.genet.2103139. At the *Journal of the History of Medicine and Allied Sciences*, I appreciate the thoughtful feedback provided by editor Laura Hirshbein, associate editor Jacob Steere-Williams, and the anonymous reviewers. At *OBM Genetics*, I am grateful for the helpful feedback provided by editor Wendy Zhi and the anonymous reviewers.

Special thanks go to Dr. Michael Apstein, who is the most caring, dedicated, and skilled physician I have ever had the pleasure of knowing. He is a model for how to support patients in the face of uncertainty, and I feel incredibly lucky to have met him.

Finally, I would like to express my sincere gratitude to my friends and family for their tremendous support and encouragement, beginning long before I contemplated going back to school in the history of science. Carrie Oelberger, Kelly Bromfield Cha, and Leah Mallory have been wonderful friends, providing thoughtful encouragement and many enjoyable distractions over the years. My mom, Lynne O'Riorden, who has always made time to support me in various ways, provided invaluable comments on the full manuscript. I am continually in awe of her ability to persevere in the face of adversity, and I will be forever grateful for her strength after my dad died and her decision to go back to school not to pursue something that she loved, but so she could make money to support me and my brother as a single parent. I continue to be thankful for the time I had with my dad, who showed me unconditional love and kindness and who has continually inspired me to follow my own path. Alison LaBonte has been a wonderful source of support as I have worked on this book, always asking how the writing is going, sending words of encouragement, and providing me with such thoughtful and detailed feedback on the full manuscript. I am also incredibly grateful for the consistent support and encouragement provided by Derek O'Riorden, Bob Day, Gail Morgan, Rex Morgan, Gary LaBonte, Shirley Ng, and my aunts, uncles, cousins, niece, nephew, and extended family.

I am especially grateful to my kids, Emily and Jack, for bringing me endless joy and laughter and doing a wonderful job helping me to keep things in perspective. I look forward to continuing to see where their own paths lead them. Finally, I would like to express my utmost gratitude to my husband Jason, for his unwavering love, support, and encouragement, and for enthusiastically providing me with thoughtful feedback on numerous drafts of every chapter. Since the time we were students together in college, he has consistently supported my academic pursuits while making sure that there is always time set aside for fun. This book would not have been possible without him.

Notes

Introduction

1. E. Dolgin, "Mystery Disease Sleuthing Grows—With and Without NIH Funding," *Nature Medicine* 20, no. 2 (2014), https://doi.org/10.1038/nm0214-108; R. C. Spillmann et al., "A Window into Living with an Undiagnosed Disease: Illness Narratives from the Undiagnosed Diseases Network," *Orphanet Journal of Rare Diseases* 12, no. 1 (2017), https://doi.org/10.1186/s13023-017-0623-3.

2. Charles E. Rosenberg and Janet Lynne Golden, *Framing Disease: Studies in Cultural History* (Rutgers University Press, 1992); Robert Aronowitz, *Unnatural History: Breast Cancer and American Society* (Cambridge University Press, 2007); Charles E. Rosenberg, "The Tyranny of Diagnosis: Specific Entities and Individual Experience," *Milbank Quarterly* 80, no. 2 (2002), https://doi.org/10.1111/1468-0009.t01-1-00003.

3. B. M. Kuehn, "US Launches Undiagnosed Diseases Program," *JAMA* 300, no. 1 (2008): 27, https://doi.org/10.1001/jama.300.1.27; National Institutes of Health, "Undiagnosed Diseases Program," press release, May 19, 2008, https://www.genome.gov/Pages/Newsroom/CurrentNewsReleases/MediaCallTranscript.pdf.

4. Julie Steenhuysen, "U.S. Agency Taps Medical Centers to Investigate Rare Diseases," *Reuters*, July 1, 2014, https://www.reuters.com/article/markets/u-s-agency-taps-medical-centers-to-investigate-rare-diseases-idUSL2N0PC17A/; "Facts and Figures," Undiagnosed Diseases Network, https://undiagnosed.hms.harvard.edu/about-us/facts-and-figures/.

5. "The Landscape for Rare Diseases in 2024," *Lancet Global Health* 12, no. 3 (2024), https://doi.org/10.1016/S2214-109X(24)00056-1.

6. For more on the notion of "passing" in the setting of disability or other marginalized identities, see Erving Goffman, *Stigma: Notes on the Management of Spoiled Identity* (Prentice-Hall, 1963); Tobin Siebers, "Disability as Masquerade," *Literature and Medicine* 23, no. 1 (2004), https://doi.org/10.1353/lm.2004.0010.

7. Physician note from November 3, 1999.

8. Physician note from February 9, 2000.

9. James C. Cunningham and Lynn M. Taussig, *An Introduction to Cystic Fibrosis for Patients and Families*, 3rd ed. (Cystic Fibrosis Foundation), 7.

10. Physician note from February 9, 2000.

11. D. H. Andersen and R. G. Hodges, "Celiac Syndrome: V. Genetics of Cystic Fibrosis of the Pancreas, with a Consideration of Etiology," *American Journal of Diseases of Children* 72 (1946), https://doi.org/10.1001/archpedi.1946.02020300069004.

12. Physician note from May 8, 2001.

13. Anne Kerr, "(Re)Constructing Genetic Disease: The Clinical Continuum between Cystic Fibrosis and Male Infertility," *Social Studies of Science* 30, no. 6 (2000): 856, https://www.jstor.org/stable/285789.

14. Rosenberg, "Tyranny of Diagnosis," 243.

15. Instead of "atypical CF," the current terms used to describe people who do not meet the diagnostic criteria for CF include CFTR-related metabolic syndrome (CRMS)/cystic fibrosis screen positive, inconclusive diagnosis (CFSPID), and CFTR-related disorder (CFTR-RD). For a discussion of "milder forms" of CF, see A. Kerr, "Understanding Genetic Disease in a Socio-Historical Context: A Case Study of Cystic Fibrosis," *Sociology of Health & Illness* 27, no. 7 (2005), https://doi.org/10.1111/j.1467-9566.2005.00462.x.

16. For example, I have had several extended bouts with *Clostridium difficile* (now reclassified as *Clostridioides difficile*) infection in the absence of typical risk factors.

17. This statement is not meant to minimize or dismiss the legitimacy of psychiatric diseases, but if a psychiatric diagnosis is given when the disease is not psychiatric in nature, then significant harm can result, including the lack of access to appropriate treatment.

18. Renée C. Fox, "The Evolution of Medical Uncertainty," *Milbank Memorial Fund Quarterly. Health and Society* 58, no. 1 (1980), https://www.ncbi.nlm.nih.gov/pubmed/6903782; S. Timmermans and M. Buchbinder, "Patients-in-Waiting: Living Between Sickness and Health in the Genomics Era," *Journal of Health and Social Behavior* 51, no. 4 (2010), https://doi.org/10.1177/0022146510386794; P. K. Han et al., "Varieties of Uncertainty in Health Care: A Conceptual Taxonomy," *Medical Decision Making* 31, no. 6 (2011), https://doi.org/10.1177/0272989X11393976; V. Bhise et al., "Defining and Measuring Diagnostic Uncertainty in Medicine: A Systematic Review," *Journal of General Internal Medicine* 33, no. 1 (2018), https://doi.org/10.1007/s11606-017-4164-1; A. Jutel, "Uncertainty and the Inconvenient Facts of Diagnosis," *Endeavour* 45, no. 1–2 (2021), https://doi.org/10.1016/j.endeavour.2021.100764.

19. Timmermans and Buchbinder, "Patients-in-Waiting," 417; T Stivers and S. Timmermans, "Negotiating the Diagnostic Uncertainty of Genomic Test Results," *Social Psychology Quarterly* 79, no. 3 (2016), https://doi.org/10.1177/01902725166587; Stefan Timmermans et al., "Narrating Uncertainty: Variants of Un-

certain Significance (VUS) in Clinical Exome Sequencing," *BioSocieties* 12, no. 3 (2017), https://doi.org/10.1057/s41292-016-0020-5.

20. Timmermans and Buchbinder, "Patients-in-Waiting," 417.

21. Timmermans and Buchbinder, "Patients-in-Waiting,"; Rosenberg, "Tyranny of Diagnosis"; Robert Aronowitz, *Risky Medicine: Our Quest to Cure Fear and Uncertainty* (University of Chicago Press, 2015); Jeremy A. Greene, *Prescribing by Numbers: Drugs and the Definition of Disease* (Johns Hopkins University Press, 2007).

22. On textbook science versus paradigm-challenging science, see Thomas S. Kuhn, *The Structure of Scientific Revolutions* (University of Chicago Press, 1962). For textbook examples, see Bruce Alberts et al., *Essential Cell Biology*, 4th ed. (Garland Science Taylor & Francis Group, 2014), 677; Lisa A. Urry et al., *Campbell Biology*, 11th ed. (Pearson, 2017), 286. On the history of CF, see Keith Wailoo and Stephen Pemberton, *The Troubled Dream of Genetic Medicine: Ethnicity and Innovation in Tay-Sachs, Cystic Fibrosis, and Sickle Cell Disease* (Johns Hopkins University Press, 2006); Kerr, "(Re)Constructing Genetic Disease"; Kerr, "Understanding Genetic Disease"; A. M. Hedgecoe, "Expansion and Uncertainty: Cystic Fibrosis, Classification and Genetics," *Sociology of Health & Illness* 25, no. 1 (2003), https://doi.org/10.1111/1467-9566.t01-2-00324; Stephen Pemberton, "Cystic Fibrosis," in *Encyclopedia of American Disability History*, ed. Susan Burch (Facts on File, 2009); Susan M. Lindee and Rebecca Ann Mueller, "Is Cystic Fibrosis Genetic Medicine's Canary?," *Perspectives in Biology and Medicine* 54, no. 3 (2011), https://doi.org/10.1353/pbm.2011.0035; Rachel Grob, *Testing Baby: The Transformation of Newborn Screening, Parenting, and Policy Making* (Rutgers University Press, 2011); Joëlle Vailly, *The Birth of a Genetics Policy: Social Issues of Newborn Screening* (Ashgate, 2013); Michelle LaBonte, "Addressing Uncertainty: The Emergence of the CRMS/CFSPID Diagnostic Category Following Newborn Screening for Cystic Fibrosis," *OBM Genetics* 5, no. 3 (2021), https://doi.org/10.21926/obm.genet.2103139; Michelle LaBonte, "Diagnostic Uncertainty, Microbes, and the Isolation of People with Cystic Fibrosis," *Journal of the History of Medicine and Allied Sciences* 72, no. 3 (2022), https://doi.org/10.1093/jhmas/jrab056; Rebecca Mueller, "The Impact of Transmissible Microbes: How the Cystic Fibrosis Community Mobilized Against Cepacia," *Perspectives in Biology and Medicine* 66, no. 1 (2023), https://doi.org/10.1353/pbm.2023.0005; Rebecca Mueller, "Prognostic Imagination: Genetic Counseling Amidst Therapeutic Innovation and Evolving Futures," *Journal of Genetic Counseling* 32, no. 4 (2023), https://doi.org/10.1002/jgc4.1660; Gregory Radick, *Disputed Inheritance: The Battle over Mendel and the Future of Biology* (University of Chicago Press, 2022), 352; P. M. Farrell et al., "Cystic Fibrosis Diagnostic Challenges over 4 Decades: Historical Perspectives and Lessons Learned," *Journal of Pediatrics* 181S (2017), https://doi.org/10.1016/j.jpeds.2016.09.067; Bijal P. Trivedi, *Breath from Salt: A Deadly Genetic Disease, a New Era in Science, and the Patients and Families Who Changed Medicine Forever* (BenBella Books, Inc., 2020); James Littlewood, A *History of Cystic Fibrosis,* https://cysticfibrosis.online/.

23. Vivian Tappan, "The History of Cystic Fibrosis of the Pancreas," 17, typescript prepared for *Parade*, January 3, 1957, located in Some Lay Addresses on Cystic Fibrosis by Vivian Tappan, M.D., Yale University School of Medicine, 1956–1966, Yale University.

24. Cystic Fibrosis Foundation 2024 Patient Registry Highlights, https://www.cff.org/sites/default/files/2025-05/2024-Patient-Registry-Highlights-Report.pdf. The median age of survival is for those who are eligible for CFTR modulators. Susan Lindee, "Before the Gene: Leroy Matthews and the Cleveland Comprehensive Treatment Program for Cystic Fibrosis, 1957–1961," paper presented at the History of Science Society, 2011.

25. As a group of medical professionals noted in 2017, "once the classic example of a single-gene, autosomal recessive, life-shortening condition, CF and related disorders are now known to form a phenotypic spectrum with genetic etiology rooted in more than 2000 known variants of the cystic fibrosis transmembrane conductance regulator (*CFTR*) gene." See Karen S. Raraigh et al., "Diagnosis and Treatment of Cystic Fibrosis: A (Not-So) Simple Recessive Condition," *Current Genetic Medicine Reports* 5, no. 2 (2017), https://doi.org/10.1007/s40142-017-0122-9, 91; H. Levy and P. M. Farrell, "New Challenges in the Diagnosis and Management of Cystic Fibrosis," *Journal of Pediatrics* 166, no. 6 (2015), https://doi.org/10.1016/j.jpeds.2015.03.042; Peadar G. Noone and Michael R. Knowles, "'CFTR-Opathies': Disease Phenotypes Associated with Cystic Fibrosis Transmembrane Regulator Gene Mutations," *Respiratory Research* 2, no. 6 (2001), https://doi.org/10.1186/rr82. As Anne Kerr notes, "an alternative discourse of CF as a collection of related disorders, as opposed to a single disease entity, also ran alongside these discussions of classic disease, mild variants and heterozygosity." Kerr, "Understanding Genetic Disease," 885. We might apply Mol's concept of the body multiple to the issue of diagnostic uncertainty in CF, such that the varied CF ontologies enacted by different actors all "hang together" not as one distinct object, but as a set of sometimes coordinating and sometimes contradicting objects. Annemarie Mol, *The Body Multiple: Ontology in Medical Practice* (Duke University Press, 2002), 83.

26. Draft Summary of the First Workshop of the Joint Working Group on the Ethical, Legal and Social Issues Related to Mapping and Sequencing the Human Genome, Williamsburg, Virginia, February 5–6, 1990, HGP-DO-005, NHGRI Human Genome Project (HGP) Archive.

27. Cystic Fibrosis Foundation, "Health Equity in Cystic Fibrosis," January 25, 2024, https://www.youtube.com/watch?v=8mAhxmtvM2M; Wright Cystic Fibrosis Screening Tool, ©2021 by Michele Wright, Ph.D., and Terry Wright, https://noaacf.org/the-wright-cystic-fibrosis-screening-tool/.

28. Cystic Fibrosis Foundation, "About Cystic Fibrosis," https://www.cff.org/intro-cf/about-cystic-fibrosis.

29. Charles E. Rosenberg, "Introduction: Framing Disease: Illness, Society, and History," in *Framing Disease: Studies in Cultural History*, ed. Charles E. Rosenberg and Janet Lynne Golden (Rutgers University Press, 1992), xiii.

30. Stivers and Timmermans, "Uncertainty of Genomic Test Results."

31. Dorothy H. Andersen, "Cystic Fibrosis of the Pancreas and Its Relation to Celiac Disease: A Clinical and Pathologic Study," *American Journal of Diseases of Children* 56, no. 2 (1938), https://doi.org/10.1001/archpedi.1938.01980140114013. Andersen described the disease as "cystic fibrosis of the pancreas," and descriptions consistent with CF go back several centuries or more.

32. For a discussion of early definitions of CF, see Wailoo and Pemberton, *Troubled Dream of Genetic Medicine*; Kerr, "Understanding Genetic Disease."

33. Rosenberg, "Tyranny of Diagnosis"; Michel Foucault, *The Birth of the Clinic: An Archaeology of Medical Perception*, (Pantheon Books, 1973); Erwin H. Ackerknecht, *Medicine at the Paris Hospital, 1794–1848* (Johns Hopkins Press, 1967); Stanley Joel Reiser, *Medicine and the Reign of Technology* (Cambridge University Press, 1978), 8; Jacalyn Duffin, *Lovers and Livers: Disease Concepts in History* (University of Toronto Press, 2005); Margaret M. Lock, *The Alzheimer Conundrum: Entanglements of Dementia and Aging* (Princeton University Press, 2013); Peter Keating and Alberto Cambrosio, *Biomedical Platforms: Realigning the Normal and the Pathological in Late-Twentieth-Century Medicine* (MIT Press, 2003); Alvan Feinstein, *Clinical Judgment* (Robert E. Kreiger, 1985; original edition 1967).

34. Andersen, "Cystic Fibrosis of the Pancreas."

35. John Harley Warner, *The Therapeutic Perspective: Medical Practice, Knowledge, and Identity in America, 1820–1885* (Harvard University Press, 1986); Rosenberg, "Tyranny of Diagnosis." As Jacalyn Duffin notes, "some diseases are still classified and identified in this symptom-based way, especially those of unknown cause." Duffin, *Lovers and Livers*, 9.

36. Rosenberg, "Tyranny of Diagnosis," 242; Georges Canguilhem, *The Normal and the Pathological* (Zone Books, 1989).

37. Rosenberg, "Tyranny of Diagnosis," 243.

38. A. M. Brandt and M. Gardner, "Antagonism and Accommodation: Interpreting the Relationship Between Public Health and Medicine in the United States During the 20th Century," *American Journal of Public Health* 90, no. 5 (2000), https://doi.org/10.2105/ajph.90.5.707; Rosenberg, "Tyranny of Diagnosis," 242; Andrew Cunningham, "Transforming Plague: The Laboratory and the Identity of Infectious Disease," in *The Laboratory Revolution in Medicine*, ed. Andrew Cunningham and Perry Williams (Cambridge University Press, 2002), 209. The shift to viewing diseases as specific entities was not absolute, as Robert Aronowitz points out. Robert A. Aronowitz, *Making Sense of Illness: Science, Society, and Disease* (Cambridge University Press, 1998), 8–9.

39. Rosenberg, "Tyranny of Diagnosis"; Reiser, *Medicine and the Reign of Technology*; Joel D. Howell, *Technology in the Hospital: Transforming Patient Care in the Early Twentieth Century* (Johns Hopkins University Press, 1995); H. Evans, "Losing Touch: The Controversy over the Introduction of Blood Pressure Instruments into Medicine," *Technology and Culture* 34, no. 4 (1993), https://doi

.org/10.2307/3106415; Edward A. Dominguez et al., "Adoption of Thermometry into Clinical Practice in the United States," *Clinical Infectious Diseases* 9, no. 6 (1987), https://doi.org/10.1093/clinids/9.6.1193; Jacalyn Duffin, *To See with a Better Eye: A Life of R. T. H. Laennec*, (Princeton University Press, 2014).

40. Rosenberg, "Tyranny of Diagnosis." Rosenberg also points to the EKG and the EEG at this time period. For a discussion of the use of trained judgment for the interpretation of electroencephalograms, and the notion that "accuracy should not be sacrificed to objectivity," see Lorraine Daston and Peter Galison, *Objectivity* (Zone Books, Distributed by MIT Press, 2007), 321–329. For a history of the electrocardiogram, see Robert G. Frank Jr., "The Telltale Heart: Physiological Instruments, Graphic Methods, and Clinical Hopes 1854–1914," in *The Investigative Enterprise: Experimental Physiology in Nineteenth-Century Medicine*, ed. William Coleman and Frederic L. Holmes (University of California Press, 1988). For a discussion of the social context in which medical technologies were introduced and conceived by physicians, patients, and hospital administrators, see Howell, *Technology in the Hospital*; Nancy Tomes, *Remaking the American Patient: How Madison Avenue and Modern Medicine Turned Patients into Consumers* (University of North Carolina Press, 2016); Bettyann Kevles, *Naked to the Bone: Medical Imaging in the Twentieth Century* (Rutgers University Press, 1997).

41. Brandt and Gardner, "Antagonism and Accommodation," 711; Rosenberg, "Tyranny of Diagnosis," 247.

42. Andersen, "Cystic Fibrosis of the Pancreas"; Dorothy H. Andersen, "Pancreatic Enzymes in the Duodenal Juice in the Celiac Syndrome," *American Journal of Diseases of Children* 63, no. 4 (1942), https://doi.org/10.1001/archpedi.1942.02010040011001.

43. Adele E. Clarke et al., "Biomedicalization: Technoscientific Transformations of Health, Illness, and U.S. Biomedicine," *American Sociological Review* 68, no. 2 (2003): 168, https://doi.org/10.2307/1519765.

44. B. Kerem et al., "Identification of the Cystic Fibrosis Gene: Genetic Analysis," *Science* 245, no. 4922 (1989), https://doi.org/10.1126/science.2570460; J. R. Riordan et al., "Identification of the Cystic Fibrosis Gene: Cloning and Characterization of Complementary DNA," *Science* 245, no. 4299 (1989), https://doi.org/10.1126/science.2475911; J. M. Rommens et al., "Identification of the Cystic Fibrosis Gene: Chromosome Walking and Jumping," *Science* 245, no. 4922 (1989), https://doi.org/10.1126/science.2772657; D. E. Koshland Jr., "The Cystic Fibrosis Gene Story," *Science* 245, no. 4922 (1989), https://doi.org/10.1126/science.245.4922.1029. Even with the availability of genetic testing for CF, the "sweat test" for analyzing chloride levels remains a key diagnostic.

45. Dorothy Nelkin and Laurence R. Tancredi, *Dangerous Diagnostics: The Social Power of Biological Information* (University of Chicago Press, 1994), 22. For more on computer-aided diagnostics, see Andrew S. Lea, *Digitizing Diagnosis: Medicine, Minds, and Machines in Twentieth-Century America* (Johns Hopkins

University Press, 2023); Jeremy A. Greene and Andrew S. Lea, "Digital Futures Past—the Long Arc of Big Data in Medicine," *New England Journal of Medicine* 381, no. 5 (2019), https://doi.org/10.1056/NEJMms1817674.

46. For a discussion of meconium ileus as an indicator of possible CF on prenatal ultrasound, see Meghana Sathe and Roderick Houwen, "Meconium Ileus in Cystic Fibrosis," *Journal of Cystic Fibrosis* 16, suppl. 2 (2017), https://doi.org/10.1016/j.jcf.2017.06.007. For a discussion of lung changes on X-ray prompting diagnostic testing for CF, see Dorothy E. Roberts, *Fatal Invention: How Science, Politics, and Big Business Re-Create Race in the Twenty-First Century* (New Press, 2011); Richard S. Garcia, "The Misuse of Race in Medical Diagnosis," *Journal of Children's Health* 1, no. 2 (2003).

47. Reiser, *Medicine and the Reign of Technology*, 162. This trust in the objectivity and decisiveness of diagnostic technology went beyond doctors, as "many patients believed that when physicians applied elaborate diagnostic procedures, an answer to their problems was almost certain," 163.

48. Reiser, *Medicine and the Reign of Technology*; Keating and Cambrosio, *Biomedical Platforms*, 43–44; Howell, *Technology in the Hospital.*

49. Rosenberg, "Tyranny of Diagnosis," 244.

50. Keith Wailoo, *Drawing Blood: Technology and Disease Identity in Twentieth-Century America* (Johns Hopkins University Press, 1997); Keating and Cambrosio, *Biomedical Platforms*. According to Keating and Cambrosio, the ability to determine the CD4 count shifted the diagnostic criteria for AIDS away from symptoms.

51. Reiser, *Medicine and the Reign of Technology*, 230; Howell, *Technology in the Hospital*; N. D. Jewson, "The Disappearance of the Sick-Man from Medical Cosmology, 1770–1870," *Sociology* 10, no. 2 (1976), https://doi.org/10.1177/003803857601000202; P. Underwood, "On Certainty and Uncertainty," *Social Science & Medicine* 23, no. 6 (1986), https://doi.org/10.1016/0277-9536(86)90158-9.

52. Aronowitz, *Risky Medicine*; Greene, *Prescribing by Numbers*; Rosenberg, "Tyranny of Diagnosis"; Nelkin and Tancredi, *Dangerous Diagnostics*. Joseph Dumit's ethnographic work also highlights the role of thresholds and risk reduction in disease definition. Joseph Dumit, *Drugs for Life: How Pharmaceutical Companies Define Our Health* (Duke University Press, 2012).

53. Rosenberg, "Tyranny of Diagnosis," 254; Evans, "Introduction of Blood Pressure Instruments"; Greene, *Prescribing by Numbers*.

54. Duffin, *Lovers and Livers*, 19.

55. Duffin, *Lovers and Livers*, 19.

56. Reflecting on this issue, Duffin notes that "lacking a material proof of bodily change, the patient's sensations appear to be less serious, and, sometimes, less credible, as if they had been fabricated . . . in other words, now it is possible to feel very sick and be denied the dignity of a diagnosis." Duffin, *Lovers and Livers*, 21; L. Stone, "Schrödinger's Disease and the Ethics of (Non)Diagnosis: The Problem of Medically Unexplained Symptoms in Contemporary Medical Practice," *American*

Journal of Bioethics 18, no. 5 (2018): 18, https://doi.org/10.1080/15265161.2018.1445318.

57. For reflections on advantages of diagnostic uncertainty, see Stefan Timmermans and Mara Buchbinder, *Saving Babies?: The Consequences of Newborn Genetic Screening* (University of Chicago Press, 2013), 15; I. Whitmarsh et al., "A Place for Genetic Uncertainty: Parents Valuing an Unknown in the Meaning of Disease," *Social Science & Medicine* 65, no. 6 (2007), https://doi.org/10.1016/j.socscimed.2007.04.034; Timmermans et al., "Narrating Uncertainty," 441; A. J. Hogan, "Making the Most of Uncertainty: Treasuring Exceptions in Prenatal Diagnosis," *Studies in History and Philosophy of Science Part C: Studies in History and Philosophy of Biological and Biomedical Sciences* 57 (2016), https://doi.org/10.1016/j.shpsc.2016.02.020; Janneke M. L. Kuiper et al., "The Social Shaping of a Diagnosis in Next Generation Sequencing," *New Genetics and Society* 40, no. 4 (2021): 431, https://doi.org/10.1080/14636778.2020.1853514.

58. Renée C. Fox, "Training for Uncertainty," in *The Student-Physician: Introductory Studies in the Sociology of Medical Education*, ed. Robert K. Merton, George G. Reader, and Patricia L. Kendall (Harvard University Press, 1957). Fox was influenced by the work of Talcott Parsons. Talcott Parsons, *The Social System* (Free Press, 1951), 449.

59. Fox, "Training for Uncertainty"; Fox, "The Evolution of Medical Uncertainty."

60. Fox, "Training for Uncertainty," 213.

61. Fox, "Training for Uncertainty," 221. Italics in original.

62. Renée C. Fox, "Training for Uncertainty in the Pre-Clinical Years of Medical School," *Columbia University Pre-Med: The National Pre-Medical Journal* 1, no. 1 (Autumn 1961). Journal located in box 1, Production Files: Volume I, Number I, Pre-Med journal records, 1960–1970, CP2 P91, University Archives, Rare Book & Manuscript Library, Columbia University Libraries. Renee C. Fox, "Training for Uncertainty in the Clinical Years of Medical School," *Pre-Med: A National Pre-Medical Journal* 1, no. 2 (Winter 1961). Journal located in box 6, folder Training for Uncertainty, Renee C. Fox Papers, 1912–2018 (inclusive), H MS c569, Countway Library of Medicine, Center for the History of Medicine, Harvard Medical School. Renee C. Fox, "Training for Uncertainty in the Pre-Clinical Years of Medical School," *Journal of the Pre-Medical Society Columbia University* (Spring 1960). Journal located in box 6, folder Training for Uncertainty, Renee C. Fox Papers, 1912–2018 (inclusive), H MS c569, Countway Library of Medicine, Center for the History of Medicine, Harvard Medical School. "Med Student Is Object of New Magazine," *Daily News*, October 8, 1961.

63. Fox, "Training for Uncertainty"; Han et al., "Varieties of Uncertainty in Health Care," 828; Fox, "The Evolution of Medical Uncertainty." For accounts by physicians on the importance of recognizing and properly addressing diagnostic uncertainty in medicine, see D. B. Reuben, "Learning Diagnostic Restraint," *New England Journal of Medicine* 310, no. 9 (1984), https://doi.org/10.1056/NEJM198403013100911; L. Rosenbaum, "Living Unlabeled—Diagnosis and Disorder," *New*

England Journal of Medicine 359, no. 16 (2008), https://doi.org/10.1056/NEJMp0804984; A. L. Simpkin and R. M. Schwartzstein, "Tolerating Uncertainty—the Next Medical Revolution?," *New England Journal of Medicine* 375, no. 18 (2016), https://doi.org/10.1056/NEJMp1606402. For more on "natural kinds" and kind-making, see Ian Hacking, *The Social Construction of What?* (Harvard University Press, 1999); Geoffrey C. Bowker and Susan Leigh Star, *Sorting Things Out: Classification and Its Consequences* (MIT Press, 1999).

64. Wailoo, *Drawing Blood*; Charles E. Rosenberg, *Our Present Complaint: American Medicine, Then and Now* (Johns Hopkins University Press, 2007); C. Feudtner, "Minds the Dead Have Ravished—Shell Shock, History, and the Ecology of Disease-Systems," *History of Science* 31, no. 94 (1993): 406, https://doi.org/10.1177/007327539303100402; Aronowitz, *Making Sense of Illness*; Keating and Cambrosio, *Biomedical Platforms*.

65. Wailoo, *Drawing Blood*; Stephen Pemberton, *The Bleeding Disease: Hemophilia and the Unintended Consequences of Medical Progress* (Johns Hopkins University Press, 2011), 99. Charles Rosenberg also points out the range of factors that can influence disease definition, such as insurance codes, hospital layout, and response to therapeutics. Rosenberg, *Our Present Complaint*.

66. Kuiper et al., "The Social Shaping of a Diagnosis," 429; Bowker and Star, *Sorting Things Out*; Robert A. Aronowitz, "When Do Symptoms Become a Disease?," *Annals of Internal Medicine* 134, no. 9, part 2 (2001), https://doi.org/10.7326/0003-4819-134-9_Part_2-200105011-00002; Annemarie Jutel, *Putting a Name to It: Diagnosis in Contemporary Society* (Johns Hopkins University Press, 2011); Lara Keuck, "Diagnosing Alzheimer's Disease in Kraepelin's Clinic, 1909–1912," *History of the Human Sciences* 31, no. 2 (2018), https://doi.org/10.1177/0952695118758879.

67. Barton Childs, *Genetic Medicine: A Logic of Disease* (Johns Hopkins University Press, 1999), 46.

68. Kerr, "Understanding Genetic Disease," 890; Hedgecoe, "Expansion and Uncertainty"; Wailoo and Pemberton, *Troubled Dream of Genetic Medicine*; Grob, *Testing Baby*; Vailly, *Birth of a Genetics Policy*; Anne Kerr, *Genetics and Society: A Sociology of Disease* (Routledge, 2004), chapter 3.

69. Renée C. Fox, "Chapter 13: Medical Uncertainty Revisited," in *Gender, Health, and Healing: The Public/Private Divide*, ed. Gill Bendelow et al. (Routledge, 2001); Stefan Timmermans and Marc Berg, *The Gold Standard: The Challenge of Evidence-Based Medicine and Standardization in Health Care* (Temple University Press, 2003); Han et al., "Varieties of Uncertainty in Health Care"; Hogan, "Making the Most of Uncertainty"; Bhise et al., "Defining and Measuring Diagnostic Uncertainty"; N. Bochatay and N. M. Bajwa, "Learning to Manage Uncertainty: Supervision, Trust and Autonomy in Residency Training," *Sociology of Health & Illness* 42, suppl. 1 (2020), https://doi.org/10.1111/1467-9566.13070.

70. D. Light Jr., "Uncertainty and Control in Professional Training," *Journal of Health and Social Behavior* 20, no. 4 (1979): 310–12, https://www.ncbi.nlm.nih.gov/pubmed/541485; Martha S. Gerrity et al., "Uncertainty and Professional Work:

Perceptions of Physicians in Clinical Practice," *American Journal of Sociology* 97, no. 4 (1992), https://doi.org/10.1086/229860.

71. P. Atkinson, "Training for Certainty," *Social Science & Medicine* 19, no. 9 (1984): 954, https://doi.org/10.1016/0277-9536(84)90324-1; Donald W Light, "Letter to the Editor," *Social Science & Medicine* 21, no. 9 (1985): 1051; Underwood, "On Certainty and Uncertainty."

72. Timmermans and Buchbinder, *Saving Babies?*, 13; L. Diamond-Brown, "The Doctor-Patient Relationship as a Toolkit for Uncertain Clinical Decisions," *Social Science & Medicine* 159 (2016): 109, https://doi.org/10.1016/j.socscimed.2016.05.002; Renée C. Fox, *Experiment Perilous: Physicians and Patients Facing the Unknown* (Routledge, 2019 [1959]), 36; Fox, "Chapter 13: Medical Uncertainty Revisited," 250.

73. Wailoo, *Drawing Blood*, 2.

74. Nelkin and Tancredi, *Dangerous Diagnostics*, 36.

75. Ludwik Fleck, *Genesis and Development of a Scientific Fact* (University of Chicago Press, 1979); Ilana Löwy, "Testing for a Sexually Transmissible Disease, 1907–1970: The History of the Wassermann Reaction," in *AIDS and Contemporary History*, ed. Virginia Berridge and Philip Strong (Cambridge University Press, 1993); K. Kameda et al., "Imperfect Diagnosis: The Truncated Legacies of Zika Testing," *Social Studies of Science* 51, no. 5 (2021), https://doi.org/10.1177/03063127211035492.

76. Reiser, *Medicine and the Reign of Technology*. According to the abstract of the discussion that followed, Philadelphia physician E. R. Long noted that his mentor, H. Gideon Wells, had once told him that "the diagnosis of tumors is a matter of taste." Carl C. Birkelo et al., "Tuberculosis Case Finding: A Comparison of the Effectiveness of Various Roentgenographic and Photofluorographic Methods," *JAMA* 133, no. 6 (1947): 366, https://doi.org/10.1001/jama.1947.02880060001001.

77. Michelle Murphy, *Sick Building Syndrome and the Problem of Uncertainty: Environmental Politics, Technoscience, and Women Workers* (Duke University Press, 2006).

78. Nelkin and Tancredi, *Dangerous Diagnostics*, 46; Amos Tversky and Daniel Kahneman, "Judgment Under Uncertainty: Heuristics and Biases: Biases in Judgments Reveal Some Heuristics of Thinking Under Uncertainty," *Science* 185, no. 4157 (1974), https://doi.org/10.1126/science.185.4157.1124. Also related to the interpretation of diagnostic tests, Eden Medina and Ilan Sandberg Wiener's study of the misidentification of remains from disappeared individuals during the Chilean dictatorship demonstrates how changes in technology (from initial craniofacial matching to subsequent DNA analysis) can lead to troubling uncertainty about the identity of human remains. Eden Medina and Ilan Sandberg Wiener, "Science and Harm in Human Rights Cases: Preventing the Revictimization of Families of the Disappeared," *Yale Law Review* 125 (2016), http://www.yalelawjournal.org/forum/science-and-harm-in-human-rights-cases; Keating and Cambrosio, *Biomedical Platforms*, 9.

79. Sheila Rothman, *Living in the Shadow of Death: Tuberculosis and the Social Experience of Illness in American History* (Johns Hopkins University Press, 1995); Evelynn Maxine Hammonds, *Childhood's Deadly Scourge: The Campaign to Control Diphtheria in New York City, 1880–1930* (Johns Hopkins University Press, 1999); Daniel J. Wilson, *Living with Polio: The Epidemic and Its Survivors* (University of Chicago Press, 2005).

80. "Covid-19, Cold, Allergies and the Flu: What Are the Differences?," https://www.mayoclinic.org/diseases-conditions/coronavirus/in-depth/covid-19-cold-flu-and-allergies-differences/art-20503981; "Is It Flu, Covid-19, Allergies, or a Cold?," *NIH News in Health*, January 2022, https://newsinhealth.nih.gov/sites/nihNIH/files/2022/January/NIHNiHJan2022.pdf.

81. See Chapter 1 of *Challenging Diagnosis*.

82. A. R. Feinstein, "Boolean Algebra and Clinical Taxonomy. I. Analytic Synthesis of the General Spectrum of a Human Disease," *New England Journal of Medicine* 269 (1963), https://doi.org/10.1056/NEJM196310312691801; Feinstein, *Clinical Judgment*. For more on what prompts someone to seek medical attention, see Alvan R. Feinstein, "Clinical Epidemiology: II. The Identification of Rates of Disease," *Annals of Internal Medicine* 69, no. 5 (1968), https://doi.org/10.7326/0003-4819-69-5-1037. For a discussion of how the introduction of new diagnostic technologies can influence survival rates, see Alvan R. Feinstein et al., "The Will Rogers Phenomenon: Stage Migration and New Diagnostic Techniques as a Source of Misleading Statistics for Survival in Cancer," *New England Journal of Medicine* 312, no. 25 (1985), https://doi.org/10.1056/NEJM198506203122504.

83. Feinstein, *Clinical Judgment*, 216–217; Mol, *The Body Multiple*; Duffin, *Lovers and Livers*.

84. Stivers and Timmermans, "Uncertainty of Genomic Test Results," 201.

85. Aronowitz, *Unnatural History*, 70; Rosenberg, "Introduction: Framing Disease," xiii. As Rosenberg explains, diagnosis comes with social legitimacy, and as such "even a dangerous, but familiar and understandable, disease can be emotionally more manageable than a mysterious and unpredictable affliction," xvii.

86. Sandra G. Boodman, "For Decades, She Was Told She Was 'Just Anxious.' A Midair Incident Uncovered the Truth," *Washington Post*, January 12, 2019, https://www.washingtonpost.com/national/health-science/for-decades-she-was-told-she-was-just-anxious-a-midair-incident-uncovered-the-truth/2019/01/11/33329f90-f5a3-11e8-bc79-68604ed88993_story.html.

87. Boodman, "Just Anxious." Devlin's experience calls to mind Charles Rosenberg's description of diagnosis as a "ritual of disclosure: a curtain is pulled aside, and uncertainty is replaced—for better or worse—by a structured narrative." Rosenberg, "Tyranny of Diagnosis," 255. In Devlin's case, the replacement of uncertainty with a diagnosis was "for better," as she finally had an explanation that came with social legitimacy, and she was able to benefit from therapeutic interventions. For an account of diagnostic uncertainty and contested illness, see Ross Gregory Douthat, *The Deep Places: A Memoir of Illness and Discovery*, (Convergent, 2021).

88. C. G. K. Atkins, "Why Bioethics Should Pay Attention to Patients Who Suffer Medically Unexplained (Physical) Symptoms—a Discussion of Uncertainty, Suffering, and Risk," *American Journal of Bioethics* 18, no. 5 (2018), https://doi.org/10.1080/15265161.2018.1445319; D. O'Leary, "Why Bioethics Should Be Concerned with Medically Unexplained Symptoms," *American Journal of Bioethics* 18, no. 5 (2018), https://doi.org/10.1080/15265161.2018.1445312; M. H. Arnold and I. Kerridge, "Rejecting Reality and Substituting One's Own: Why Bioethics Should Be Concerned with Medically Unexplained Symptoms," *American Journal of Bioethics* 18, no. 5 (2018): 27, https://doi.org/10.1080/15265161.2018.1445315; T. E. Eriksen et al., "At the Borders of Medical Reasoning: Aetiological and Ontological Challenges of Medically Unexplained Symptoms," *Philosophy, Ethics, and Humanities in Medicine* 8 (2013), https://doi.org/10.1186/1747-5341-8-11; M. J. Redinger et al., "Conversion Disorder Diagnosis and Medically Unexplained Symptoms," *American Journal of Bioethics* 18, no. 5 (2018): 32, https://doi.org/10.1080/15265161.2018.1445317; A. K. Swartz, "A Feminist Bioethics Approach to Diagnostic Uncertainty," *American Journal of Bioethics* 18, no. 5 (2018), https://doi.org/10.1080/15265161.2018.1447046; A. Schwab, "Calibrating Confident Judgments About Medically Unexplained Symptoms," *American Journal of Bioethics* 18, no. 5 (2018): 37, https://doi.org/10.1080/15265161.2018.1445313; Stone, "Schrödinger's Disease and the Ethics of (Non)Diagnosis"; Maria R. Dahm and Carmel Crock, "Understanding and Communicating Uncertainty in Achieving Diagnostic Excellence," *JAMA* 327, no. 12 (2022), https://doi.org/10.1001/jama.2022.2141; Monica Greco, "Pragmatics of Explanation: Creative Accountability in the Care of 'Medically Unexplained Symptoms,'" *Sociological Review* 65, no. 2, suppl. (2017), https://doi.org/10.1177/0081176917710425.

89. Rosenberg, *Our Present Complaint*; Kristin Kay Barker, *The Fibromyalgia Story: Medical Authority and Women's Worlds of Pain* (Temple University Press, 2005); Murphy, *Sick Building Syndrome*; H. J. Roberts, *Difficult Diagnosis: A Guide to the Interpretation of Obscure Illness* (Saunders, 1958), 2.

90. Katie K., "Finding Truth and Facing It: My Late CF Diagnosis," *Cystic Fibrosis Foundation CF Community Blog*, October 26, 2016, https://www.cff.org/CF-Community-Blog/Posts/2016/Finding-Truth-and-Facing-It-My-Late-CF-Diagnosis/.

91. Katie K., "Finding Truth and Facing It."

92. P. M. Farrell et al., "Guidelines for Diagnosis of Cystic Fibrosis in Newborns Through Older Adults: Cystic Fibrosis Foundation Consensus Report," *Journal of Pediatrics* 153, no. 2 (2008), https://doi.org/10.1016/j.jpeds.2008.05.005.

93. Katie K., "Finding Truth and Facing It."

94. Other early cases of dismissal by physicians can be seen as well. For example, one child described in the 1950s was initially thought to have "no organic disease" and the health concerns were attributed to "maternal anxiety," yet the child was later diagnosed with cystic fibrosis. See H. Shwachman et al., "Mucovisci-

dosis," *Advances in Pediatrics* 7 (1955): 257, https://www.ncbi.nlm.nih.gov/pubmed/14349778.

95. Maryanne O'Hara, oral history interview with the author, May 11, 2022; Maryanne O'Hara *Little Matches: A Memoir of Grief and Light* (HarperOne, 2021).

96. Lucy Lester, oral history interview with the author, June 2, 2021.

97. Lester, interview.

98. Lester, interview.

99. Reiser, *Medicine and the Reign of Technology*; Howell, *Technology in the Hospital*; Wailoo, *Drawing Blood*; Rosenberg, "Tyranny of Diagnosis"; Keating and Cambrosio, *Biomedical Platforms*; M. Susan Lindee, *Moments of Truth in Genetic Medicine* (Johns Hopkins University Press, 2005); Greene, *Prescribing by Numbers*; Roberts, *Fatal Invention*; Lundy Braun, *Breathing Race into the Machine: The Surprising Career of the Spirometer from Plantation to Genetics* (University of Minnesota Press, 2014); Aronowitz, *Risky Medicine*; Ilana Löwy, *Tangled Diagnoses: Prenatal Testing, Women, and Risk* (The University of Chicago Press, 2018); Arleen Tuchman, *Diabetes: A History of Race and Disease* (Yale University Press, 2020); Lea, *Digitizing Diagnosis*.

100. J. Barben, "First Description of Cystic Fibrosis," *Journal of Cystic Fibrosis* 20, no. 1 (2021), https://doi.org/10.1016/j.jcf.2020.08.008.

101. Andersen, "Cystic Fibrosis of the Pancreas," 344 (emphasis mine).

102. "The National Association of African Americans with Cystic Fibrosis: Terry Wright's CF Story," 2021, https://noaacf.org/terry-wrights-cf-story/.

103. Roberts, *Fatal Invention*; Michael J. Montoya, *Making the Mexican Diabetic: Race, Science, and the Genetics of Inequality* (University of California Press, 2011).

104. "Kiss Your Baby to Detect CF," *Chicago Defender*, September 13, 1973, 13.

105. R. B. Elliott, "Wrinkling of Skin in Cystic Fibrosis," *Lancet* 2, no. 7872 (1974): 108, https://doi.org/10.1016/S0140-6736(74)91675-4.

106. Renewed interest in the bucket test would emerge in the twenty-first century, as discussed in the epilogue.

107. Philip Farrell, oral history interview with the author, July 22, 2021.

108. For more on newborn screening for CF, see Grob, *Testing Baby*; Vailly, *Birth of a Genetics Policy*.

109. For a discussion of the terms variant and mutation, see G. R. Cutting, "Annotating DNA Variants Is the Next Major Goal for Human Genetics," *American Journal of Human Genetics* 94, no. 1 (2014), https://doi.org/10.1016/j.ajhg.2013.12.008.

110. G. E. Palomaki et al., "Clinical Sensitivity of Prenatal Screening for Cystic Fibrosis via *CFTR* Carrier Testing in a United States Panethnic Population," *Genetics in Medicine* 6, no. 5 (2004), https://doi.org/10.1097/01.gim.0000139505.06194.39.

111. Cystic Fibrosis Mutation Database, http://www.genet.sickkids.on.ca/StatisticsPage.html; J. E. Ideozu et al., "Diversity of *CFTR* Variants Across Ancestries Characterized Using 454,727 UK Biobank Whole Exome Sequences," *Genome Medicine* 16, no. 1 (2024), https://doi.org/10.1186/s13073-024-01316-5.

112. LaBonte, "Diagnostic Uncertainty, Microbes, and Isolation"; Mueller, "Impact of Transmissible Microbes."

113. In contrast, carrier status has been more widely associated with clinical consequences, at least in some contexts, in diseases such as sickle cell anemia, thalassemia, and some bleeding disorders. For a discussion of different conceptions of disease manifestations in those with sickle cell trait in Senegal, Europe, and North America, see Duana Fullwiley, *The Enculturated Gene: Sickle Cell Health Politics and Biological Difference in West Africa* (Princeton University Press, 2011). For a discussion about discrimination of those with sickle cell trait, see Troy Duster, *Backdoor to Eugenics*, 2nd ed. (Routledge, 2003); Keith Wailoo, "Inventing the Heterozygote: Molecular Biology, Racial Identity, and the Narratives of Sickle Cell Disease, Tay-Sachs, and Cystic Fibrosis," in *Race, Nature, and the Politics of Difference*, ed. Moore et al. (Duke University Press, 2003); Keith Wailoo, *Dying in the City of the Blues: Sickle Cell Anemia and the Politics of Race and Health* (University of North Carolina Press, 2001). For more on bleeding disorders, see Pemberton, *The Bleeding Disease*.

114. Radick, *Disputed Inheritance*.

115. Kristen M. Beckett, "The Cystic Fibrosis Heterozygote Advantage: A Synthesis of Ideas," *Anthropologica* 39, no. 1/2 (1997), https://doi.org/10.2307/25605860; P. M. Polgreen and A. P. Comellas, "Clinical Phenotypes of Cystic Fibrosis Carriers," *Annual Review of Medicine* 73 (2022), https://doi.org/10.1146/annurev-med-042120-020148. Sickle cell anemia carriers are also referred to as individuals with sickle cell trait.

116. A. C. Miller et al., "Cystic Fibrosis Carriers Are at Increased Risk for a Wide Range of Cystic Fibrosis-Related Conditions," *Proceedings of the National Academy of Sciences* 117, no. 3 (2020), https://doi.org/10.1073/pnas.1914912117.

117. Chenjie Zeng et al., "Diseases Common in Persons with Cystic Fibrosis Among *CFTR* Heterozygotes," *JAMA Internal Medicine* 185, no. 8 (2025), https://doi.org/10.1001/jamainternmed.2025.1853.

118. D. Fisman, "Cystic Fibrosis Heterozygosity: Carrier State or Haploinsufficiency?," *Proceedings of the National Academy of Sciences* 117, no. 6 (2020), https://doi.org/10.1073/pnas.1921730117.

119. R. Porter, "The Patient's View: Doing Medical History from Below," *Theory and Society* 14 (1985), https://www.jstor.org/stable/657089; Flurin Condrau, "The Patient's View Meets the Clinical Gaze," *Social History of Medicine* 20, no. 3 (2007); Howell, *Technology in the Hospital*; Wilson, *Living with Polio*; Jaipreet Virdi, *Hearing Happiness: Deafness Cures in History* (University of Chicago Press,

2020); Emily K. Abel, *Sick and Tired: An Intimate History of Fatigue* (University of North Carolina Press, 2021); Rothman, *Living in the Shadow of Death*.

Chapter One

1. "One More Cold, Doctor Said, May Be His Last," *Miami Herald*, July 14, 1953, C-1; "Early Birthday Party Is Planned for Doomed Boy," *Fort Lauderdale News*, July 12, 1953, 10-A.

2. Pat Murphy, "He Might Be Home Next Week: Bell Baby Won't Die, Doctors Report," *Miami Herald*, July 24, 1953, 17; "One More Cold," C-1.

3. "National Cystic Fibrosis Research Foundation: Its Aims and Activities," 1956, Bureau of Community Health/General Records, 1916–1979 (Additions, 1937–1977), box 2, folder 5/Cystic Fibrosis, Wisconsin Historical Society.

4. "Little Byron Is Dying: Tot Enjoys Early 'Birthday' Doctors Say Will Be His Last," *Fort Lauderdale News*, July 18, 1953, 1-B.

5. "Little Byron Is Dying," 1-B; "Early Birthday Party," 10-A; "One More Cold," C-1.

6. "'Doomed' Boy to See Boston Specialist: Byron Bell May Yet Have Many Birthdays," *Fort Lauderdale News*, July 19, 1953, 1.

7. "'Doomed' Boy to See Boston Specialist," 1.

8. Murphy, "He Might Be Home," 17.

9. Murphy, "He Might Be Home," 17.

10. For a description of the procedure as it was carried out in 1952, see Mary Ellen Avery, Reflections on 'What I Do Not Know About Cystic Fibrosis,' Dr. Shwachman's Day, 7 April 1976, box 15, folder 5, H MS c201, Mary Ellen Avery Papers, Francis A. Countway Library of Medicine, Center for the History of Medicine, Harvard Medical Library and Boston Medical Library.

11. Frank Hogan, "'Complete Recovery' Seen for Byron," *Fort Lauderdale News*, July 24, 1953, 1-A.

12. Murphy, "He Might Be Home," 17.

13. Hogan, "Complete Recovery," 1-B.

14. Hogan, "Complete Recovery," 1-B.

15. Hogan, "Complete Recovery," 1-A; "Byron 'Happy as a Lark': Bell Family Holds Reunion; Dad, Son Burn Midnight Oil," *Fort Lauderdale News*, August 1, 1953, 1.

16. Hogan, "Complete Recovery," 1-B.

17. E. K. Abel, "The Rise and Fall of Celiac Disease in the United States," *Journal of the History of Medicine and Allied Sciences* 65, no. 1 (2010), https://doi.org/10.1093/jhmas/jrp018; Emily K. Abel, *Gluten Free for Life: Celiac Disease, Medical Recognition, and the Food Industry* (New York University Press, 2024); Sydney A. Halpern, *American Pediatrics: The Social Dynamics of Professionalism,*

1880–1980 (University of California Press, 1988); Richard A. Meckel, *Save the Babies: American Public Health Reform and the Prevention of Infant Mortality, 1850–1929* (Johns Hopkins University Press, 1990); A. McGehee Harvey, *Science at the Bedside: Clinical Research in American Medicine 1905–1945* (Johns Hopkins University Press, 1981). When the hospital associated with the Rockefeller Institute for Medical Research opened in 1906, "one of the five priority diseases under study" was " 'intestinal infantilism' (celiac disease)." Howard Markel, *The Secret of Life: Rosalind Franklin, James Watson, Francis Crick, and the Discovery of DNA's Double Helix* (W. W. Norton, 2021), 26.

18. Sidney Valentine Haas and Merrill Patterson Haas, *Management of Celiac Disease* (J. B. Lippincott, 1951), 7. Gee gave a lecture on the topic in 1887, followed by a published account in 1888. M. S. Losowsky, "A History of Coeliac Disease," *Digestive Diseases* 26, no. 2 (2008), https://doi.org/10.1159/000116768.

19. Samuel Gee, "On the Coeliac Affection," *St. Bartholomew's Hospital Reports* 24 (1888): 17, 18. Other physicians would describe a syndrome consistent with the "coeliac affection" over the subsequent decades, with names such as "chronic intestinal indigestion," "infantilism from chronic intestinal infection," "Gee-Herter disease," and "celiac disease." Part of Gee's quote was included in Abel, "The Rise and Fall of Celiac Disease," 82.

20. Gee, "On the Coeliac Affection," 20; J. Greenberg, "An Attempt to Reproduce Coeliac Disease Experimentally in Young Animals by Excluding the External Pancreatic Secretion from the Intestine," *Yale Journal of Biology and Medicine* 6, no. 2 (1933), https://www.ncbi.nlm.nih.gov/pubmed/21433594; Leonard G. Parsons, "Celiac Disease: Rachford Memorial Lectures," *American Journal of Diseases of Children* 43, no. 5 (1932), https://doi.org/10.1001/archpedi.1932.01950060001001.

21. Andersen, "Cystic Fibrosis of the Pancreas"; Kenneth D. Blackfan and Charles D. May, "Inspissation of Secretion, Dilation of the Ducts and Acini, Atrophy and Fibrosis of the Pancreas in Infants," *Journal of Pediatrics* 13, no. 5 (1938), https://doi.org/10.1016/S0022-3476(38)80155-4.

22. Andersen, "Cystic Fibrosis of the Pancreas"; Murphy, "He Might Be Home," 17.

23. For a discussion of Farber's work on cancer in children, see Robin Wolfe Scheffler, *A Contagious Cause: The American Hunt for Cancer Viruses and the Rise of Molecular Medicine* (University of Chicago Press, 2019), 89–91; Siddhartha Mukherjee, *The Emperor of All Maladies: A Biography of Cancer* (Scribner, 2010).

24. When Gee characterized the "coeliac affection" in 1888, he noted that "nothing unnatural can be seen in the stomach, intestines, or other digestive organs" on autopsy. Gee, "On the Coeliac Affection," 18. In contrast, two Chicago physicians pointed out in 1935 that "changes in almost every organ of the digestive tract and in the glands of internal secretion have been held responsible for celiac disease from time to time." Julius H. Hess and Otto Saphir, "Celiac Disease (Chronic Intestinal Indigestion): A Report of Three Cases with Autopsy Findings,"

Journal of Pediatrics 6, no. 1 (1935): 4, https://doi.org/10.1016/S0022-3476(35)80071-1.

25. R. A. Gibbons, "The Coeliac Affection in Children (Continued)," *Edinburgh Medical Journal* 35, no. 5 (1889): 424; F. J. Poynton et al., "A Contribution to the Study of a Group of Cases of Chronic Recurrent Diarrhoea in Childhood," *Proceedings of the Royal Society of Medicine* 7, Med. Sect. (1914), https://doi.org/10.1177/003591571400700803; Joseph H. Pratt et al., "The Effect of Excluding Pancreatic Juice from the Intestine," *Transactions of the Association of American Physicians Twenty-Fourth Session* XXIV (1909): 279; Greenberg, "Attempt to Reproduce Coeliac Disease"; G. F. Still, "The Lumleian Lectures on CŒliac Disease. Lecture II," *Lancet* 192 (1918): 195, https://doi.org/10.1016/S0140-6736(00)53675-7; Hess and Saphir, "Celiac Disease (Chronic Intestinal Indigestion)," 13.

26. Robert Coleman Kemp, *Diseases of the Stomach, Intestines, and Pancreas*, 3rd ed. (W. B. Saunders, 1917), 955.

27. Michael Bliss, *The Discovery of Insulin* (University of Chicago Press, 1982); John Christopher Feudtner, *Bittersweet: Diabetes, Insulin, and the Transformation of Illness* (University of North Carolina Press, 2003). For historical accounts of the exocrine pancreas, see Frederic Lawrence Holmes, *Claude Bernard and Animal Chemistry: The Emergence of a Scientist* (Harvard University Press, 1974); Anna Cecilia de Romo, "Tallow and the Time Capsule: Claude Bernard's Discovery of the Pancreatic Digestion of Fat," *History and Philosophy of the Life Sciences* 11, no. 2 (1989), http://www.jstor.org/stable/23330351; E. R. Ragland, "Experimenting with Chymical Bodies: Reinier De Graaf's Investigations of the Pancreas," *Early Science and Medicine* 13, no. 6 (2008), https://doi.org/10.1163/157338208x362705. Some people with CF also develop cystic fibrosis–related diabetes. M. E. Hodson, "Diabetes Mellitus and Cystic Fibrosis," *Baillière's Clinical Endocrinology and Metabolism* 6, no. 4 (1992), https://doi.org/10.1016/S0950-351X(05)80166-1.

28. Martin Bodian, *Fibrocystic Disease of the Pancreas: A Congenital Disorder of Mucus Production—Mucosis* (Grune & Stratton, 1953), 4; G. Fanconi, *Der intestinale Infantilismus und ahnliche Formen der chronischen Verdauungsstorung* (Verlag von S. Karger, 1928); Cecil Clarke and Geoffrey Hadfield, "Congenital Pancreatic Disease with Infantalism," *Quarterly Journal of Medicine* 17, no. 68 (1924); Hess and Saphir, "Celiac Disease (Chronic Intestinal Indigestion)"; Margaret H. Harper, "Two Cases of Congenital Pancreatic Steatorrhoea with Infantilism," *Medical Journal of Australia* 2, no. 20 (1930).

29. A. H. Parmelee, "The Pathology of Steatorrhea," *American Journal of Diseases of Children* 50, no. 6 (1935), https://doi.org/10.1001/archpedi.1935.01970120070006; G. Fanconi et al., "Das Coeliakiesyndrom bei angeborener Zystischer Pankreasfibromatose und Bronchiektasien," *Wiener Medizinische Wochenschrift* 86 (1936). Some physicians presented similar cases that did not include the celiac label. See Kenneth D. Blackfan and S. Burt Wolbach, "Vitamin A Deficiency in Infants," *Journal of Pediatrics* 3, no. 5 (1933), https://doi.org/10.1016

/S0022-3476(33)80022-9; Clarke and Hadfield, "Congenital Pancreatic Disease with Infantalism," 358. Fanconi, "Der Intestinale Infantilismus," 158.

30. Keith Wailoo points out that the availability of antibiotics around this time "had a dramatic impact on the way many diseases . . . were visualized," as some children continued to have health challenges even after antibiotic treatment because "they had developed infectious diseases primarily because of underlying or preexisting disorders like diabetes, cystic fibrosis, or sickle cell anemia." Wailoo, *Dying in the City of the Blues*, 115–116.

31. Andersen, "Cystic Fibrosis of the Pancreas"; Dorothy H. Andersen, "Cystic Fibrosis of the Pancreas and Its Relation to Coeliac Disease: A Clinical and Pathological Study," typescript, 1938, box 2, folder 3, Dorothy Andersen Papers, Archives & Special Collections, Health Sciences Library, Columbia University.

32. John Scott Baird, *Dorothy Hansine Andersen: The Life and Times of the Pioneering Physician-Scientist Who Identified Cystic Fibrosis* (Springer, 2022).

33. Benjamin F. Shearer and Barbara S. Shearer, *Notable Women in the Life Sciences: A Biographical Dictionary* (Greenwood Press, 1996), 8, 344–51; Baird, *Dorothy Hansine Andersen*; "Dorothy Andersen (1901–1963)," Embryo Project Encyclopedia, Arizona State University, http://embryo.asu.edu/handle/10776/11772. During this time, women physicians were more likely to work within certain specialties, including pediatrics. George Weisz, *Divide and Conquer: A Comparative History of Medical Specialization* (Oxford University Press, 2006), 194.

34. Baird, *Dorothy Hansine Andersen*. According to Baird, Andersen's own health challenges may have contributed to her transition from surgery to pathology.

35. Baird, *Dorothy Hansine Andersen*; *Lost Women of Science*, podcast, season 1, "The Pathologist in the Basement," November 4, 2021, https://lostwomenofscience.org/season-1-1.

36. Baird, *Dorothy Hansine Andersen*. See Andersen's collection of correspondence related to her patients, box 1, folders 5–8, Dorothy Andersen Papers, Archives & Special Collections, Health Sciences Library, Columbia University.

37. Dorothy H. Andersen, "Cystic Fibrosis of the Pancreas, Vitamin A Deficiency, and Bronchiectasis," *Journal of Pediatrics* 15, no. 6 (1939): 763, https://doi.org/10.1016/S0022-3476(39)80077-4; Andersen, "Cystic Fibrosis of the Pancreas."

38. Sidney V. Haas, "Celiac Disease and Its Ultimate Prognosis," *Journal of Pediatrics* 13, no. 3 (1938), https://doi.org/10.1016/S0022-3476(38)80148-7; Hess and Saphir, "Celiac Disease (Chronic Intestinal Indigestion)"; Williams McKim Marriott, *Infant Nutrition a Textbook of Infant Feeding for Students and Practitioners of Medicine*, 2nd. ed (C.V. Mosby, 1935); Jonathan Campbell Meakins, *The Practice of Medicine* (C. V. Mosby, 1936); Langley Porter and William Elmer Carter, *Management of the Sick Infant and Child*, 5th rev. ed. (C. V. Mosby, 1938); F. Shippam, "Coeliac Disease," *Canadian Medical Association Journal* 34, no. 3 (1936), https://pmc.ncbi.nlm.nih.gov/articles/PMC1561556/; Arthur E. Wade, "Celiac Disease:

Intestinal Absorption and Gastrointestinal Motility," *Journal of Pediatrics* 8, no. 5 (1936), https://doi.org/10.1016/S0022-3476(36)80154-1.

39. Andersen, "Cystic Fibrosis, Vitamin A Deficiency, and Bronchiectasis," 763; Stefano Guandalini, "A Brief History of Celiac Disease," *Impact*, 7 (2007): 2; Haas, "Celiac Disease and Its Ultimate Prognosis"; Abel, "The Rise and Fall of Celiac Disease."

40. Andersen, "Cystic Fibrosis, Vitamin A Deficiency, and Bronchiectasis," 763.

41. S. F. Dowell et al., "Mortality from Pneumonia in Children in the United States, 1939 through 1996," *New England Journal of Medicine* 342, no. 19 (2000), https://doi.org/10.1056/NEJM200005113421904; S. H. Podolsky, "The Changing Fate of Pneumonia as a Public Health Concern in 20th-Century America and Beyond," *American Journal of Public Health* 95, no. 12 (2005), https://doi.org/10.2105/AJPH.2004.048397. Serotherapy was the standard of care for pneumonia in the late 1930s, yet it is unclear what type of therapeutic intervention was attempted on the girl. Scott H. Podolsky, *Pneumonia Before Antibiotics: Therapeutic Evolution and Evaluation in Twentieth-Century America* (Johns Hopkins University Press, 2006), chapter 5.

42. Andersen also noted changes in the liver and lungs on autopsy. Andersen, "Cystic Fibrosis of the Pancreas," 344.

43. "Hospital Service in the United States: Eighteenth Annual Presentation of Hospital Data by the Council on Medical Education and Hospitals of the American Medical Association," *JAMA* 112, no. 10 (1939): 925, https://doi.org/10.1001/jama.1939.02800100019007; D. E. Brown, "High Autopsy-Percentage," *New England Journal of Medicine* 251, no. 21 (1954), https://doi.org/10.1056/NEJM195411182512106.

44. Charles E. Rosenberg, *The Care of Strangers: The Rise of America's Hospital System* (Basic Books, 1987), 82, 87; Erwin Heinz Ackerknecht, *Medicine at the Paris Hospital, 1794–1848* (Johns Hopkins University Press, 1967).

45. Foucault, *Birth of the Clinic*. For the role of autopsy in efforts to identify signs of sanctity, see Katharine Park, *Secrets of Women: Gender, Generation, and the Origins of Human Dissection* (Zone Books, 2006); Bradford Bouley, *Pious Postmortems: Anatomy, Sanctity, and the Catholic Church in Early Modern Europe* (University of Pennsylvania Press, 2017).

46. "The Case Record of the Massachusetts General Hospital," *The Boston Medical and Surgical Journal* 189, no. 2 (1923), https://doi.org/10.1056/NEJM192307121890216; "The Case Records of the Massachusetts General Hospital," *New England Journal of Medicine* 239, no. 18 (1948), https://doi.org/10.1056/NEJM194810282391810; S. H. Podolsky et al., "The Evolving Roles of the Medical Journal," *New England Journal of Medicine* 366, no. 16 (2012), https://doi.org/10.1056/NEJMp1113567; A. M. Brandt, "A Reader's Guide to 200 Years of the New England Journal of Medicine," *New England Journal of Medicine* 366, no. 1 (2012), https://doi.org/10.1056/NEJMp1112812; "'C.P.C.'—Clinical Analysis or Guessing

Game?," *New England Journal of Medicine* 245, no. 21 (1951), https://doi.org/10.1056/NEJM195111222452110.

47. Andersen, "Cystic Fibrosis of the Pancreas," 393.

48. Steven J. Peitzman, *Dropsy, Dialysis, Transplant: A Short History of Failing Kidneys* (Johns Hopkins University Press, 2007), 59.

49. Andersen, "Cystic Fibrosis of the Pancreas," 344.

50. Andersen, "Cystic Fibrosis of the Pancreas," 344–45.

51. Foucault, *Birth of the Clinic.*

52. Andersen, "Cystic Fibrosis of the Pancreas," 344–45.

53. Andersen, "Cystic Fibrosis of the Pancreas," 344–45.

54. Andersen, "Cystic Fibrosis of the Pancreas," 351. The earliest case of cystic fibrosis of the pancreas that Andersen identified from the published literature was described by Karl Landsteiner in 1905. K. Landsteiner, "Darmverschluss Durch Eingedicktes Meconium; Pankreatitis," *Das Zentralblatt für allgemeine Pathologie u. pathologische Anatomie* 16 (1905). Many physicians believe that Landsteiner provided the first characterization of the pancreatic changes seen in cystic fibrosis. Bodian, *Fibrocystic Disease of the Pancreas*, 10, and G. B. S. Roberts, "Fibrocystic Disease of the Pancreas: A Histological Study of the Pancreas in Childhood with a Survey of the Clinical, Epidemiological, and Genetic Features of the Disease" (Doctor of Medicine, University of Glasgow, 1957), 7.

55. This statement is from a 1939 publication. Andersen, "Cystic Fibrosis, Vitamin A Deficiency, and Bronchiectasis," 766. For example, Frank Deford, whose daughter had CF, explained in 1986, "Basically, it's a white disease." Patricia Brennan, "His Daughter's Legacy: 'Alex: The Life of a Child,'" *Washington Post*, April 19, 1986. Quoted in Wailoo and Pemberton, *Troubled Dream of Genetic Medicine.*, 112.

56. Walter Greason, "Blackness and Whiteness as Historical Forces in the 20th Century United States," *Multicultural Perspectives* 11, no. 1 (2009), https://doi.org/10.1080/15210960902717650.

57. Andersen, "Cystic Fibrosis of the Pancreas."

58. Peitzman, *Dropsy, Dialysis, Transplant*, 58.

59. Andersen, "Cystic Fibrosis of the Pancreas," 358–59.

60. Andersen, "Cystic Fibrosis of the Pancreas."

61. Bodian, *Fibrocystic Disease of the Pancreas*, 4–5; "Fibrocystic Disease of the Pancreas," *British Medical Journal* 2, no. 4642 (1949): 1462, http://www.jstor.org/stable/25374576; "Fibrocystic Disease of the Pancreas," *Lancet* 250, no. 6487 (1947): 951, https://doi.org/10.1016/S0140-6736(47)91334-2; L. S. Goin, "Fibrocystic Disease of the Pancreas," *Radiology* 51, no. 1 (1948): 36, https://doi.org/10.1148/51.1.36; D. Pitt, "Fibrocystic Disease of the Pancreas: A Review of 14 Cases," *Medical Journal of Australia* 1, no. 4 (1948): 91, https://doi.org/10.5694/j.1326-5377.1948.tb96948.x; Charles D. May, *Cystic Fibrosis of the Pancreas in Infants and Children* (Charles C. Thomas, 1954), 6; D. A. Christie and E. M. Tansey, Cystic Fibrosis, Wellcome

Witnesses to Twentieth Century Medicine, Volume 20, June 11, 2002, witness seminar transcript, Wellcome Trust Center for the History of Medicine, University College London, 2004, 3.

62. Andersen, "Cystic Fibrosis of the Pancreas."

63. Andersen, "Cystic Fibrosis of the Pancreas," 380; May, *Cystic Fibrosis of the Pancreas*, 6.

64. Aronowitz, *Making Sense of Illness*.

65. Andersen, "Cystic Fibrosis of the Pancreas," 397; Haas and Haas, *Management of Celiac Disease*, 2.

66. Andersen, "Cystic Fibrosis of the Pancreas," 397; "Fibrocystic Disease of the Pancreas," 952; Solomon Rauch et al., "Congenital Familial Steatorrhea with Fibromatosis of the Pancreas and Bronchiolectasis," *Journal of Pediatrics* 14, no. 4 (1939): 462, https://doi.org/10.1016/S0022-3476(39)80166-4.

67. Abel, "The Rise and Fall of Celiac Disease," 100.

68. Andersen, "Cystic Fibrosis of the Pancreas," 397.

69. Blackfan and May, "Inspissation of Secretion," 633; Tracy B. Mallory, "Case Records of the Massachusetts General Hospital Case 26331," *New England Journal of Medicine* 223, no. 7 (1940): 256, https://doi.org/10.1056/NEJM194008152230705.

70. Blackfan and May, "Inspissation of Secretion," 627.

71. They identified two groups of patients consistent with Andersen's group I and group II/III. Baird, *Dorothy Hansine Andersen*, 80.

72. Blackfan and May, "Inspissation of Secretion," 627.

73. Blackfan and May, "Inspissation of Secretion," 628. The prioritization of the pancreatic lesion was reinforced by Ottawa physician F. W. Jeffrey in 1941 in his report of ninety cases of cystic fibrosis. F. W. Jeffrey, "Cystic Fibrosis of the Pancreas," *Canadian Medical Association Journal* 45, no. 3 (1941): 224, https://www.ncbi.nlm.nih.gov/pubmed/20322203.

74. Sidney Farber, "Pancreatic Insufficiency and the Celiac Syndrome" *New England Journal of Medicine* 229, no. 17 (1943): 654, https://doi.org/10.1056/NEJM194310212291705. The framing of CF as a pancreas disease was reinforced by previous studies done in dogs. Andersen, "Cystic Fibrosis of the Pancreas," 372. Particularly striking was Sidney Farber's 1943 claim that "children with pancreatic fibrosis behave as do dogs in which the pancreatic juices have been excluded from the intestines." Sidney Farber, "Pancreatic Insufficiency and the Celiac Syndrome (Concluded)," *New England Journal of Medicine* 229, no. 18 (1943): 683–84, https://doi.org/10.1056/NEJM194310282291804.

75. Rosenberg, *The Care of Strangers*, 153. Andersen cites Benoit, Tiling, and Siwe when describing the examination of "duodenal contents" in three patients in her series. Andersen, "Cystic Fibrosis of the Pancreas," 357. A. E. Garrod, "The Schorstein Lecture on the Diagnosis of Disease of the Pancreas: Delivered at the London Hospital Medical College on February 20th, 1920," *British Medical Journal* 1, no. 3092 (1920), https://doi.org/10.1136/bmj.1.3092.459.

76. Peitzman, *Dropsy, Dialysis, Transplant*, 66; Rosenberg, *The Care of Strangers*, 154. For example, this type of connection between postmortem findings and changes in a bodily fluid during life was also noted by physician Richard Bright in his characterization of "certain morbid changes of the kidney" on autopsy and associated alterations in urine composition. Steven J. Peitzman, "From Bright's Disease to End-Stage Renal Disease," in *Framing Disease*, ed. Rosenberg and Golden, 9; C. E. Rosenberg, "Disease in History: Frames and Framers," *Milbank Quarterly* 67, suppl. 1 (1989): 5, https://doi.org/10.2307/3350182.

77. Andersen, "Pancreatic Enzymes in the Duodenal Juice," 643. Andersen pointed to the work of Alfred Hess as significant for the analysis of duodenal contents in infants.

78. Max Einhorn, *The Duodenal Tube and Its Possibilities* (Saunders, 1920), 23; John C Hemmeter, "The History of the Discovery of Duodenal Intubation," *Medical Record (1866–1922)*, Feb. 26 (1921): 341; Julius Friedenwald and Samuel Morrison, "The History of the Development of the Stomach Tube with Some Notes on the Duodenal Tube," *Bulletin of the Institute of the History of Medicine* 4 (1936), http://www.jstor.com/stable/44438280.

79. Alfred F. Hess, "A Duodenal Tube for Infants," *American Journal of Diseases of Children* 1, no. 5 (1911), https://doi.org/10.1001/archpedi.1911.04100050041003. The tube developed by Hess was a modified version of the duodenal tube first described in 1910 by New York physician M. Gross for studies in adults.

80. Hess, "Duodenal Tube," 360, 365.

81. Andersen, "Pancreatic Enzymes in the Duodenal Juice," 643; Alfred F. Hess, "The Pancreatic Ferments in Infants," *American Journal of Diseases of Children* 4, no. 4 (1912), https://doi.org/10.1001/archpedi.1912.04100220010002; Herbert F. Philipsborn et al., "An Analysis of the Duodenal Drainage in the Steatorrheas," *Journal of Pediatrics* 26, no. 2 (1945), https://doi.org/10.1016/S0022-3476(45)80164-6.

82. Jacques Loeb, *The Dynamics of Living Matter* (Columbia University Press, 1906), 9, 11, 23.

83. Hess, "Pancreatic Ferments," 206.

84. Hess, "Pancreatic Ferments," 218.

85. Andersen, "Pancreatic Enzymes in the Duodenal Juice," 644; A. C. Ivy, "Certain Aspects of the Applied Physiology of External Pancreatic Secretion," *American Journal of Digestive Diseases* 3, no. 9 (1936): 682, https://doi.org/10.1007/BF02999189.

86. Andersen, "Cystic Fibrosis, Vitamin A Deficiency, and Bronchiectasis," 765, 771.

87. Blackfan and May, "Inspissation of Secretion," 633.

88. Farber, "Pancreatic Insufficiency and the Celiac Syndrome (Concluded)," 685.

89. Farber, "Pancreatic Insufficiency and the Celiac Syndrome (Concluded)," 685; R. L. Kennedy, "Cystic Fibrosis of the Pancreas," *Nebraska State Medical Journal* 31, no. 12 (1946): 493–94, https://www.ncbi.nlm.nih.gov/pubmed/20274916.

90. For more on the use of the X-ray for diagnostic purposes, see M. C. Sosman, "The Shattuck Lecture: The Specificity and Reliability of Roentgenographic Diagnosis," *New England Journal of Medicine* 242, no. 22 (1950), https://doi.org/10.1056/NEJM195006012422201.

91. Tracy B. Mallory et al., "Case Records of the Massachusetts General Hospital Case 29431," *New England Journal of Medicine* 229, no. 18 (1943):689, https://doi.org/10.1056/NEJM194310282291805; Philipsborn et al., "Duodenal Drainage in the Steatorrheas," 107.

92. William D. Bevis, "Stool Analysis in Pancreatic Fibrosis and Celiac Disease" (Doctor of Medicine, Yale University, 1949), 14.

93. *Fifty-Eighth Annual Report for the Year 1940 Infants' Hospital 300 Longwood Avenue Boston* (The Children's Hospital, 1940), 5. They referred to cystic fibrosis as "pancreatic fibrosis."

94. Mallory, "Case 26331." Comment by Ralph Daffinee, 254. For more on the history of clinicopathological conferences, see Christopher Crenner, *Private Practice in the Early Twentieth-Century Medical Office of Dr. Richard Cabot* (Johns Hopkins University Press, 2005), chapter 3.

95. Mallory, "Case 26331," 256. Other physicians reinforced this point. Jeffrey, "Cystic Fibrosis of the Pancreas," 225; "Fibrocystic Disease of the Pancreas," 952; Haas and Haas, *Management of Celiac Disease*, 2.

96. Murphy, "He Might Be Home," 17.

97. Farber, "Pancreatic Insufficiency and the Celiac Syndrome (Concluded)," 682; Charlotte L. Maddock et al., "Pancreatic Function and Disease in Early Life. II. Effect of Secretin on Pancreatic Function of Infants and Children," *American Journal of Diseases of Children* 66, no. 4 (1943), https://doi.org/10.1001/archpedi.1943.02010220023003; Harry Shwachman et al., "Pancreatic Function and Disease in Early Life: III. Methods of Analyzing Pancreatic Enzyme Activity," *American Journal of Diseases of Children* 66, no. 4 (1943): 418, https://doi.org/10.1001/archpedi.1943.02010220071008.

98. Shwachman et al., "Analyzing Pancreatic Enzyme Activity," 418.

99. Statement by Boston physician Edward Neuhauser. Goin, "Fibrocystic Disease of the Pancreas," 43.

100. J. H. Fanos, "'We Kept Our Promises': An Oral History of Harry Shwachman, M.D.," *American Journal of Medical Genetics Part A* 146A, no. 3 (2008): 288, https://doi.org/10.1002/ajmg.a.32113. For another account of duodenal intubation, see William W. Waring, "Center Directors Remember: New Orleans," in *Cystic Fibrosis in the 20th Century*, ed. Carl F. Doershuk (AM Publishing, 2001), 278–79.

101. Andersen and Hodges, "Celiac Syndrome: V." In 1946, Andersen and Hodges noted that "although the incidence among siblings approximates the 25 per cent expected of a mendelian recessive trait, the distribution of the cases in families suggests that the disease, although hereditary, requires more than one factor for its expression," 80. "Cystic Fibrosis of the Pancreas," pamphlet prepared for

doctors by the Children's Exocrine Research Foundation, November 1955, box 2, folder 1, Printed Matter, 1955, 1960, Dorothy Andersen Papers, Archives and Special Collections, Health Sciences Library, Columbia University.

102. Helen Bullock, "Her Children Victims: Mother Waging Fight on Disease," *Dallas Morning News*, May 22, 1955, 4. At that time, Sharples referred to cystic fibrosis as mucoviscidosis. Ian Menzies, "Doctor-Mother Fights for Children's Lives," *Daily Boston Globe*, January 27, 1957. Ronald M. Deutsch, "Cystic Fibrosis . . . Enemy of Our Children," *Ladies' Home Journal* 72, no. 11 (1955).

103. Letter from Wynne Sharples to Joseph W. St. Geme on October 2, 1955, box 204, folder Cystic Fibrosis #1 1955–1967 May, Joseph Stokes, Jr. Papers: Series VI. Diseases and Treatment, Mss.B.St65p, American Philosophical Society; "Exocrine Research Foundation," *New England Journal of Medicine* 253, no. 6 (1955), https://doi.org/10.1056/NEJM195508112530613; "A Mother's Campaign," *Newsweek* 45, no. 24 (1955). For more on the history of the Cystic Fibrosis Foundation, see Evelyn Graub and Milton Graub, "Origin and Development of the Cystic Fibrosis Foundation," in *Cystic Fibrosis in the 20th Century*; Robert J. Beall and Sherry L. Keramidas, "The Cystic Fibrosis Foundation," in *Textbook of Cystic Fibrosis*, ed. John D. Lloyd-Still (John Wright and PSG, 1983); Trivedi, *Breath from Salt*, Chapters 8 and 9.

104. Doris F. Tulcin, *Memoirs of a Monarch: A Chronicle of My Life* (iUniverse, 2008), 30.

105. Tulcin, *Memoirs of a Monarch*, 30.

106. Cystic Fibrosis Foundation, "Reflections from Doris Tulcin," 2020, https://www.youtube.com/watch?v=wKxzijDUD1w.

107. Greene, *Prescribing by Numbers*, 226–27; I. S. Campbell et al., "Visceral Vistas: Basil Hirschowitz and the Birth of Fiberoptic Endoscopy," *Annals of Internal Medicine* 165, no. 3 (2016), https://doi.org/10.7326/M16-0025. As Campbell and colleagues note, the implementation of the fiberscope had more to do with patient satisfaction and ease of use than the diagnostic accuracy of the instrument compared to the earlier technology (semiflexible gastroscopy).

108. H. F. Philipsborn et al., "The Diagnosis of Fibrocystic Disease of the Pancreas," *Journal of Pediatrics* 25, no. 4 (1944): 289; Edward L. Pratt and Kathleen R. Fahey, "Clinical Adequacy of a Single Measurement of Vitamin A Absorption," *American Journal of Diseases of Children* 68, no. 2 (1944).

109. Andersen, "Pancreatic Enzymes in the Duodenal Juice," 645.

110. Andersen, "Pancreatic Enzymes in the Duodenal Juice," 645.

111. Andersen, "Pancreatic Enzymes in the Duodenal Juice," 645.

112. Andersen, "Pancreatic Enzymes in the Duodenal Juice," 645.

113. Andersen, "Pancreatic Enzymes in the Duodenal Juice," 645.

114. B. P. York et al., "Cystic Fibrosis of the Pancreas," *Southern Medicine and Surgery* 111, no. 1 (1949): 43, https://www.ncbi.nlm.nih.gov/pubmed/18109852; J. O. Collins and J. Standard, "Cystic Fibrosis of Pancreas," *Connecticut State Medical Journal* 11, no. 3 (1947): 178, https://www.ncbi.nlm.nih.gov/pubmed/20285294.

115. H. Shwachman et al., "Significance of Altered Viscosity of Duodenal Content in Pancreatic Fibrosis (Mucoviscidosis)," *AMA American Journal of Diseases of Children* 80, no. 5 (1950): 864, https://www.ncbi.nlm.nih.gov/pubmed/14777167.

116. Steven Shapin and Simon Schaffer, *Leviathan and the Air-Pump: Hobbes, Boyle, and the Experimental Life* (Princeton University Press, 2011); H. M. Collins, *Changing Order: Replication and Induction in Scientific Practice* (University of Chicago Press, 1992).

117. Lewis E. Gibson, "A New Era in Diagnosis: The Sweat Test," in *Cystic Fibrosis in the 20th Century*, 56.

118. Gibson, "A New Era in Diagnosis," 56–57.

119. Dorothy Andersen "kindly demonstrated" the duodenal intubation test to Boston physician Charlotte Maddock. Shwachman et al., "Analyzing Pancreatic Enzyme Activity," 418.

120. Goin, "Fibrocystic Disease of the Pancreas," 39; H. N. Christensen and H. Shwachman, "Determination of the Plasma Glycine After Gelatin Feeding as a Diagnostic Procedure for Pancreatic Fibrosis," *Journal of Clinical Investigation* 28, no. 2 (1949): 319, https://doi.org/10.1172/JCI102074; Bevis, "Stool Analysis," 2.

121. Ralph Brien, "Cystic Fibrosis Strikes Family—Killer Loose in R.I. House," *Moline Dispatch*, June 13, 1958, 21.

122. Pitt, "Fibrocystic Disease of the Pancreas," 93; "Fibrocystic Disease of the Pancreas," 1462.

123. They used the term "duodenal catheterization." H. Shwachman et al., "Studies in Pancreatic Fibrosis: A Simple Diagnostic Gelatin Film Test for Stool Trypsin," *Pediatrics* 4, no. 2 (1949): 222, https://doi.org/10.1542/peds.4.2.222.

124. Andersen previously used the viscosimetric method (which examined viscosity) to determine trypsin activity in duodenal fluid because of its "reliability and sensitivity." Dorothy H. Andersen and Marialuise V. Early, "Method of Assaying Trypsin Suitable for Routine Use in Diagnosis of Congenital Pancreatic Deficiency," *American Journal of Diseases of Children* 63, no. 5 (1942): 891, https://doi.org/10.1001/archpedi.1942.02010050055005.

125. They used a "modified Fermi method," which used gelatin as a substrate to assess trypsin activity in duodenal fluid. Andersen and Early, "Method of Assaying Trypsin," 891, 892.

126. Ivy, "Applied Physiology of External Pancreatic Secretion," 680; Philipsborn et al., "Duodenal Drainage in the Steatorrheas," 116; Andersen and Early, "Method of Assaying Trypsin."

127. Farber, "Pancreatic Insufficiency and the Celiac Syndrome (Concluded)," 683.

128. Andersen, "Pancreatic Enzymes in the Duodenal Juice," 658; Philipsborn et al., "Duodenal Drainage in the Steatorrheas," 117; G. E. Gibbs, "Some Diagnostic and Therapeutic Techniques in Cystic Fibrosis of the Pancreas," *California Medicine* 69, no. 5 (1948), https://www.ncbi.nlm.nih.gov/pubmed/18731569; D. E.

Johnstone and E. Neter, "Studies on the Laboratory Diagnosis of Cystic Fibrosis of the Pancreas. Positive Gelatin Film Tests Due to Gelatin-Liquefying Bacteria in Feces and Duodenal Juice," *Pediatrics* 7, no. 4 (1951), https://doi.org/10.1542/peds.7.4.483; H. Shwachman, "Progress in the Study of 'Mucoviscidosis' (Pancreatic Fibrosis); with Illustrative Case Presentations," *Pediatrics* 7, no. 2 (1951), https://doi.org/10.1542/peds.7.2.153.

129. Farber, "Pancreatic Insufficiency and the Celiac Syndrome (Concluded)," 686; S. Farber and L. K. Diamond, "Temporary Remissions in Acute Leukemia in Children Produced by Folic Acid Antagonist, 4-Aminopteroyl-Glutamic Acid," *New England Journal of Medicine* 238, no. 23 (1948), https://doi.org/10.1056/NEJM194806032382301; Farber, "Pancreatic Insufficiency and the Celiac Syndrome."

130. Farber, "Pancreatic Insufficiency and the Celiac Syndrome (Concluded)," 686; Mallory, "Case 26331," 256.

131. Mallory et al., "Case 29431," 691.

132. Mallory et al., "Case 29431," 691. Farber disagreed with other physicians who believed that the vitamin A deficiency seen in patients with CF was the cause of the lung changes.

133. Mallory et al., "Case 29431," 692.

134. Mallory et al., "Case 29431," 692; Farber, "Pancreatic Insufficiency and the Celiac Syndrome (Concluded)," 686, 687; Sidney Farber, "Pancreatic Function and Disease in Early Life. V. Pathologic Changes Associated with Pancreatic Insufficiency in Early Life," *Archives of Pathology* 37, no. 4 (1944): 249.

135. Farber, "Pathologic Changes Associated with Pancreatic Insufficiency," 250.

136. Katharine Dodd, "Intestinal Obstruction Due to Meconium Ileus in a Newborn Infant," *Journal of Pediatrics* 9, no. 4 (1936), https://doi.org/10.1016/S0022-3476(36)80232-7.

137. Farber, "Pathologic Changes Associated with Pancreatic Insufficiency," 238. For another view, see M. Harper, "Congenital Steatorrhoea Due to Defect of the Pancreas," *Medical Journal of Australia* 1, no. 5 (1949): 138, https://doi.org/10.5694/j.1326-5377.1949.tb28307.x; Farber, "Pathologic Changes Associated with Pancreatic Insufficiency," 249.

138. Farber, "Pathologic Changes Associated with Pancreatic Insufficiency," 249.

139. Farber, "Pathologic Changes Associated with Pancreatic Insufficiency," 249.

140. Bodian, *Fibrocystic Disease of the Pancreas*; Harper, "Congenital Steatorrhoea," 140.

141. S. Farber, "Some Organic Digestive Disturbances in Early Life," *Journal of the Michigan State Medical Society* 44 (1945): 592. Italics in original. As Farber noted, the term *mucoviscidosis* was "proposed for temporary convenience only and should be dropped as soon as a diagnostic term based on etiology can be found," 592.

142. Farber, "Some Organic Digestive Disturbances in Early Life," 593.

143. Mallory et al., "Case 29431," 691.

144. Shwachman et al., "Significance of Altered Viscosity," 865.

145. Shwachman et al., "Significance of Altered Viscosity," 865. The term *mucoviscidosis* has continued to be used in some contexts and regions.

146. W. Sinclair Jr., "Cystic Fibrosis of the Pancreas," *Ohio State Medical Journal* 44, no. 10 (1948): 1024, https://www.ncbi.nlm.nih.gov/pubmed/18885090.

147. Sinclair, "Cystic Fibrosis of the Pancreas," 1024.

148. Sinclair, "Cystic Fibrosis of the Pancreas," 1024.

149. G. E. Gibbs et al., "Incomplete Pancreatic Deficiency in Cystic Fibrosis of the Pancreas," *Journal of Pediatrics* 37, no. 3 (1950): 321, https://doi.org/10.1016/S0022-3476(50)80150-6.

150. Shwachman, "Progress in the Study of 'Mucoviscidosis' "; "E. Mead Johnson Award for Research in Pediatrics," *Pediatric Research* 43, no. 4 (1998), https://doi.org/10.1203/00006450-199804001-00015. The speech was given on October 17, 1950, at the annual meeting of the American Academy of Pediatrics in Chicago, and physician Charles D. May was the other recipient of the award. Dorothy Andersen was honored with the E. Mead Johnson Award in 1939.

151. Shwachman, "Progress in the Study of 'Mucoviscidosis,' " 155.

152. Shwachman, "Progress in the Study of 'Mucoviscidosis,' " 155. CF was also referred to as pancreatic fibrosis or mucoviscidosis.

153. Shwachman, "Progress in the Study of 'Mucoviscidosis,' " 155.

154. Shwachman, "Progress in the Study of 'Mucoviscidosis,' " 155, 156. In his examination of duodenal fluid over a three-year period, Shwachman found that 90 percent of patients with CF had significantly increased viscosity of the duodenal fluid.

155. Shwachman, "Progress in the Study of 'Mucoviscidosis,' " 154.

156. Carl F. Doershuk, *Cystic Fibrosis in the 20th Century: People, Events, and Progress* (AM Publishing, 2001); Wailoo and Pemberton, *Troubled Dream of Genetic Medicine*; P. A. di Sant'Agnese and D. H. Andersen, "Celiac Syndrome IV; Chemotherapy in Infections of the Respiratory Tract Associated with Cystic Fibrosis of the Pancreas; Observations with Penicillin and Drugs of the Sulfonamide Group, with Special Reference to Penicillin Aerosol," *American Journal of Diseases of Children* 72 (1946), https://doi.org/10.1001/archpedi.1946.02020300024003. On the early use of pancreatin in CF, see Andersen, "Cystic Fibrosis, Vitamin A Deficiency, and Bronchiectasis," 770.

157. H. Shwachman et al., "Aureomycin Therapy in the Pulmonary Involvement of Pancreatic Fibrosis (Mucoviscidosis)," *New England Journal of Medicine* 241, no. 5 (1949): 185, https://doi.org/10.1056/NEJM194908042410501. For more on the history of these early antibiotics, see Harry M. Marks, *The Progress of Experiment: Science and Therapeutic Reform in the United States, 1900–1990* (Cambridge University Press, 1997); Robert Bud, *Penicillin: Triumph and Tragedy* (Oxford University Press, 2007).

158. Fanos, "We Kept Our Promises," 289. For more on broad-spectrum antibiotics and resistance, see Scott H. Podolsky, *The Antibiotic Era: Reform, Resistance, and the Pursuit of a Rational Therapeutics* (Johns Hopkins University Press, 2015).

159. Fanos, "We Kept Our Promises," 289.

160. Goin, "Fibrocystic Disease of the Pancreas," 38. In the same year, Melbourne physician David Pitt similarly suggested that the survival of five of the fourteen patients in his series was "perhaps due to the good fortune of early diagnosis and satisfactory treatment." Pitt, "Fibrocystic Disease of the Pancreas," 100.

161. "Case Records of the Massachusetts General Hospital: Case 34512," *New England Journal of Medicine* 239, no. 25 (1948): 977, https://doi.org/10.1056/NEJM194812162392507.

162. "Case 34512," 978. For an account of the history of concerns about antibiotic resistance, see Podolsky, *The Antibiotic Era*; Harper, "Congenital Steatorrhoea," 141.

163. Bodian, *Fibrocystic Disease of the Pancreas*, 7.

164. Gibbs et al., "Incomplete Pancreatic Deficiency," 324.

165. Shwachman, "Progress in the Study of 'Mucoviscidosis,' " 154; Bodian, *Fibrocystic Disease of the Pancreas*, 67.

166. May, *Cystic Fibrosis of the Pancreas*, 4.

167. May, *Cystic Fibrosis of the Pancreas*, 4.

168. May, *Cystic Fibrosis of the Pancreas*, 16, 17.

169. Shwachman et al., "Mucoviscidosis," 272.

170. Shwachman et al., "Mucoviscidosis," 272.

171. Shwachman et al., "Mucoviscidosis," 259.

172. "Cystic Fibrosis—Diagnosis, Management and Prognosis," *Medical News*, November 17, 1958, 14, box 2, cystic fibrosis folder, Collection AC12, Boston Children's Hospital Archives.

173. "Cystic Fibrosis—Diagnosis, Management and Prognosis," 14.

174. National Cystic Fibrosis Research Foundation, Medical Information: Cystic Fibrosis Description Symptoms Diagnosis Treatment, 1965, 2–3, box 2, cystic fibrosis folder, Collection AC12, Boston Children's Hospital Archives.

175. National Cystic Fibrosis Research Foundation, Medical Information, 1965, 3.

176. National Cystic Fibrosis Research Foundation, Your Child and Cystic Fibrosis, undated, 1, box 2, cystic fibrosis folder, Collection AC12, Boston Children's Hospital Archives.

177. National Cystic Fibrosis Research Foundation, Medical Information, 1965, 12–13; Cystic Fibrosis Teaching, Research and Care Center Program grant application July 1, 1968–June 30, 1969, submitted to the Cleveland Cystic Fibrosis Foundation, MS 4245, container 4, folder 102, Health Fund of Greater Cleveland Records, Western Reserve Historical Society, Cleveland. Consistent with the foundation's assessment, Cleveland physicians were using the duodenal intubation test "only to resolve diagnostic problems" in the late 1960s, 2.

178. Aronowitz, *Unnatural History*; Greene, *Prescribing by Numbers*.

179. Shwachman et al., "Mucoviscidosis," 273.

180. Jim Gay, "Byron Is Fine Now: Another Birthday for 'Doomed' Boy," *Fort Lauderdale News*, September 19, 1957, 15.

Chapter Two

1. Karma Smith Belnap, *Not to Worry, Mom, I'm OK: Lessons in Living from a Beloved Son* (Covenant Communications, 1996), 3; Karma Smith Belnap, "Lee's Story," *Reader's Digest*, December 1998, 183.

2. Belnap, *Not to Worry, Mom*, 5.

3. Belnap, *Not to Worry, Mom*, 5.

4. Belnap, *Not to Worry, Mom*, 6.

5. Belnap, *Not to Worry, Mom*, 6. This recollection of the interpretation of the test highlights how even when parents or patients don't have the training required to interpret a test, they do have the ability to read the affect of the individuals carrying out the test.

6. *Guide to Diagnosis and Management of Cystic Fibrosis: A Syllabus for Physicians* (National Cystic Fibrosis Research Foundation, 1963), 1, 3.

7. P. B. Davis, "Cystic Fibrosis since 1938," *American Journal of Respiratory and Critical Care Medicine* 173, no. 5 (2006): 479, https://doi.org/10.1164/rccm.200505-840OE.

8. Belnap, *Not to Worry, Mom*, 7.

9. For a different example of a mismatch between clinical findings and test results, see D. Hilfiker, "Facing Our Mistakes," *New England Journal of Medicine* 310, no. 2 (1984), https://doi.org/10.1056/NEJM198401123100211.

10. Belnap, *Not to Worry, Mom*, 8. Additional sources of uncertainty distinct from the test itself included the age of the person undergoing the test, the time of year, and the existence of other medical conditions. For example, other conditions that can be associated with elevated electrolytes include "untreated adrenal insufficiency and untreated hypothyroidism." Marian W. Godbey, "Cystic Fibrosis in Adults," *Journal of the Mississippi State Medical Association* (June 1985): 162. P. B. Davis and P. A. di Sant'Agnese, "Diagnosis and Treatment of Cystic Fibrosis. An Update," *Chest* 85, no. 6 (1984): 803, https://doi.org/10.1016/s0012-3692(16)62421-2; B. J. Rosenstein et al., "Cystic Fibrosis: Diagnostic Considerations," *Johns Hopkins Medical Journal* 150, no. 3 (1982): 118, https://www.ncbi.nlm.nih.gov/pubmed/7038245; Maurice Kibel, "Sweat Tests in Cystic Fibrosis," *Lancet* 312, no. 8098 (1978), https://doi.org/10.1016/S0140-6736(78)92373-5. For more on time of year and salt intake, see P. Siegenthaler et al., "Salt Excretion in Sweat in Cystic Fibrosis," *JAMA* 186 (1963): 1178, https://doi.org/10.1001/jama.1963.03710130074023.

11. Morris Schaeffer, *Federal Legislation and the Clinical Laboratory* (G. K. Hall, 1981).

12. Diagnostic tests fall under the umbrella of medical devices. Arthur A. Daemmrich and Joanna Radin, *Perspectives on Risk and Regulation: The FDA at 100* (Chemical Heritage Foundation, 2007); Daniel P. Carpenter, *Reputation and Power: Organizational Image and Pharmaceutical Regulation at the FDA* (Princeton University Press, 2010); Greene, *Prescribing by Numbers*. For a history of chemical regulation, see Colleen Lanier-Christensen, "Toxic Rules: Chemical Regulation, International Trade, and the Epistemic Consequences of Standardized Practices" (PhD diss., Harvard University, 2023).

13. Physicians also looked to electrolyte levels in the hair, nails, and saliva as additional diagnostic approaches. For a discussion of the history of the sweat test, see Kerr, "Understanding Genetic Disease," 881.

14. L. E. Gibson and R. E. Cooke, "A Test for Concentration of Electrolytes in Sweat in Cystic Fibrosis of the Pancreas Utilizing Pilocarpine by Iontophoresis," *Pediatrics* 23, no. 3 (1959), https://www.doi.org/10.1542/peds.23.3.545.

15. Some of the earliest diagnostic tools, such as the thermometer and the stethoscope, also underwent many iterations. Dominguez et al., "Adoption of Thermometry"; Reiser, *Medicine and the Reign of Technology*, chapter 2; Stanley J Reiser, "Technology and the Use of the Senses in Twentieth-Century Medicine," in *Medicine and the Five Senses*, ed. W. F. Bynum and Roy Porter (Cambridge University Press, 1993), chapter 1.

16. Cystic Fibrosis Foundation, "GAP" Conference Reports: Problems in Sweat Testing, February 6–7, 1975, 6. H MS c201, box 15, folder 5, Mary Ellen Avery Papers, Francis A. Countway Library of Medicine, Center for the History of Medicine, Harvard Medical Library and Boston Medical Library. In the Nordic region in the 1950s, antibiotic susceptibility testing for diagnostic purposes was not standardized, and different results were often obtained depending on who did the testing. A. K. Lie, "Producing Standards, Producing the Nordic Region: Antibiotic Susceptibility Testing, from 1950–1970," *Science in Context* 27, no. 2 (2014): 220, https://doi.org/10.1017/s0269889714000052.

17. W. R. Kessler and D. H. Andersen, "Heat Prostration in Fibrocystic Disease of the Pancreas and Other Conditions," *Pediatrics* 8, no. 5 (1951): 648, https://doi.org/10.1542/peds.8.5.648. They referred to CF as fibrocystic disease of the pancreas. Judy J. Newmark, "Report on War Against Cystic Fibrosis," *St. Louis Post-Dispatch*, September 12, 1975, 2D.

18. Kessler and Andersen, "Heat Prostration," 649.

19. Kessler and Andersen, "Heat Prostration," 649.

20. Kessler and Andersen, "Heat Prostration," 650.

21. Kessler and Andersen, "Heat Prostration," 655.

22. Toby A. Appel, *Shaping Biology: The National Science Foundation and American Biological Research, 1945–1975* (Johns Hopkins University Press, 2000); Caroline Hannaway, *Biomedicine in the Twentieth Century: Practices, Policies, and Politics* (IOS Press, 2008); Angela N. H. Creager, *Life Atomic: A History of*

Radioisotopes in Science and Medicine (University of Chicago Press, 2013); William H. Schneider, "The Origin of the Medical Research Grant in the United States: The Rockefeller Foundation and the NIH Extramural Funding Program," *Journal of the History of Medicine and Allied Sciences* 70, no. 2 (2014), https://doi.org/10.1093/jhmas/jrt074.

23. The United Fruit Company had been particularly invested in celiac disease for marketing purposes ever since physician Sidney Haas published a paper about the value of the banana in the treatment of the disease in 1924. Abel, "The Rise and Fall of Celiac Disease"; Abel, *Gluten Free for Life*; Leigh Cook, "Area Victim of CF Outliving Most," *Asbury Park Press*, July 23, 1978, E10; "Children Won't Live Long So Get Special Christmas," *Beaver Dam Daily Citizen*, December 8, 1950, 1; "Doomed to Die," *Star Tribune*, November 28, 1948, 31.

24. There has been some debate about the assignment of credit for the discovery of the sweat electrolyte abnormality in CF. Paul A. di Sant'Agnese, "Experiences of a Pioneer Researcher: Discovery of the Sweat Electrolyte Defect and the Early Medical History of Cystic Fibrosis," in *Cystic Fibrosis in the 20th Century*; Christie and Tansey, *Cystic Fibrosis. Wellcome Witnesses*; Baird, *Dorothy Hansine Andersen*, chapter 13; "Season 1: The Pathologist in the Basement"; Newmark, "Report on War Against Cystic Fibrosis," 2D.

25. R. C. Darling et al., "Electrolyte Abnormalities of the Sweat in Fibrocystic Disease of the Pancreas," *American Journal of the Medical Sciences* 225, no. 1 (1953), https://www.ncbi.nlm.nih.gov/pubmed/13007698, 68. The study drew in part on Darling's prior work on chloride in sweat. R. C. Darling, "Some Factors Regulating the Composition and Formation of Human Sweat," *Archives of Physical Medicine and Rehabilitation* 29, no. 3 (1948), https://www.ncbi.nlm.nih.gov/pubmed/18910439. The United Fruit Company would continue to fund work by Dorothy Andersen and Paul di Sant'Agnese on idiopathic celiac disease in the 1950s. See Box 77, Folder 70, Idiopathic Celiac Disease United Fruit Co., Grants ca. 1920–1990, Archives and Special Collections, Health Sciences Library, Columbia University.

26. Darling et al., "Electrolyte Abnormalities," 68.

27. Darling et al., "Electrolyte Abnormalities"; P. di Sant'Agnese et al., "Abnormal Electrolyte Composition of Sweat in Cystic Fibrosis of the Pancreas," *American Journal of Diseases of Children* 86, no. 5 (1953), https://www.ncbi.nlm.nih.gov/pubmed/13103781.

28. P. A. di Sant'Agnese et al., "Abnormal Electrolyte Composition of Sweat in Cystic Fibrosis of the Pancreas: Clinical Significance and Relationship to the Disease," *Pediatrics* 12, no. 5 (1953), https://doi.org/10.1542/peds.12.5.549. In addition to measuring sweat electrolyte levels in people with CF and controls, the physicians also examined the sweat composition in the families of people with CF. P. A. di Sant'Agnese et al., "Sweat Electrolyte Disturbances Associated with Childhood Pancreatic Disease," *American Journal of Medicine* 15, no. 6 (1953), https://doi.org/10.1016/0002-9343(53)90169-7.

29. P. A. di Sant'Agnese, "Fibrocystic Disease of the Pancreas with Normal or Partial Pancreatic Function: Current Views on Pathogenesis and Diagnosis," *Pediatrics* 15, no. 6 (1955):695, https://doi.org/10.1542/peds.15.6.683.

30. Di Sant'Agnese, "Fibrocystic Disease of the Pancreas," 691; "Cystic Fibrosis of the Pancreas," *United States Navy Medical News Letter* 28, no. 8 (1956): 7.

31. Shwachman et al., "Mucoviscidosis," 279.

32. Shwachman et al., "Mucoviscidosis," 279.

33. D. H. Andersen, "Cystic Fibrosis of the Pancreas," *Journal of Chronic Diseases* 7, no. 1 (1958): 75, https://doi.org/10.1016/0021-9681(58)90185-1. For Shwachman's recollections, see Fanos, "We Kept Our Promises"; Charles G. Brooks, "Simple, Quick Test Spots Cystic Fibrosis," *Evening Star*, March 10, 1957, 25.

34. Shwachman et al., "Mucoviscidosis," 297, 322, reference 114; P. Toltzis, "50 Years Ago in the Journal of Pediatrics: The Sweat Test in Cystic Fibrosis: A Comparison of Overnight Sweat Collection Versus the Pilocarpine Iontophoresis Method," *Journal of Pediatrics* 175 (2016): 73, https://doi.org/10.1016/j.jpeds.2016.02.062.

35. Shwachman et al., "Mucoviscidosis," 297.

36. G. J. Barbero et al., "A Simplified Technique for the Sweat Test in the Diagnosis of Fibrocystic Disease of the Pancreas," *Pediatrics* 18, no. 2 (1956): 189, https://doi.org/10.1542/peds.18.2.189.

37. Barbero et al., "Simplified Technique for the Sweat Test," 191.

38. Andersen, "Cystic Fibrosis of the Pancreas," 75.

39. K. A. Misch and H. M. Holden, "Sweat Test for the Diagnosis of Fibrocystic Disease of the Pancreas: Report of a Fatality," *Archives of Disease in Childhood* 33, no. 168 (1958): 179, https://doi.org/10.1136/adc.33.168.179.

40. Misch and Holden, "Report of a Fatality," 180.

41. G. J. Barbero, "Diagnosis of Cystic Fibrosis of the Pancreas," *Pediatrics* 24 (1959): 664, https://www.ncbi.nlm.nih.gov/pubmed/13796594; Gibson, "A New Era in Diagnosis."

42. H. Shwachman and N. Gahm, "Studies in Cystic Fibrosis of the Pancreas: A Simple Test for the Detection of Excessive Chloride on the Skin," *New England Journal of Medicine* 255, no. 21 (1956), https://doi.org/10.1056/NEJM195611222552107. In addition to the chloride plate test, other simple screening tests for CF were developed in the 1950s. Barbero, "Diagnosis of Cystic Fibrosis of the Pancreas"; L. Gluck, "A Patch Test for Chloride in Sweat as a Simple Screening Method for Detecting Cystic Fibrosis of the Pancreas: Preliminary Report," *Pediatrics* 23, no. 4 (1959), https://doi.org/10.1542/peds.23.4.731.

43. Shwachman and Gahm, "Simple Test for Detection of Excessive Chloride," 999.

44. In the case of an infant, the foot could be used. To prepare the chloride test medium, silver nitrate and potassium chromate were added to agar before the solution was poured into the Petri dish and allowed to solidify.

45. The chloride plate test, as described by Shwachman and Gahm, did not

include wrapping the hand in a plastic bag for one hour to induce sweating, as was recalled by Lee Smith Belnap's mother.

46. Shwachman and Gahm, "Simple Test for Detection of Excessive Chloride," 999; Roberts, *Difficult Diagnosis*, 48–49, 758.

47. As the investigators note, "the large number of +++ reactions in parents and siblings is in accord with the genetic data indicating that these individuals represent the heterozygote, assuming that one gene is involved in the transmission of this disease as a mendelian recessive," and "in 2 previously unrecognized cases a +++ reaction in siblings led to the diagnosis of the disease." Shwachman and Gahm, "Simple Test for Detection of Excessive Chloride," 999, 1001.

48. Shwachman and Gahm, "Simple Test for Detection of Excessive Chloride," 1000. By 1981, Shwachman clearly considered the chloride plate test to be a screening test that needed to be followed by a quantitative sweat test. H. Shwachman and A. Mahmoodian, "Reappraisal of the Chloride Plate Test as Screening Test for Cystic Fibrosis," *Archives of Disease in Childhood* 56, no. 2 (1981), https://doi.org/10.1136/adc.56.2.137.

49. Commission on Chronic Illness, *Chronic Illness in the United States, Volume I, Prevention of Chronic Illness* (Harvard University Press, 1957), 45. For more on the commission, see George Weisz, *Chronic Disease in the Twentieth Century: A History* (Johns Hopkins University Press, 2014).

50. "Clues to Disease Found: Here Are Symptoms of Cystic Fibrosis," *Linton Daily Citizen*, July 4, 1957, 4B; "Sweating Is Clue to Deadly Child's Malady," *Portsmouth Times*, August 1, 1957; "New Test 'Fingerprints' a Ruthless Disease of Childhood," *Ladies' Home Journal*, May 1957.

51. Trivedi, *Breath from Salt*; Steven Epstein, "Patient Groups and Health Movements," in *Handbook of Science and Technology Studies*, ed. E. J. Hackett (MIT Press, 2008). Basil O'Connor, president of the National Foundation for Infantile Paralysis (NFIP), provided guidance to those involved in the early years of the National Cystic Fibrosis Research Foundation. Graub and Graub, "Origin and Development of the Cystic Fibrosis Foundation." This was also a time when the American Cancer Society had messaging such as "only you can prevent cancer" and "with a check-up and a check." Aronowitz, *Unnatural History*, 163.

52. Brooks, "Simple, Quick Test Spots Cystic Fibrosis," 25.

53. National News Bulletin: Published Monthly by the National Cystic Fibrosis Research Foundation, January 1957, 4, box 204, folder Cystic Fibrosis #1 1955–1957 May, Joseph Stokes, Jr. Papers: Series VI. Diseases and Treatment, Mss.B.St65p, American Philosophical Society. The news bulletin described the chloride plate test as both a "NEW DIAGNOSTIC TEST" and something that could be used to "screen all the members of an average public school in half an hour."

54. "Clues to Disease Found," 4B. For other accounts of the chloride plate test in the US, Canada, and South Africa, see Walter C. Alvarez, "Cystic Fibrosis Foundation Established: New Test Found for Childhood's Killer," *Sante Fe New*

Mexican, April 28, 1957, 3; "Fight Aims at Disease of Children," *Austin American*, February 9, 1958, B10; Peter Desbarats, "City Doctors Battle Incurable Malady: Mark of Baby's Hand Reveals Disease," *Winnipeg Tribune*, November 24, 1956, 11; P. Catzel, "The Finger-Print Sweat Test," *South African Medical Journal* 32, no. 12 (1958), https://www.ncbi.nlm.nih.gov/pubmed/13543484.

55. J. R. Starke, "Universal Screening for Tuberculosis Infection. School's Out!," *JAMA* 274, no. 8 (1995), https://doi.org/10.1001/jama.1995.03530080068043; Barron H. Lerner, *Contagion and Confinement: Controlling Tuberculosis Along the Skid Road* (Johns Hopkins University Press, 1998).

56. Wynne Sharples, A Message from the President: Notes on Progress and Accomplishments ~1958, box 205, folder Cystic Fibrosis #3 1958 Jan-Apr, Cystic Fibrosis 1955–1964, Joseph Stokes, Jr. Papers: Series VI. Diseases and Treatment, Mss.B.St65p, American Philosophical Society, 7; National Cystic Fibrosis Research Foundation News Bulletin, October 1958, box 205, folder Cystic Fibrosis #4 1958 May-Dec, Cystic Fibrosis 1955-1964, Joseph Stokes, Jr. Papers: Series VI. Diseases and Treatment, Mss.B.St65p, American Philosophical Society, 5; "Cystic Fibrosis Tests for Tots," *Philadelphia Tribune*, November 8, 1958.

57. L. L. Kulczycki et al., "A Survey of School Children for Cystic Fibrosis," *American Journal of Diseases of Children* 10 (1960), https://doi.org/10.1001/archpedi.1960.04020040176004. Described as "a large industrial city approximately 45 miles west of Boston containing many groups of second and third generation settlers from various European countries," it is possible that the investigators chose this town because of the widespread assumptions at the time about the relationship between CF and race. Kulczycki et al., "A Survey of School Children for Cystic Fibrosis," 175. Just a few years earlier, Harry Shwachman and colleagues noted that although CF had been seen "in many racial groups," they had observed a "high incidence of the disease in children of French-Canadian, Irish, and English stock" in their Boston hospital. Shwachman et al., "Mucoviscidosis," 251. Also in the mid-1950s, Paul di Sant'Agnese had remarked that "cystic fibrosis has striking racial predilections," occurring "equally in all groups of the white race," but rarely or not at all in other racialized groups. P. A. di Sant'Agnese, "Cystic Fibrosis of the Pancreas," *American Journal of Medicine* 21, no. 3 (1956): 406, https://doi.org/10.1016/0002-9343(56)90040-7.

58. The bag sweat test was the primary quantitative test used in this study.

59. Kulczycki et al., "A Survey of School Children for Cystic Fibrosis," 179.

60. L. W. Matthews et al., "A Therapeutic Regimen for Patients with Cystic Fibrosis," *Journal of Pediatrics* 65 (1964): 559, https://doi.org/10.1016/s0022-3476(64)80290-0; Lindee, Before the Gene; M. L. LaBonte, "The Mist Tent: An Analysis of Therapeutic Change in the History of Cystic Fibrosis Care," *Bulletin of the History of Medicine* 92, no. 4 (2018), https://doi.org/10.1353/bhm.2018.0074.

61. As Andersen noted in a 1958 publication, "the simplicity of this method recommends it but the reliability has not yet been adequately tested." Andersen, "Cystic Fibrosis of the Pancreas," 75. For examples of false negative chloride plate

tests, see Misch and Holden, "Report of a Fatality," 180; "Case Records of the Massachusetts General Hospital; Case 44092," *New England Journal of Medicine* 258, no. 9 (1958): 447, https://doi.org/10.1056/NEJM195802272580909. For a discussion about challenges interpreting the chloride plate test, see Barbero, "Diagnosis of Cystic Fibrosis of the Pancreas," 661.

62. Joan Beck, "Jeannie's Fight for Life: 4 Year Old a Victim of Cystic Fibrosis," *Chicago Daily Tribune*, September 22, 1960, G3.

63. Beck, "Jeannie's Fight for Life," G3.

64. Beck, "Jeannie's Fight for Life," G3.

65. Beck, "Jeannie's Fight for Life," G3.

66. Beck, "Jeannie's Fight for Life," G3.

67. Beck, "Jeannie's Fight for Life," G3.

68. Beck, "Jeannie's Fight for Life," G3.

69. Beck, "Jeannie's Fight for Life," G3.

70. Barbero, "Diagnosis of Cystic Fibrosis of the Pancreas," 662.

71. Barbero, "Diagnosis of Cystic Fibrosis of the Pancreas," 662–63.

72. A. M. Mauer and C. D. West, "A Simple Method for Collection and Analysis of Sweat for Chloride," *JAMA Pediatrics* 92, no. 2 (1956), https://doi.org/10.1001/archpedi.1956.02060030154009.

73. Gibson and Cooke, "A Test for Electrolytes in Sweat." According to Gibson, his supervisor at the NIH "was interested in finding if CF carriers had abnormal sweat and suggested (strongly) that I sweat test some parents" using the bag sweat test. Gibson recalled that "these adventures made me think that iontophoresis might be a great advance for the diagnosis of CF." Gibson, "A New Era in Diagnosis," 58; "Johns Hopkins: Trailblazing Johns Hopkins Pediatrician Force Behind Head Start Program, Dies at Age 93," *ENP Newswire*, February 18, 2014.

74. Timmermans and Berg, *The Gold Standard*, 27.

75. D. S. Jones and S. H. Podolsky, "The History and Fate of the Gold Standard," *Lancet* 385, no. 9977 (2015): 1503, https://doi.org/10.1016/S0140-6736(15)60742-5.

76. Gibson and Cooke, "A Test for Electrolytes in Sweat."

77. Gibson and Cooke, "A Test for Electrolytes in Sweat." mEq/L, a measure of electrolyte concentration, refers to milliequivalents per liter.

78. E. Elian et al., "Intestinal Obstruction of the Newborn Infant. Usefulness of the Sweat Electrolyte Test in Differential Diagnosis," *New England Journal of Medicine* 264 (1961): 13, https://doi.org/10.1056/NEJM196101052640104. The specific adaptation was not indicated. They did mention one safety concern associated with this test, noting the development of "small superficial burns" in three cases in which the electrode directly contacted the skin.

79. Robert P. Clark, "Cystic Fibrosis Fund Drive Is Set: Mysterious Disease Kills Many Children," *Courier-Journal*, September 10, 1961, 16. While the Gibson–Cooke test was not mentioned in this newspaper article, the image suggests that this test, or an adaptation of it, was used.

80. "Big Name, Little Machine: New Unit Eases Diagnosis of CF," *Austin American*, September 17, 1961, B11.

81. "Funds Given for Unit at Hospital," *Daily Evening Item*, November 21, 1963; "Doctors to Speak at Cystic Fibrosis Meeting," *Independent-Record*, February 3, 1965; "Equipment Donated," *Shreveport Journal*, April 1, 1965; "Lab Gets Pathology Machine," *Quad-City Times*, July 12, 1968. Both of Lee's parents were involved in the formation of an Idaho chapter of the National Cystic Fibrosis Research Foundation in 1964, and his parents each served as chapter president early on. "Fight Posed on Disease of Children," *Idaho Statesman*, December 30, 1964, 8; "To New York," *Idaho Daily Statesman*, February 23, 1968, 10.

82. *Guide to Diagnosis and Management of Cystic Fibrosis*, 21.

83. *Guide to Diagnosis and Management of Cystic Fibrosis*, 25; P. M. Farrell and R. E. Koscik, "Sweat Chloride Concentrations in Infants Homozygous or Heterozygous for F508 Cystic Fibrosis," *Pediatrics* 97, no. 4 (1996), https://pubmed.ncbi.nlm.nih.gov/8632940/. Other tests, such as nasal transepithelial voltage measurements, have been used to clarify diagnoses in people with normal sweat test results in the setting of clinical symptoms and two *CFTR* gene mutations. Barbara Stewart et al., "Normal Sweat Chloride Values Do Not Exclude the Diagnosis of Cystic Fibrosis," *American Journal of Respiratory and Critical Care Medicine* 151 (1995), https://doi.org/10.1164/ajrccm/151.3_Pt_1.899.

84. Harry Shwachman and Lucas L. Kulczycki, "This Week's Citation Classic," *Current Contents/Clinical Medicine* 26, June 29 (1987), 18.

85. Maria Fátima Servidoni et al., "Sweat Test and Cystic Fibrosis: Overview of Test Performance at Public and Private Centers in the State of São Paulo, Brazil," *Jornal Brasileiro de Pneumologia* 43, no. 2 (2017), https://doi.org/10.1590/s1806-37562016000000076; Marco Salvatore et al., "The Italian Pilot External Quality Assessment Program for Cystic Fibrosis Sweat Test," *Clinical Biochemistry* 49, no. 7–8 (2016), https://doi.org/10.1016/j.clinbiochem.2015.12.014; Davide Treggiari et al., "Role of Sweat Ion Ratios in Diagnosing Cystic Fibrosis," *Pediatric Pulmonology* 56, no. 7 (2021), https://doi.org/10.1002/ppul.25395; Ambika Shenoy et al., "Newborn Screening for Cystic Fibrosis: Infant and Laboratory Factors Affecting Successful Sweat Test Completion," *International Journal of Neonatal Screening* 7, no. 1 (2020), https://doi.org/10.3390/ijns7010001.

86. "New Test Devised for Cystic Fibrosis," *JAMA* 192, no. 2 (1965): 26, https://doi.org/10.1001/jama.1965.03080150120055.

87. Vincent Gerald Stine, "Regulating Laboratory Testing: The Policy Cycle of CLIA '88" (PhD diss., University of Maryland Baltimore County, 2005), 73. Robert P. Goldman and Sid Ross, "A Scandal That Threatens Your Health," *Independent Press-Telegram*, July 11, 1961; Oscar Godbout, "Unethical Medical Laboratories Face Curbs in City Crackdown," *New York Times*, October 10, 1960.

88. Schaeffer, *Federal Legislation and the Clinical Laboratory*, xvi, xvii. Schaeffer

was the assistant commissioner of health and general director of laboratories in the City of New York from 1959 to 1971. Discussing concerns about the lack of proper regulation of laboratories in most states in 1967, Schaeffer noted that "in some cases, [laboratories] are doing a so-called sink test, which means they pour the patient's sample down the sink and turn in a negative report." Faye Marley, "Official Asks Laws for Medical Labs," *The Record*, February 11, 1967, A27; Wolfgang Saxon, "Morris Schaeffer, 89, Virologist Who Tightened Controls on Labs," *New York Times*, March 25, 1997, B7.

89. Stine, "Regulating Laboratory Testing," 71.

90. Schaeffer, *Federal Legislation and the Clinical Laboratory*, xxiii; Clinical Laboratories Improvement Act of 1967, Publ. L. 90-174, 81 Stat. 536, Sec. 5.

91. Furthermore, according to historian Christoph Gradmann, the FDA was attempting to regulate diagnostics at least as early as the 1960s in the context of discs for antibiotic susceptibility determination. Despite pushback that such regulation was not within the FDA's jurisdiction, a 1969 Supreme Court ruling that the FDA could regulate the discs used for antibiotic susceptibility testing suggests that the court was acknowledging the FDA's role in regulating diagnostics at that point. Christoph Gradmann, "Sensitive Matters: The World Health Organisation and Antibiotic Resistance Testing, 1945–1975," *Social History of Medicine* 26, no. 3 (2013): 561, https://doi.org/10.1093/shm/hkt018.

92. According to Timmermans and Berg, the first few decades of the twentieth century focused on standardizing the environment in which medical practice occurred, followed by a relative lull in interest in standardization until the late 1980s, when "standardization gradually reemerged as a focal point of interest in the health care field" as it related to the practice of medicine. Timmermans and Berg, *The Gold Standard*, 13. Referring to the Pap smear, Casper and Clark note that "the search for means of standardization has been long, arduous and not particularly successful." M. J. Casper and A. E. Clarke, "Making the Pap Smear into the 'Right Tool' for the Job," *Social Studies of Science* 28, no. 2 (1998): 273, https://doi.org/10.1177/030631298028002003.

93. J. D. Cece et al., "Pancreatic Cystic Fibrosis in an Adult," *JAMA* 181 (1962): 32, https://doi.org/10.1001/jama.1962.03050270033006.

94. Based on this patient, as well as other cases in the medical literature, the investigators noted that "a spectrum of severity may be present as shown by *formes frustes* of the disease and varying degrees of organ involvement." Cece et al., "Pancreatic Cystic Fibrosis in an Adult," 31.

95. Cece et al., "Pancreatic Cystic Fibrosis in an Adult," 33. The sweat chloride concentration was 162 mEq/L and the sweat sodium concentration was 180 mEq/L.

96. The Children's Hospital Medical Center Annual Report, 1964, https://archive.org/details/childrenshospita1964chil/, 41.

97. "New Test Devised for Cystic Fibrosis," 26. The CF gene was not characterized until 1989, but its existence was inferred.

98. "New Test Devised for Cystic Fibrosis," 26. "Diagnostic Aids," *Naugatuck Daily News*, October 21, 1966, 2. As Lewis Gibson noted years later, "it is not generally appreciated that the measurement of the concentration of salt in fingernails is actually a modified sweat test" because the "salt in the nails comes primarily from sweat glands and may be eluted out with distilled water." L. E. Gibson, "The Decline of the Sweat Test. Comments on Pitfalls and Reliability," *Clinical Pediatrics* 12, no. 7 (1973): 450, https://doi.org/10.1177/000992287301200817.

99. W. J. Warwick and L. Hansen, "The Silver Electrode Method for Rapid Analysis of Sweat Chloride," *Pediatrics* 36, no. 2 (1965), https://doi.org/10.1542/peds.36.2.261.

100. Warwick and Hansen, "Silver Electrode Method," 262. With this method, controls were found to have chloride concentrations of 30 mEq/L or lower, whereas people with CF had chloride concentrations of 55 mEq/L or higher. W. J. Warwick, "Cystic Fibrosis Sweat Test for Newborns," *JAMA* 198, no. 1 (1966), https://doi.org/10.1001/jama.198.1.177.

101. Walter Eldot, "Free Sweat Test for Ely Children Almost Like Party," *Duluth News Tribune*, May 15, 1966.

102. Eldot, "Almost Like Party," 7.

103. Eldot, "Almost Like Party."

104. Warwick and Hansen, "Silver Electrode Method."

105. Cystic Fibrosis, revised shooting script for a motion picture for the National Cystic Fibrosis Research Foundation by John Mackenzie, January 16, 1967, Shwachman 2/2, vertical subject and biographical files, Boston Children's Hospital Archives. For an account of the film, including images, see George J. Mannina, "NIAMD Scientists Featured in Training Film on Cystic Fibrosis," *NIH Record*, April 18, 1967, 8.

106. Mannina, "NIAMD Scientists Featured in Training Film," 8.

107. Narration based on the film transcript (not the film itself). "Cystic Fibrosis Revised Shooting Script," 14. Emphasis added.

108. "Dr. Jack Masur Escorts Presidential Party on Tour of Clinical Center Facilities," *NIH Record*, August 10, 1967, 5.

109. Frank Deford, *Alex: The Life of a Child* (Viking Press, 1983), 20.

110. Gibson, "The Decline of the Sweat Test." 450.

111. Gibson, "The Decline of the Sweat Test," 452. Emphasis added.

112. Gibson, "The Decline of the Sweat Test," 450.

113. "Cystic Fibrosis Revised Shooting Script," 13. It is unclear who wrote this note on the film transcript.

114. "GAP Problems in Sweat Testing," 6. According to an earlier GAP conference report on the CF factor, the "purpose of the GAP Conference Program" was "to assemble a limited group of investigators to informally discuss their own studies, as well as to point up possible new leads arising from their own work or from that of others, and to consider the application of new techniques to existent

problems." National Cystic Fibrosis Research Foundation, GAP Conference Reports: Cystic Fibrosis Factor, February 19–20, 1971, 4, Countway Library, Harvard Medical School; Reflections: 1975–1976 Annual Financial Report, Cystic Fibrosis Foundation, Bethesda.

115. In the opening remarks, conference chair Lewis Gibson emphasized that the sweat test had gained "widespread acceptance" in the 1960s, yet it had been associated with an increasing number of "erroneous results" since that time. "GAP Problems in Sweat Testing," 6.

116. "GAP Problems in Sweat Testing," 5.

117. It also appears that the use of the Gibson–Cooke test was declining over the first half of the 1970s. According to a 1970 questionnaire study done by physician Alexander Spock involving physicians in North Carolina, South Carolina, Tennessee, and Virginia, 10 percent used bag tests, 13 percent used Orion ion specific electrodes, 21 percent used a heat lab, 28 percent used the palm test, and 29 percent used the quantitative pilocarpine iontophoresis test. "GAP Problems in Sweat Testing."

118. The chloride plate test was referred to as the palm test in the conference report. In addition, although Warren Warwick presented evidence that the electrode test was of comparable accuracy to the Gibson–Cooke method, many conference attendees found that the electrode was not reliable in their hands, and its use was discouraged. "GAP Problems in Sweat Testing."

119. Underlining in original. "GAP Problems in Sweat Testing," 13.

120. *Clinical Laboratories Improvement Act, Hearings on S. 1737 Before the Subcommittee on Health of the Committee on Labor and Public Welfare*, 94th Congress, 1st Sess. (September 8–9, 1975). For a critique of government regulation of laboratory testing, see F. W. Sunderman, Sr., "The History of Proficiency Testing/Quality Control," *Clinical Chemistry* 38, no. 7 (1992), https://doi.org/10.1093/clinchem/38.7.1205.

121. "Report of the Committee for a Study for Evaluation of Testing for Cystic Fibrosis," *Journal of Pediatrics* 88, no. 4 (1976), https://doi.org/10.1016/S0022-3476(76)81041-4.

122. "Study for Evaluation of Testing," 724. In fact, the committee convened a workshop "for engineers, manufactures, and clinicians to discuss the intricacies of performing and interpreting the test and ideas for improving its instrumentation," 720.

123. "Study for Evaluation of Testing," 712.

124. The term "sweat test" was often used in a general sense to refer to a wide range of tests, including the Gibson–Cooke test, that measured sweat electrolyte concentrations. In addition to noting problems with sweat test method or technique, some physicians pointed out that "the sweat test, even if carried out by an experienced technician, sometimes lacks reproducibility owing presumably to physiological variations (patient's diet, temperature, and other factors at

present unrecognized)." V. Schwarz et al., "Limitations of Diagnostic Value of the Sweat Test," *Archives of Disease in Childhood* 52, no. 11 (1977): 870, https://doi.org/10.1136/adc.52.11.870. However, other physicians stressed that patient variation was only a very minor factor accounting for error in sweat testing and instead pointed to laboratory error as the most significant problem. C. A. Smalley et al., "Limitations of the Sweat Test," *Archives of Disease in Childhood* 53, no. 4 (1978), https://doi.org/10.1136/adc.53.4.351.

125. B. J. Rosenstein et al., "Cystic Fibrosis. Problems Encountered with Sweat Testing," *JAMA* 240, no. 18 (1978), https://doi.org/10.1001/jama.240.18.1987. The majority of these misdiagnoses were false positive results.

126. Rosenstein et al., "Problems Encountered with Sweat Testing," 1988. Misdiagnoses came with significant health implications.

127. G. Timothy Johnson, "Health," *Atlanta Constitution*, January 5, 1979, 3B.

128. Johnson, "Health," 3B.

129. Johnson, "Health," 3B.

130. John L. Columbo and Gordon E. Gibbs, "Cystic Fibrosis and Erroneous Sweat Tests," *Nebraska Medical Journal* (June 1979): 164.

131. Columbo and Gibbs, "Erroneous Sweat Tests," 164. The same CF center noted that a child who had a negative sweat test at another facility tested positive using the Gibson–Cooke method at their facility, and a "non-CF child with a previous result of 155 done elsewhere" had a result at the Nebraska CF center of 17 mEq/L.

132. Columbo and Gibbs, "Erroneous Sweat Tests," 165.

133. In 1981, a Rhode Island physician noted that "inaccurate collection, analysis, or interpretation of sweat electrolytes continues to be a significant clinical problem" in the diagnosis of CF. Mary Ann Passero, "Physician Responsibility for Sweat Test Accuracy," *Rhode Island Medical Journal* 64 (1981), 23. Despite referring to the sweat test as "the best method," Shwachman and colleagues note that "unfortunately, the sweat test, whether performed by the recommended method or by other methods, has been shown to be unreliable in many instances." H. Shwachman et al., "The Sweat Test: Sodium and Chloride Values," *Journal of Pediatrics* 98, no. 4 (1981): 576, https://doi.org/10.1016/s0022-3476(81)80764-0; Rosenstein et al., "Cystic Fibrosis: Diagnostic Considerations."

134. H. Lewis Webster and Clark A. Rundell, "Laboratory Diagnosis of Cystic Fibrosis," *CRC Critical Reviews in Clinical Laboratory Sciences* 18, no. 4 (1982), https://doi.org/10.3109/10408368209085074.

135. Webster and Rundell, "Laboratory Diagnosis of Cystic Fibrosis," 314.

136. K. B. Hammond et al., "Clinical Evaluation of the Macroduct Sweat Collection System and Conductivity Analyzer in the Diagnosis of Cystic Fibrosis," *Journal of Pediatrics* 124, no. 2 (1994): 255, https://doi.org/10.1016/s0022-3476(94)70314-0.

137. S. B. Fitzpatrick et al., "Diagnosis of Cystic Fibrosis During Adolescence," *Journal of Adolescent Health Care* 7, no. 1 (1986): 39, https://doi.org/10.1016/s0197-0070(86)80093-6.

138. *P & S: The Yearbook of the College of Physicians and Surgeons, Columbia University*, 1960, https://babel.hathitrust.org/cgi/pt?id=nnc2.ark:/13960/t6f202000, 68.

139. Jerry E. Hendon, *It's Been a Good Life, Dad: My Son's Struggle with Cystic Fibrosis* (iUniverse, 2016), 4.

140. Hendon, *It's Been a Good Life, Dad*, 4.

141. Hendon, *It's Been a Good Life, Dad*, 4.

142. Hendon, *It's Been a Good Life, Dad*, 5, 7.

143. La Versa Motes, "Costly Treatments, Rigorous Care for Xenia Baby with CF," *Xenia Daily Gazette*, November 5, 1971, 20.

144. Motes, "Costly Treatments, Rigorous Care," 20.

145. Charles F. Orthwein, "Mucoviscidosis: A Study of Its Clinical Features and a Review of 51 Cases," *Journal of the Kansas Medical Society* (February 1957), 122; Virginia S. and John S., oral history interview with the author, June 19, 2020; O'Hara, interview.

146. Peter N. Stearns, *Anxious Parents: A History of Modern Childrearing in America* (New York University Press, 2003), 32–34; Brittany Cowgill, Rest Uneasy: Sudden Infant Death Syndrome in Twentieth-Century America (Rutgers University Press, 2018). Wynne Sharples may have had a different experience given her training as a physician. As she noted in 1960, "let [the mother] be sure to tell her baby doctor of symptoms that worry her," and "together they may know the satisfaction of saving a child's life." Tom Sellers, "Child Killer Hits Here," *Columbus Ledger*, June 26, 1960, 4.

147. For more on race and CF, see Wailoo and Pemberton, *Troubled Dream of Genetic Medicine*. For "medical stereotyping" in CF based on race, see Roberts, *Fatal Invention*, 99.

148. L. L. Kulczycki et al., "Cystic Fibrosis in Negro Children: Results of a Search," *Clinical Pediatrics* 3 (1964): 699, https://doi.org/10.1177/000992286400301202. For assumptions about the relationship between CF and race, see W. W. Zuelzer and W. A. Newton Jr., "The Pathogenesis of Fibrocystic Disease of the Pancreas: A Study of 36 Cases with Special Reference to the Pulmonary Lesions," *Pediatrics* 4, no. 1 (1949): 53, https://doi.org/10.1542/peds.4.1.53; "Cystic Fibrosis of the Pancreas," 6; Warwick, "Cystic Fibrosis Sweat Test for Newborns," 177; James C. G. Conniff, "Child Killer at Bay," *Austin American*, January 30, 1966, SM4. For an example of CF initially not being considered in a patient with symptoms consistent with the disease because of assumptions about race, see A. Pileggi, "Cystic Fibrosis in a Negro," *Delaware Medical Journal* 34 (1962): 98, https://www.ncbi.nlm.nih.gov/pubmed/14486627.

149. Kulczycki et al., "Cystic Fibrosis in Negro Children," 699; Shwachman et al., "Mucoviscidosis," 251.

150. Kulczycki et al., "Cystic Fibrosis in Negro Children." Lucas Kulczycki, who had been involved in the Worcester school study in 1958, was one of the physicians involved in this study.

151. Kulczycki et al., "Cystic Fibrosis in Negro Children," 701. In the years following the DC study, other physicians also sought to identify CF in underrepresented groups. Ella H. Oppenheimer and John R. Esterly, "Cystic Fibrosis in Non-Caucasian Patients," *Pediatrics* 42 (1968), https://doi.org/10.1542/peds.42.3.547a; E. T. Heffer, "Cystic Fibrosis in Black Population," *New York State Journal of Medicine* 74, no. 13 (1974), https://www.ncbi.nlm.nih.gov/pubmed/4530924; L. L. Kulczycki and V. Schauf, "Cystic Fibrosis in Blacks in Washington, DC: Incidence and Characteristics," *American Journal of Diseases of Children* 127, no. 1 (1974), https://doi.org/10.1001/archpedi.1974.02110200066009; R. C. Stern et al., "Course of Cystic Fibrosis in Black Patients," *Journal of Pediatrics* 89, no. 3 (1976), https://doi.org/10.1016/S0022-3476(76)80538-0; C. W. Lober et al., "Cystic Fibrosis in a Black Woman," *JAMA* 235, no. 11 (1976), https://doi.org/10.1001/jama.1976.03260370048034.

152. Kulczycki et al., "Cystic Fibrosis in Negro Children," 701.

153. Wailoo and Pemberton, *Troubled Dream of Genetic Medicine*; Roberts, *Fatal Invention*; Braun, *Breathing Race into the Machine*.

154. "National Association of African Americans with Cystic Fibrosis," https://noaacf.org; Rita Rubin, "Tackling the Misconception That Cystic Fibrosis Is a 'White People's Disease,'" *JAMA* 325, no. 23 (2021), https://doi.org/10.1001/jama.2021.5086.

155. "Terry Wright's CF Story," https://noaacf.org/terry-wrights-cf-story.

156. Rubin, "Tackling the Misconception," E1.

157. Rubin, "Tackling the Misconception."

158. Conniff, "Child Killer at Bay," SM4.

159. Conniff, "Child Killer at Bay," SM4.

160. Conniff, "Child Killer at Bay," SM4.

161. Karma Belnap, "How She Faces a Frightening Present and Future: Boise Mother Writes About Cystic Fibrosis," *Idaho Statesman*, April 3, 1969, 11.

162. Belnap, "How She Faces a Frightening Present and Future," 11.

163. Belnap, "How She Faces a Frightening Present and Future," 11.

164. Karma Belnap, "Organizing Available Resources: The Fight Against Cystic Fibrosis," *Idaho Daily Statesman*, April 8, 1969, 9.

165. Karma Belnap, "Doctors Learn How to Detect Cystic Fibrosis," *Idaho Daily Statesman*, April 4, 1969, 9.

Chapter Three

Some material in this chapter was originally published in Michelle Lynne LaBonte, "Addressing Uncertainty: The Emergence of the CRMS/CFSPID Diagnostic Category Following Newborn Screening for Cystic Fibrosis," *OBM Genetics* 5, no. 3 (2021), https://doi.org/10.21926/obm.genet.2103139.

1. Jim Nichols, "Ignorance Isn't Bliss," *Dayton Daily News*, April 20, 1980, 93.

2. Nichols, "Ignorance Isn't Bliss," 93.

3. Nichols, "Ignorance Isn't Bliss," 93.

4. Nichols, "Ignorance Isn't Bliss," 93.

5. Nichols, "Ignorance Isn't Bliss," 93.

6. Nichols, "Ignorance Isn't Bliss," 93. Nikki's name appears to be spelled incorrectly (as Nicki) in the 1980 article. Bucky Albers, "Sopga Readies for 4 Opens," *Dayton Daily News*, May 23, 1998, 5D; Bucky Albers, "Hickman Returns to Play U.S. Open Qualifier," *Dayton Daily News*, May 19, 1996, 5D.

7. Cystic Fibrosis Foundation Annual Report, 1980, Cystic Fibrosis Foundation, Bethesda.

8. Nichols, "Ignorance Isn't Bliss," 93.

9. Nichols, "Ignorance Isn't Bliss," 93.

10. Nichols, "Ignorance Isn't Bliss," 93.

11. Reiser, *Medicine and the Reign of Technology*; B. H. Lerner, "Great Expectations: Historical Perspectives on Genetic Breast Cancer Testing," *American Journal of Public Health* 89, no. 6 (1999), https://doi.org/10.2105/ajph.89.6.938; Gerald N. Grob, *Aging Bones: A Short History of Osteoporosis* (Johns Hopkins University Press, 2014); Aronowitz, *Risky Medicine*; B. Linker, "A Dangerous Curve: The Role of History in America's Scoliosis Screening Programs," *American Journal of Public Health* 102, no. 4 (2012), https://doi.org/10.2105/AJPH.2011.300531.

12. S. J. Reiser, "The Emergence of the Concept of Screening for Disease," *Milbank Memorial Fund Quarterly. Health and Society* 56, no. 4 (1978): 403, https://www.ncbi.nlm.nih.gov/pubmed/366456; Stanley Joel Reiser, *Technological Medicine: The Changing World of Doctors and Patients* (Cambridge University Press, 2009), 145.

13. Reiser, "Screening for Disease," 405.

14. Reiser, "Screening for Disease," 414.

15. Reiser, "Screening for Disease," 416.

16. Diane B. Paul and Jeffrey P. Brosco, *The PKU Paradox: A Short History of a Genetic Disease* (Johns Hopkins University Press, 2013).

17. Lindee, *Moments of Truth*, chapter 2; Grob, *Testing Baby*; Michael S. Watson et al., "Newborn Screening: Toward a Uniform Screening Panel and System," *Genetics in Medicine* 8, suppl. 1, no. 5 (2006), https://doi.org/10.1097/01.gim.0000223891.82390.ad; Michael S. Watson et al., "Main Report," *Genetics in Medicine* 8, suppl. 1, no. 5 (2006), https://doi.org/10.1097/01.gim.0000223467.60151.02; Timmermans and Buchbinder, *Saving Babies?*; Vailly, *Birth of a Genetics Policy*; "State Looking into Screening Programs," *Daily Press*, June 8, 1977, A4.

18. J. M. G. Wilson and Gunnar Jungner, *Principles and Practice of Screening for Disease* (World Health Organization, 1968), 7.

19. Wilson and Jungner, *Screening for Disease*, 21. For a discussion of criteria for screening for "asymptomatic disease" in adults, see P. S. Frame and S. J. Carlson,

"A Critical Review of Periodic Health Screening Using Specific Screening Criteria. Part 1: Selected Diseases of Respiratory, Cardiovascular, and Central Nervous Systems," *Journal of Family Practice* 2, no. 1 (1975).

20. Wilson and Jungner, *Screening for Disease*, 21.

21. Wilson and Jungner, *Screening for Disease*, 26, 27.

22. Paul and Brosco, *PKU Paradox, 193*.

23. John D. Lloyd-Still, "Newborn Screening Tests," in *Textbook of Cystic Fibrosis*, ed. Lloyd-Still (John Wright and PSG, 1983); P. G. Robinson and R. B. Elliott, "Rapid Semiquantitative Tests for Trypsin and Chymotrypsin Application to Screening for Cystic Fibrosis, Enterokinase Deficiency and Pancreatic Hypoplasia in Neonates," *New Zealand Medical Journal* 79, no. 517 (1974), https://www.ncbi.nlm.nih.gov/pubmed/4527956; Farrell et al., "Cystic Fibrosis Diagnostic Challenges"; B. S. Danes and A. G. Bearn, "Oyster Ciliary Inhibition by Cystic Fibrosis Culture Medium," *Journal of Experimental Medicine* 136, no. 5 (1972), https://doi.org/10.1084/jem.136.5.1313; Robert J. Beall and Sherry L. Keramidas, "The Role of a Voluntary Health Agency in Public and Professional Education in Genetic Diseases and Genetic Screening," *Perspectives in Genetic Counseling* 4, no. 3 (1982).

24. "Study for Evaluation of Testing," 711. Recall from Chapter 2 that the committee was also tasked with evaluating diagnostic sweat tests.

25. "Study for Evaluation of Testing," 731.

26. "Kiss Your Baby to Detect CF," 13.

27. Elliott, "Wrinkling of Skin," 108.

28. J. R. Crossley et al., "Dried-Blood Spot Screening for Cystic Fibrosis in the Newborn," *Lancet* 1, no. 8114 (1979), https://doi.org/10.1016/s0140-6736(79)90825-0.

29. Cystic Fibrosis: A Plea for a Future. Volume 3. Appendices, Appendix 1: Working Group Reports, 1978, Cystic Fibrosis Foundation, 1. For more about the role of the NIH in the history of this report, see Cystic Fibrosis: A Plea for a Future. Volume 1. Exectuive Summary, 1.

30. "A Plea for a Future," 1.

31. Heinrich Fischer, *Das Buch vom Aberglauben* (im Schwickertschen Verlage, 1790), 137; Hermann Heinrich Ploss, *Das Kind in Brauch und Sitte der Völker* (A. Auerbach, 1876), 142. For more on early accounts of salty skin, see P. Trouvé et al., "Cystic Fibrosis: A Journey Through Time and Hope," *International Journal of Molecular Sciences* 25, no. 17 (2024), https://doi.org/10.3390/ijms25179599.

32. Hortense Myers, "Salty Kiss Is Symptom," *The Republic*, September 21, 1962, 7.

33. Conniff, "Child Killer at Bay," SM5. Italics in original.

34. For a discussion of the use of taste in diagnostics, see Robert Tattersall, *Diabetes: The Biography* (Oxford University Press, 2009), chapter 1.

35. Aronowitz, *Unnatural History*, chapter 6; Barron H. Lerner, *The Breast Cancer Wars: Hope, Fear, and the Pursuit of a Cure in Twentieth-Century America* (Oxford University Press, 2001), chapter 3. Information about Kiss Your Baby campaigns was included in the Cystic Fibrosis Health Education Unit that immediately

preceded the Breast Self-Examination unit in the 1980 Medical and Health Annual. Alvin N. Eden, "Health Education Unit 14: Cystic Fibrosis," in *1980 Medical and Health Annual*, ed. Ellen Bernstein (Encyclopaedia Britannica, 1979).

36. "Kissing Your Baby Is Cystic Fibrosis Test," *Rock Island Argus*, May 4, 1978, 17; Jan Plamper, *The History of Emotions: An Introduction* (Oxford University Press, 2015).

37. Elaine Tyler May, *Homeward Bound: American Families in the Cold War Era* (Basic Books, 2008).

38. "'Healthy' Kisses," *Frederick News Post*, May 2, 1977, 5.

39. "Kiss Baby Week," *Journal and Courier*, April 26, 1973, 4; Proclamation for Cystic Fibrosis Kiss Your Baby Week, May 6–13, 1973, executive order signed April 23, 1973, Otis R. Bowen and Larry A. Conrad, State of Indiana, Executive Department, Indianapolis, Otis Bowen Museum and Archives.

40. "'Kiss Your Baby Week' Aids Cystic Fibrosis," *Times-Mail*, May 10, 1973, 22. As noted in an article in the *Times-Mail* in 1974, the Indiana chapter "was given the 'Best Public Education Award' by the National Foundation in May, 1974," for its Kiss Your Baby Week. "Cystic Fibrosis Group Changes Corporate Name," *Times-Mail*, November 20, 1974, 22.

41. This claim is based on a search of newspapers.com in 2025.

42. "Kiss Your Baby to Detect CF," 13; "Chairperson Named," *New Journal and Guide*, December 1, 1978.

43. "Kiss Your Baby to Detect CF," 13. For similar language, see "Kiss Can Detect Cystic Fibrosis," *Dixon Evening Telegraph*, August 10, 1974, 6; "CF Diagnosis: Early Is Best," *Austin Statesman*, September 23, 1973, B9.

44. Bonnie Britton, "Early Diagnosis Vital: Kiss Can Spot Cystic Fibrosis," *Indianapolis Star*, May 5, 1974, 112; "Cystic Fibrosis Group to Direct Fund Drive," *Jackson Sun*, September 22, 1975, 3; "Mrs. Roberts Is Chairman of 'Kiss Your Baby Week,'" *Kokomo Tribune*, April 16, 1975, 9; "When Is a Kiss Not Just a Kiss?," *PR Newswire*, February 2, 1989.

45. Pam Peglow, "Treat 250 Iowans for Cystic Fibrosis," *Carrol Daily Times Herald*, March 4, 1975, 8. For additional accounts in the mid-1970s, see "Awareness Needed to Prevent Cystic Fibrosis," *Opinion-Tribune*, May 8, 1974, 2; "Kiss Your Baby; It Could Save His Life," *Cuero Daily Record*, August 22, 1975, 3; Herbert Black, "'Dr. Cystic Fibrosis' to Retire, but His Search Will Go On," *Boston Globe*, April 11, 1976, 46; and "Mrs. Miller to Head Local Kiss a Baby Campaign," *Williamson County Sun*, July 29, 1976, 8.

46. Jean Tyson, "The Kiss Test: Salty Taste of Baby's Skin May Mean CF," *Atlanta Constitution*, November 13, 1977, 5G.

47. Tyson, "The Kiss Test," 5G. For other accounts of the "nervous mother," see Portia Scott-Brookins, "CF Patients Speak Out on Their Problems," *Atlanta Daily World*, September 12, 1982, 1; Jenn Whinnem, "I Have Cystic Fibrosis and This Is What I Have to Say About Five Feet Apart," *Medium.com*, November 26, 2018.

48. Tyson, "The Kiss Test," 5G.

49. Mickey Flowers, "Mother's Kiss Helped Diagnosis of CF," *The Sentinel*, June 12, 1975, 22.

50. Flowers, "Mother's Kiss," 22.

51. Flowers, "Mother's Kiss," 22.

52. Flowers, "Mother's Kiss," 22.

53. For examples, see "Cystic Fibrosis Foundation," advertisement, *The Exceptional Parent*, June 1975, 23, "Naegle Gets State Award," *Columbus Times*, April 18, 1984, 6 (poster), Bob Talbert, "Namedrops: George and Athena Hanzakos," *Detroit Free Press*, February 12, 1981, 31 (bumper sticker), and "Daytime Programs: Good Morning, Detroit," *Detroit Free Press*, February 12, 1979, 9B, and "Detroit Today," *Detroit Free Press* (1981), 44 (TV broadcast), "'A Kiss for Life,'" *The Daily Item*, November 24, 1977, E4 (dinner dance). For additional awareness efforts, see "Kiss Your Baby," advertisement, *Detroit Free Press*, February 8, 1982, 7A; "A Kiss Can Save a Life," advertisement, *Washington Post*, February 2, 1983, B5; and "It's Kiss Your Baby Week," advertisement, *Detroit Free Press*, February 13, 1984, 7. "Parental Alert to Cystic Fibrosis Set," *Thousand Oaks Star*, September 12, 1984, 31.

54. Display ad 42, *Hartford Courant*, September 9, 1975, 13.

55. Display ad 42, 13. A similar advertisement was placed in the *Los Angeles Times* in 1980, in which the same baby and woman were featured in a slightly different position, with the baby's hand lowered and the woman kissing the baby's forehead. See Display ad 40, *Los Angeles Times*, September 9, 1980, OC_A4. For similar ads placed in the *Los Angeles Times*, see Display ad 93, *Los Angeles Times*, September 11, 1979, OC_C7, and Display ad 57, *Los Angeles Times*, September 8, 1981, OC_A6.

56. "'A Kiss for Life,'" E4.

57. Leanne Ciampa Hadley, *Touching Heaven: Real Stories of Children, Life, and Eternity* (Revell, 2013), 65. This account is not dated, but the event likely occurred in the 1970s or 1980s.

58. Hadley, *Touching Heaven*, 65.

59. Tyson, "The Kiss Test," 5G.

60. Stand-alone photo 3, *Chicago Tribune*, October 26, 1977, 16. President Jimmy Carter met with Cystic Fibrosis Foundation poster child Robbyn Foxx in June 1977 in the Oval Office of the White House (and he met with several other poster children in the years before and after). Joseph A. Lastelic, "Poster Girl Gets a Peek into Amy's Tree House," *Kansas City Times*, June 9, 1977, 14A.

61. "People: Baby-Kissing for Health," *Newsday*, October 26, 1977, 9.; "Names in the News," *The Gazette*, October 27, 1977, 41; "Kiss Can Signal Cystic Fibrosis," *York Daily Record*, October 27, 1977, 13; "Rosalynn Demonstrates the Kiss Test," *Honolulu Advertiser*, October 26, 1977, 52.

62. "Kiss Your Baby," *Honolulu Star-Bulletin*, November 18, 1977, 53; "Insurance Women Receive Recognition," *Laurel Leader Call*, June 28, 1980, 7; Cystic Fibrosis Foundation Annual Report 1982, 15, Cystic Fibrosis Foundation, Bethesda.

63. "People: Kissing for a Record, and a Cause," *Newsday*, May 7, 1978, 11; Michael Kernan, "The Kiss," *Washington Post*, February 14, 1984; Steven Prokesch, "Longest Kiss Time Recorded," *New Castle News*, May 8, 1978.

64. Earl Bohn, *Associated Press*, May 6, 1978; "Smoochers Break a World Record," *Valley Morning Star*, May 7, 1978, 11. The event was sponsored by the Western Pennsylvania chapter of the CF Foundation.

65. "A Kiss for Cystic Fibrosis," *Washington Post*, October 8, 1981; "Naegle Gets State Award," 6; Cheryl Fincher, "Cystic Fibrosis Testing Is Simply a Kiss," *Macon News*, September 23, 1982, 2B; Luiane Lee, "Rivers Unpacks Her Salty Humor Once More," *Kokomo Tribune*, August 24, 1989, 11; Bob Talbert, "A Hot Detroiter and Some Sizzling Sounds," *Detroit Free Press*, January 17, 1987, 10C; "CF? Detroit Lions Star Urges 'Kiss Your Baby,' " *Marshall Chronicle*, February 5, 1987, 3.

66. Benjamin Spock, *Baby and Child Care* (Hawthorn Books, 1976), 538; Benjamin Spock and Michael B. Rothenberg, *Baby and Child Care* (Pocket Books, 1985), 620. While cystic fibrosis is described in the 1968 and 1991 editions, kissing a baby to detect elevated salt is not referenced. In addition, Spock's texts directed parents to the Cystic Fibrosis Foundation for additional information.

67. "ABC's Rebecca Jarvis Interviews Emily," https://www.youtube.com/watch?v=PQiJ1QzGt-E, September 20, 2021.

68. Robert Beall, email message to Michelle LaBonte, August 30, 2025.

69. Judy B. Rollins, "Cystic Fibrosis Camp Gives 'Family' Support," *Salt Lake Tribune*, September 21, 1980, 4W.

70. "A Salty-Tasting Kiss Was Warning Sign That Alerted Sharps to Cystic Fibrosis," *Union Appeal*, September 17, 1980, 1.

71. Jan Aylsworth, "Family Learns to Accept, Cope with Cystic Fibrosis," *Evansville Courier*, September 21, 1980, 6B.

72. Bob Talbert, "Kiss Your Baby," *Detroit Free Press*, February 8, 1980, 11B.

73. Talbert, "Kiss Your Baby," 11B.

74. Talbert, "Kiss Your Baby," 11B.

75. Asia McDonald, "One of Our Bravest Students," *Detroit Free Press*, October 21, 2003, 2C.

76. Consumer Health Education: A Directory by the U.S. Department of Health, Education, and Welfare, 1976, DHEW Publication (HRA) 77–607, 29. The CF Foundation was also involved in campaigns to educate physicians about CF in the 1950s. Ben Zinser, "Children's Malady: Expert Reveals Progress in Cystic Fibrosis," *Independent*, September 13, 1957, C1.

77. Wanda Walker, "Gayla and Cystic Fibrosis: A Salty Kiss Was Her Salvation," *Marshall News Messenger*, November 13, 1977, C1(17).

78. Walker, "Gayla and Cystic Fibrosis," C1.

79. Walker, "Gayla and Cystic Fibrosis," C1.

80. Walker, "Gayla and Cystic Fibrosis," C1.

81. Mary McCarty, "His Spirit Persevered Despite His 'Relentless Disease,'" *Dayton Daily News*, November 18, 2001, 1B.

82. McCarty, "His Spirit Persevered," 1B.

83. Robert Beall, email message to Michelle LaBonte, August 30, 2025.

84. Robert Beall, email message to Michelle LaBonte, August 30, 2025.

85. For examples of additional awareness efforts, see "Kiss Your Baby," advertisement, 7A, "A Kiss Can Save a Life," display ad 28, B5; "It's Kiss Your Baby Week," advertisement, 7; "Parental Alert to Cystic Fibrosis Set," 31. For more on subjectivity and taste, see S. Shapin, "The Sciences of Subjectivity," *Social Studies of Science* 42, no. 2 (2012), https://doi.org/10.1177/0306312711435375; S. Shapin, "A Taste of Science: Making the Subjective Objective in the California Wine World," *Social Studies of Science* 46, no. 3 (2016), https://doi.org/10.1177/0306312716651346.

86. Lucius Duncan Bulkley, *On the Relations of Diseases of the Skin to Internal Disorders, with Observations on Diet, Hygiene and General Therapeutics* (Rebman, 1906); Kurt Wiener, *Skin Manifestations of Internal Disorders (Dermadromes)* (Mosby, 1947), 7.

87. Bulkley, *Diseases of the Skin*, 152; "Lucius Duncan Bulkley, M.D. 1845–1928," *Archives of Dermatology* 18, no. 5 (1928), https://doi.org/10.1001/archderm.1928.02380170111011.

88. J. Maxwell Rogoski, *Skins of Commerce: An Epidermal Tour through American Medicine and Markets, 1900–1970* (PhD diss, University of Pennsylvania, 2019), 15. Italics in original.

89. Wiener, *Skin Manifestations of Internal Disorders*; Maurice J. Reuter, "Kurt Wiener, M.D. 1891–1960," *Archives of Dermatology* 82, no. 3 (1960), https://doi.org/10.1001/archderm.1960.01580030125028.

90. Wiener, *Skin Manifestations of Internal Disorders*, 8. Wiener defined dermadrome as "literally, fellow traveler on the skin."

91. For reviews, see "Book of the Month—A Report: Skin Manifestations of Internal Disorders," *Postgraduate Medicine*, no. 6 (1947); H. Haldin-Davis, "Reviews: Dermadromes," *British Medical Journal* 1, no. 4563 (1948); "Book Notices: Skin Manifestations of Internal Disorders (Dermadromes) by Kurt Wiener," *JAMA* 136, no. 1 (1948); I. Davidsohn, "Skin Manifestations of Internal Disorders (Dermadromes)," *American Journal of Clinical Pathology* 18, no. 5 (1948), https://doi.org/10.1093/ajcp/18.5.406; J. G. Downing, "Dermatology," *New England Journal of Medicine* 240, no. 8 (1949), https://doi.org/10.1056/NEJM194902242400805.

92. P. A. di Sant'Agnese, "Book Reviews: Skin Manifestations of Internal Disorders (Dermadromes) by Kurt Wiener," *Pediatrics* 2, no. 6 (1948), 750. At that time, di Sant'Agnese was a physician at Babies Hospital in New York. Baird, *Dorothy Hansine Andersen*.

93. For more on the heat wave, see Kessler and Andersen, "Heat Prostration." For additional examples of the value of skin changes in the diagnostic process, see J. S. Collings and D. M. Clark, "General Practice, Today and

Tomorrow," *New England Journal of Medicine* 248, no. 5 (1953), https://doi.org/10.1056/NEJM195301292480505; H. Beerman and C. H. Greenbaum, "Some Aspects of the Relationship of Cutaneous and Gastrointestinal Disorders; A Review of Recent Literature," *American Journal of the Medical Sciences* 234, no. 4 (1957), https://www.ncbi.nlm.nih.gov/pubmed/13469812; "Book Reviews: Difficult Diagnosis: A Guide to the Interpretation of Obscure Illness by H. J. Roberts," *JAMA* 172, no. 2 (1960); "Book Review of the Skin and Internal Disease by Sture A. M. Johnson," *Archives of Internal Medicine* 122, no. 2 (1968); Harry B. Greenberg, "The Book Forum: The Skin and Internal Disease by Sture A. M. Johnson," *JAMA* 205, no. 3 (1968); Robert W. Goltz, "Book Review: Skin Signs of Systemic Disease by Irwin Braverman," *New England Journal of Medicine* 287, no. 14 (1972), https://doi.org/10.1056/NEJM197210052871427.

94. H. Beerman, "The Skin and Internal Disease," *Southern Medical Journal* 59, no. 5 (1966): 528, https://doi.org/10.1097/00007611-196605000-00005.

95. Robert A. Aronowitz, "Lyme Disease: The Social Construction of a New Disease and Its Social Consequences," *Milbank Quarterly* 69, no. 1 (1991), https://www.ncbi.nlm.nih.gov/pubmed/2034186, 80; Arthur M. Ginzler and T. T. Fox, "Disseminated Lupus Erythematosus: A Cutaneous Manifestation of a Systemic Disease (Libman-Sacks): Report of a Case," *Archives of Internal Medicine* 65, no. 1 (1940), https://doi.org/10.1001/archinte.1940.00190070036003; Jerome E. Groopman and Michael S. Gottlieb, "Kaposi's Sarcoma: An Oncologic Looking Glass," *Nature* 299, no. 5879 (1982), https://doi.org/10.1038/299103a0; Claudia Hernandez and Anna L. Bruckner, "Focus on 'Covid Toes,'" *Archives of Dermatology* 156, no. 9 (2020), https://doi.org/10.1001/jamadermatol.2020.2062. For an analysis of skin color and dermatological findings, see LaShyra Nolen, "How Medical Education Is Missing the Bull's-Eye," *New England Journal of Medicine* 382, no. 26 (2020), https://doi.org/10.1056/NEJMp1915891, 2491.

96. Lisa Arkin, oral history interview with the author, October 19, 2021.

97. R. B. Elliott, "A 60 Year Voyage in Cystic Fibrosis," Cystic Fibrosis NZ, October 31, 2018, https://www.cfnz.org.nz/news-and-events/latest-news/a-60-year-voyage-in-cystic-fibrosis.

98. Elliott, "60 Year Voyage."

99. Elliott, "Wrinkling of Skin," 108; Robinson and Elliott, "Rapid Semiquantitative Tests for Trypsin and Chymotrypsin."

100. Elliott, "60 Year Voyage."

101. A. P. Norman et al., "Skin Wrinkling in Cystic Fibrosis," *Lancet* 2, no. 7876 (1974): 358, https://doi.org/10.1016/S0140-6736(74)91746-2.

102. Norman et al., "Skin Wrinkling in Cystic Fibrosis," 358. Children in this study were exposed to "hot water."

103. L. Park et al., "Aquagenic Wrinkling of the Palms and the Potential Role for Genetic Testing," *Pediatric Dermatology* 29, no. 3 (2012): 237, https://doi.org/10.1111/j.1525-1470.2011.01609.x. Park and colleagues specifically referenced a

1975 paper by Martin Johns (see below), who studied children from the Hospital for Sick Children in London described in the 1974 Norman et al. paper.

104. E. J. Moynahan, "Skin Wrinkling in Cystic Fibrosis," *Lancet* 2, no. 7885 (1974), https://doi.org/10.1016/s0140-6736(74)91249-5, 907; M. Weinstein et al., "Skin Wrinkling and Nerve Function," *Lancet* 2, no. 7885 (1974), https://doi.org/10.1016/s0140-6736(74)91250-1, 907.

105. C. Economou-Mavrou et al., "Skin Wrinkling in Cystic Fibrosis," *Lancet* 2, no. 7886 (1974): 953, https://doi.org/10.1016/s0140-6736(74)91155-6.

106. Economou-Mavrou et al., "Skin Wrinkling in Cystic Fibrosis," 953.

107. R. B. Elliott, "Skin Wrinkling in Cystic Fibrosis," *Lancet* 2, no. 7893 (1974): 1383, https://doi.org/10.1016/s0140-6736(74)92249-1.

108. Elliott, "Skin Wrinkling in Cystic Fibrosis," 1383. Elliott also noted that "Mr. P. Nobbs, a student of mine, kindly observed the wrinkling to eliminate bias."

109. Elliott, "Skin Wrinkling in Cystic Fibrosis," 1383.

110. M. K. Johns, "Skin Wrinkling in Cystic Fibrosis," *Medical & Biological Illustration* 25, no. 4 (1975), https://www.ncbi.nlm.nih.gov/pubmed/1228347. Johns' credentials are listed as AIIP, ARPS, AIMBI.

111. Johns, "Skin Wrinkling in Cystic Fibrosis," 207. Of interest, "initially experiments were carried out with cold water, when it was found that the phenomenon occurred in the same way but took longer to do so."

112. Johns, "Skin Wrinkling in Cystic Fibrosis," 207, 209.

113. Johns, "Skin Wrinkling in Cystic Fibrosis," 210.

114. As Johns noted, "the greatest difficulty in producing these pictures was in the case of neonates, and here the problem was solved by testing the feet and photographing the plantar surface." However, "the wrinkling was very slight in all the neonates tested and it was very difficult to assess it at the time of the test" such that "the photographs very often reversed the initial assessment of presence and degree of wrinkling" of newborn's feet." Johns, "Skin Wrinkling in Cystic Fibrosis," 209–10.

115. It is unclear whether CF physicians in other regions were aware of Elliott's article. Reflecting on the mid-1970s studies more than three decades later, German dermatologists noted that "at that time, large-scale studies on the relevance of this cutaneous symptom were not performed, and over the last 30 years the association had been neglected." C. S. Seitz et al., "Painful Wrinkles in the Bathtub: Association with Hyperhidrosis and Cystic Fibrosis," *Dermatology* 216, no. 3 (2008): 225–26, https://doi.org/10.1159/000112929. In 1984, investigators from Scotland noted that skin wrinkling following water exposure was decreased in people with diabetes. C. V. Clark et al., "Decreased Skin Wrinkling in Diabetes Mellitus," *Diabetes Care* 7, no. 3 (1984), https://doi.org/10.2337/diacare.7.3.224.

116. Crossley et al., "Dried-Blood Spot Screening"; J. R. Crossley et al., "Neonatal Screening for Cystic Fibrosis, Using Immunoreactive Trypsin Assay in Dried Blood Spots," *Clinica Chimica Acta* 113, no. 2 (1981), https://doi.org/10.1016/0009-08981(81)90145-5.

117. E. Elias et al., "Diagnostic Importance of Changes in Circulating Concentrations of Immunoreactive Trypsin," *Lancet* 2, no. 8028 (1977), https://doi.org/10.1016/s0140-6736(77)90066-6.

118. Elias et al., "Diagnostic Importance," 66.

119. The radioimmunoassay test could detect both "trypsin or its pro-enzyme trypsinogen." Elias et al., "Diagnostic Importance," 67.

120. Creager, *Life Atomic*, chapter 8; Angela Creager, "Molecular Surveillance: A History of Radioimmunoassays," in *Crafting Immunity: Working Histories of Clinical Immunology* (Taylor & Francis, 2008), 201.

121. Elias et al., "Diagnostic Importance," 68.

122. Crossley et al., "Dried-Blood Spot Screening."

123. Elliott, "60 Year Voyage."

124. Elliott, "60 Year Voyage"; D. J. H. Brock, "Screening," in *Cystic Fibrosis*, ed. M. Hodson and D. Geddes (Oxford University Press, 2000), 189.

125. Crossley et al., "Dried-Blood Spot Screening," 472.

126. Joanna Radin, *Life on Ice: A History of New Uses for Cold Blood* (University of Chicago Press, 2017).

127. Crossley et al., "Dried-Blood Spot Screening," 473.

128. J. R. Crossley et al., "Cystic-Fibrosis Screening in the Newborn," *Lancet* 2, no. 8048 (1977), https://doi.org/10.1016/s0140-6736(77)90543-8; P. M. Farrell et al., "The Impact of the *CFTR* Gene Discovery on Cystic Fibrosis Diagnosis, Counseling, and Preventive Therapy," *Genes* 11, no. 4 (2020), https://doi.org/10.3390/genes11040401; G. Travert et al., "History of Newborn Screening for Cystic Fibrosis-the Early Years," *International Journal of Neonatal Screening* 6, no. 1 (2020), https://doi.org/10.3390/ijns6010008; U. Stephan et al., "Cystic Fibrosis Detection by Means of a Test-Strip," *Pediatrics* 55, no. 1 (1975), https://www.ncbi.nlm.nih.gov/pubmed/803309; H. Kollberg and K. Hellsing, "Screening for Cystic Fibrosis by Analysis of Albumin in Meconium," *Acta Paediatrica Scandinavica* 64, no. 3 (1975), https://doi.org/10.1111/j.1651-2227.1975.tb03868.x.

129. Travert et al., "The Early Years."

130. D. N. King et al., "Sensitive Trypsin Assay for Dried-Blood Specimens as a Screening Procedure for Early Detection of Cystic Fibrosis," *Lancet* 2, no. 8154 (1979), https://doi.org/10.1016/s0140-6736(79)92336-5.

131. Jeanette Crossley, Neonatal Screening—All Aspects, comment to James Littlewood, https://cysticfibrosis.online/neonatal-screening.

132. Crossley, comment to Littlewood.

133. Crossley, comment to Littlewood.

134. Crossley et al., "Neonatal Screening for Cystic Fibrosis." Their assay measured the level of trypsinogen.

135. Crossley et al., "Neonatal Screening for Cystic Fibrosis," 114.

136. Crossley et al., "Neonatal Screening for Cystic Fibrosis," 116.

137. A second blood sample was requested only if two independent measurements of the original bloodspot at five days following birth registered an

immunoreactive trypsinogen value of greater than 250 AU/l. AU stands for arbitrary unit.

138. Crossley et al., "Neonatal Screening for Cystic Fibrosis," 118.

139. They referred to rates of false positive and false negative test results.

140. N. Binney et al., "On the Origin of Sensitivity and Specificity," *Annals of Internal Medicine* 174, no. 3 (2021), https://doi.org/10.7326/M20-5028; Löwy, "Testing for a Sexually Transmissible Disease."

141. Wilson and Jungner, *Screening for Disease*.

142. Wilson and Jungner, *Screening for Disease*, 22.

143. A. M. Brandt, "AIDS in Historical Perspective: Four Lessons from the History of Sexually Transmitted Diseases," *American Journal of Public Health* 78, no. 4 (1988), https://doi.org/10.2105/ajph.78.4.367; P. D. Cleary et al., "Compulsory Premarital Screening for the Human Immunodeficiency Virus. Technical and Public Health Considerations," *JAMA* 258, no. 13 (1987), https://www.ncbi.nlm.nih.gov/pubmed/3476759; L. O. Gostin et al., "The Case Against Compulsory Casefinding in Controlling AIDS—Testing, Screening and Reporting," *American Journal of Law & Medicine* 12, no. 1 (1987), https://doi.org/10.1017/S0098858800007401.

144. Crossley et al., "Neonatal Screening for Cystic Fibrosis," 119.

145. Crossley et al., "Neonatal Screening for Cystic Fibrosis," 111. Their assay measured the level of trypsinogen.

146. Crossley et al., "Neonatal Screening for Cystic Fibrosis," 120.

147. K. B. Hammond et al., "Efficacy of Statewide Neonatal Screening for Cystic Fibrosis by Assay of Trypsinogen Concentrations," *New England Journal of Medicine* 325, no. 11 (1991), https://doi.org/10.1056/nejm199109123251104; Joanne Cono et al., "Newborn Screening for Cystic Fibrosis: A Paradigm for Public Health Genetics Policy Development. Proceedings of a 1997 Workshop," *Morbidity and Mortality Weekly Report* 46, no. RR-16 (1997), https://www.ncbi.nlm.nih.gov/pubmed/9408048; Farrell, interview; S. D. Grosse et al., "Newborn Screening for Cystic Fibrosis: Evaluation of Benefits and Risks and Recommendations for State Newborn Screening Programs," *Morbidity and Mortality Weekly Report* 53, no. RR-13 (2004), https://www.ncbi.nlm.nih.gov/pubmed/15483524.

148. "Neonatal Screening for Cystic Fibrosis: Position Paper," *Pediatrics* 72, no. 5 (1983), https://www.ncbi.nlm.nih.gov/pubmed/6634283.

149. "Neonatal Screening for Cystic Fibrosis," 743.

150. "Neonatal Screening for Cystic Fibrosis," 743.

151. "Neonatal Screening for Cystic Fibrosis," 742, 744. Capitalization in original.

152. J. K. Sharp and M. J. Rock, "Newborn Screening for Cystic Fibrosis," *Clinical Reviews in Allergy & Immunology* 35, no. 3 (2008): 109, https://doi.org/10.1007/s12016-008-8082-1; S. Chatfield et al., "Neonatal Screening for Cystic Fibrosis in Wales and the West Midlands: Clinical Assessment after Five Years of Screening," *Archives of Disease in Childhood* 66, no. 1 (1991), https://doi.org/10.1136/adc.66.1_spec_no.29; Jennifer L. Macalister-Hall, "The Development of a Low-

Cost Immunoradiometric Assay for the Early Detection of Cystic Fibrosis Using Monoclonal Antibodies" (PhD diss., University of Aberdeen, 1988).

153. B. Wilcken et al., "Cystic Fibrosis Screening by Dried Blood Spot Trypsin Assay: Results in 75,000 Newborn Infants," *Journal of Pediatrics* 102, no. 3 (1983): 386, https://doi.org/10.1016/s0022-3476(83)80653-2.

154. Beryl J. Rosenstein and Terry S. Langbaum, "Diagnosis," in *Cystic Fibrosis*, ed. Lynn M. Taussig (Thieme-Stratton, 1984), 109.

155. Rosenstein and Langbaum, "Diagnosis," 105.

156. Philip M Farrell, "Chapter 9: Neonatal Screening: Toward Earlier Diagnosis and Improved Outcomes," in *Cystic Fibrosis in the 20th Century*, ed. Carl F. Doershuk (AM Publishing, 2001). The study was funded by the Cystic Fibrosis Foundation and the National Institutes of Health. N. Fost and P. M. Farrell, "A Prospective Randomized Trial of Early Diagnosis and Treatment of Cystic Fibrosis: A Unique Ethical Dilemma," *Clinical Research* 37, no. 3 (1989), https://www.ncbi.nlm.nih.gov/pubmed/2673641; "CF Receives Grant to Develop Neonatal Testing," *Baraboo News Republic*, December 18, 1984; 6. Philip M. Farrell, "Reflections on 50 Years of Cystic Fibrosis Newborn Screening Experience with Critical Perspectives, Assessment of Current Status, and Predictions for Future Improvements," *International Journal of Neonatal Screening* 11, no. 4 (2025), https://doi.org/10.3390/ijns11040088. A study in the UK was also initiated in 1985. Sharp and Rock, "Newborn Screening for Cystic Fibrosis," 109.

157. Philip Farrell, oral history interview with Clement Ren, American Academy of Pediatrics Section on Pediatric Pulmonology and Sleep Medicine, January 20, 2021, 13.

158. Norman Fost, oral history interview with Robert Lange, April 3, 2009, UW-Madison Oral History Program, http://Digital.Library.Wisc.Edu/1793/82616. For more on the controversy surrounding the trial, see Sharon Begley, "Case Involving Tests on Newborns Shows Need for Strict Ethics," *Wall Street Journal*, May 3, 2002; J. Menikoff, "The Involuntary Research Subject," *Cambridge Quarterly of Healthcare Ethics* 13, no. 4 (2004), https://doi.org/10.1017/s0963180104134051; M. P. Gordon, "A Legal Duty to Disclose Individual Research Findings to Research Subjects?," *Food and Drug Law Journal* 64, no. 1 (2009).

159. Farrell interview with Clement Ren, 12.

160. *Healthy Children: Investing in the Future*, OTA-H-345, Office of Technology Assessment, US Congress, US Government Printing Office, 1988; Travert et al., "The Early Years."

161. Thomas P. Carter and Ann M. Willey, *Genetic Disease: Screening and Management: Proceedings of the 1985 Albany Birth Defects Symposium* (Liss, 1986), xii.

162. Doris L. Wethers, "Screening the Newborn for Sickle Cell Disease: Is It Worth the Effort?," in *Genetic Disease: Screening and Management: Proceedings of the 1985 Albany Birth Defects Symposium* (Liss, 1986), 123. For more on concerns

about sickle cell screening programs, see *Genetic Screening: Procedural Guidance and Recommendations*, Committee for the Study of Inborn Errors of Metabolism, National Research Council, National Academy of Sciences, 1975; Wailoo, *Dying in the City of the Blues*.

163. Wethers, "Screening the Newborn for Sickle Cell Disease: Is It Worth the Effort?," 123.

164. Robert Guthrie, "Newborn Screening: Past, Present and Future," in *Genetic Disease: Screening and Management: Proceedings of the 1985 Albany Birth Defects Symposium* (Liss, 1986), 334.

165. Guthrie, "Newborn Screening," 334.

166. M. J. Rock et al., "Immunoreactive Trypsinogen Screening for Cystic Fibrosis: Characterization of Infants with a False-Positive Screening Test," *Pediatric Pulmonology* 6, no. 1 (1989): 42, https://doi.org/10.1002/ppul.1950060111.

167. M. J. Rock et al., "Newborn Screening for Cystic Fibrosis Is Complicated by Age-Related Decline in Immunoreactive Trypsinogen Levels," *Pediatrics* 85, no. 6 (1990): 1004, https://doi.org/10.1542/peds.85.6.1001. For an account of international discussions about IRT-based screening around this time, see Travert et al., "The Early Years."

168. Rock et al., "Age-Related Decline in Immunoreactive Trypsinogen," 1004.

169. Rock et al., "Age-Related Decline in Immunoreactive Trypsinogen," 1004–1005.

170. Rock et al., "Age-Related Decline in Immunoreactive Trypsinogen"; B. L. Therrell Jr. et al., "Immunoreactive Trypsinogen (IRT) as a Biomarker for Cystic Fibrosis: Challenges in Newborn Dried Blood Spot Screening," *Molecular Genetics and Metabolism* 106, no. 1 (2012), https://doi.org/10.1016/j.ymgme.2012.02.013.

171. Beryl J. Rosenstein, "IVth International Conference on Newborn Screening for Cystic Fibrosis: Concluding Remarks," *Pediatric Pulmonology* 11, no. S7 (1991): 85, https://doi.org/10.1002/ppul.1950110717.

172. Rosenstein, "IVth International Conference," 85; Mary E. Heeley et al., "The International Quality Assurance Program (IRTIQAS) for the Assay of Immunoreactive Trypsin in Dried Blood Spots," *Pediatric Pulmonology* 11, no. S7 (1991), https://doi.org/10.1002/ppul.1950110715.

173. A. Tluczek et al., "Parents' Knowledge of Neonatal Screening and Response to False-Positive Cystic Fibrosis Testing," *Journal of Developmental and Behavioral Pediatrics* 13, no. 3 (1992): 181, https://www.ncbi.nlm.nih.gov/pubmed/1613113. Reflecting on the state of newborn screening for CF in 1992, Philip Farrell and Elaine Mischler noted that, "thus far, the Wisconsin study has demonstrated population risks, particularly in the false-positive families, without convincing evidence of benefits." P. M. Farrell and E. H. Mischler, "Newborn Screening for Cystic Fibrosis. The Cystic Fibrosis Neonatal Screening Study Group," *Advances in Pediatrics* 39 (1992): 50, https://www.ncbi.nlm.nih.gov/pubmed/1442316.

174. For more on key events in the history of CF newborn screening, see Grosse et al., "Newborn Screening for Cystic Fibrosis, 2004 Recommendations"; P. M. Farrell

et al., "Nutritional Benefits of Neonatal Screening for Cystic Fibrosis. Wisconsin Cystic Fibrosis Neonatal Screening Study Group," *New England Journal of Medicine* 337, no. 14 (1997), https://doi.org/10.1056/NEJM199710023371403; R. E. Armstrong et al., "Constructing a Bioethical Framework to Evaluate and Optimise Newborn Bloodspot Screening for Cystic Fibrosis," *International Journal of Neonatal Screening* 6, no. 2 (2020), https://doi.org/10.3390/ijns6020040; M. Rosenfeld et al., "Cystic Fibrosis Diagnosis and Newborn Screening," *Pediatric Clinics of North America* 63, no. 4 (2016), https://doi.org/10.1016/j.pcl.2016.04.004; C. Castellani et al., "Newborn Screening for Cystic Fibrosis," *Lancet Respiratory Medicine* 4, no. 8 (2016), https://doi.org/10.1016/S2213-2600(16)00053-9; P. M. Farrell et al., "Evidence on Improved Outcomes with Early Diagnosis of Cystic Fibrosis Through Neonatal Screening: Enough Is Enough!," *Journal of Pediatrics* 147, no. 3, suppl. (2005), https://doi.org/10.1016/j.jpeds.2005.08.012; P. M. Farrell, "The Meaning of 'Early' Diagnosis in a New Era of Cystic Fibrosis Care," *Pediatrics* 119, no. 1 (2007), https://doi.org/10.1542/peds.2006-3074; P. M. Farrell et al., "Early Diagnosis of Cystic Fibrosis Through Neonatal Screening Prevents Severe Malnutrition and Improves Long-Term Growth. Wisconsin Cystic Fibrosis Neonatal Screening Study Group," *Pediatrics* 107, no. 1 (2001), https://doi.org/10.1542/peds.107.1.1; Cono et al., "Newborn Screening for Cystic Fibrosis"; M. Kharrazi et al., "Newborn Screening for Cystic Fibrosis in California," *Pediatrics* 136, no. 6 (2015), https://doi.org/10.1542/peds.2015-0811; M. K. Sontag et al., "Newborn Screening for Cystic Fibrosis: A Qualitative Study of Successes and Challenges from Universal Screening in the United States," *International Journal of Neonatal Screening* 8, no. 3 (2022), https://doi.org/10.3390/ijns8030038.

175. Vailly, *Birth of a Genetics Policy*, 50–51; Christie and Tansey, *Cystic Fibrosis. Wellcome Witnesses*, 67.

176. Rock et al., "Age-Related Decline in Immunoreactive Trypsinogen," 1006.

177. Philip M. Farrell et al., "Current Issues in Neonatal Screening for Cystic Fibrosis and Implications of the CF Gene Discovery," *Pediatric Pulmonology* 11, no. S7 (1991): 15, https://doi.org/10.1002/ppul.1950110704; David J. Hassemer et al., "Laboratory Quality Control Issues Related to Screening Newborns for Cystic Fibrosis Using Immunoreactive Trypsin," *Pediatric Pulmonology* 11, no. S7 (1991): 82, https://doi.org/10.1002/ppul.1950110716; B. Wilfond et al., "Mutation Analysis for CF Newborn Screening: A Two-Tiered Approach," *Pediatric Pulmonology* 11, no. S6 (1991): 238, https://doi.org/10.1002/ppul.1950110605.

178. Wilfond et al., "Mutation Analysis for CF Newborn Screening," 238.

179. R. B. Elliott, "Newborn Screening for Cystic Fibrosis: A Historical Perspective," *Pediatric Pulmonology* 11, no. S7 (1991): 9, https://doi.org/10.1002/ppul.1950110703.

180. Elliott, "Newborn Screening for Cystic Fibrosis," 9; Rosenstein, "IVth International Conference," 85; Farrell and Mischler, "Newborn Screening for Cystic Fibrosis," 51; Bridget Wilcken, "Newborn Screening for Cystic Fibrosis: Its Evolution and a Review of the Current Situation," *Screening* 2, no. 1 (1993): 43, https://doi.org/10.1016/0925-6164(93)90017-D.

181. Farrell and Mischler, "Newborn Screening for Cystic Fibrosis," 51.

182. Wilcken, "Newborn Screening for Cystic Fibrosis," 43. As noted in the document written by Wisconsin Department of Health and Social Services Acting Secretary Richard W. Lorang, the incorporation of DNA testing into IRT-based newborn screening for CF "will increase the accuracy of the screening and substantially reduce the number of infants who would otherwise have to be referred for further diagnostic testing." Order of the Department of Health and Social Services Amending and Creating Rules: Finding of Emergency, January 24, 1995, Wisconsin, Department of Health and Social Services, Administrative Rules, 1973–2009, box 21, folder 17, Wisconsin Historical Society, 2; Grob, *Testing Baby*; Vailly, *Birth of a Genetics Policy*.

Chapter Four

Some of the material in this chapter was originally published in Michelle Lynne LaBonte, "Addressing Uncertainty: The Emergence of the CRMS/CFSPID Diagnostic Category Following Newborn Screening for Cystic Fibrosis," *OBM Genetics* 5, no. 3 (2021), https://doi.org/10.21926/obm.genet.2103139.

1. Cambrey White, oral history interview with Michelle LaBonte, May 23, 2022.

2. Cambrey White, "Struggling to Process My Son's Rare Mutations," *Cystic Fibrosis Foundation CF Community Blog* (blog), May 10, 2022, https://www.cff.org/community-posts/2022-05/struggling-process-my-sons-rare-mutations.

3. White, "Struggling to Process"; White, interview.

4. White, interview.

5. For more on the "genetic 'carrier' of disease," see Wailoo, "Inventing the Heterozygote," 248.

6. Cambrey White, "Our Son Has Cystic Fibrosis," *Rowling with the Punches* (blog), January 3, 2022, https://rowlingwiththepunches.blogspot.com/2022/01/our-son-has-cystic-fibrosis.html.

7. Cambrey White, "Rowland's Mutations," *Rowling with the Punches* (blog), January 14, 2022, https://rowlingwiththepunches.blogspot.com/2022/01/rowlands-mutations.html.

8. Cystic Fibrosis Mutation Database, March 2, 2021, https://web.archive.org/web/20210302230028/http://genet.sickkids.on.ca/StatisticsPage.html.

9. White, interview; White, "Rowland's Mutations." California investigators pointed to a seventy-five-mutation panel in 2021. S. Sciortino et al., "Diagnostic Transitions of Cystic Fibrosis and CRMS Compared After 12 years of Newborn Screening in California," *Journal of Pediatrics* 276 (2025), https://doi.org/10.1016/j.jpeds.2024.114287; M. E. McGarry et al., "Improved Detection of Cystic Fibrosis by the California Newborn Screening Program for All Races and Ethnicities," *Pediatric Pulmonology* 59, no. 11 (2024), https://doi.org/10.1002/ppul.27155.

10. White, "Rowland's Mutations."

11. White, "Rowland's Mutations"; Yazmina Lascano-Vaca et al., "Clinical, Genetic and Microbiological Characterization of Pediatric Patients with Cystic Fibrosis in a Public Hospital in Ecuador," *BMC Pediatrics* 20, no. 1 (2020), https://doi.org/10.1186/s12887-020-2013-6; White, "Struggling to Process"; Kharrazi et al., "Newborn Screening for Cystic Fibrosis"; L. Prach et al., "Novel *CFTR* Variants Identified During the First 3 Years of Cystic Fibrosis Newborn Screening in California," *Journal of Molecular Diagnostics* 15, no. 5 (2013), https://doi.org/10.1016/j.jmoldx.2013.05.006.

12. White, "Rowland's Mutations."

13. Duster, *Backdoor to Eugenics*, 159; Troy Duster, "Buried Alive: The Concept of Race in Science," in *Genetic Nature/Culture: Anthropology and Science Beyond the Two-Culture Divide*, ed. A. Goodman et al. (University of California Press, 2003), 269–70; Wailoo and Pemberton, *Troubled Dream of Genetic Medicine*, 113. For critiques of the biological basis of race, see Evelynn Maxine Hammonds and Rebecca M. Herzig, *The Nature of Difference: Sciences of Race in the United States from Jefferson to Genomics* (MIT Press, 2008); Barbara A. Koenig et al., *Revisiting Race in a Genomic Age* (Rutgers University Press, 2008); Ian Whitmarsh and David S. Jones, *What's the Use of Race?: Modern Governance and the Biology of Difference* (MIT Press, 2010); Ruha Benjamin, "Conjuring Difference, Concealing Inequality: A Brief Tour of Racecraft," *Theory and Society* 43, no. 6 (2014), https://doi.org/10.1007/s11186-014-9238-z; Eram Alam et al., *Ordering the Human: The Global Spread of Racial Science* (Columbia University Press, 2024).

14. Dorothy Nelkin and M. Susan Lindee, *The DNA Mystique: The Gene as a Cultural Icon* (University of Michigan, 2004); Lindee, *Moments of Truth*; Nathaniel C. Comfort, *The Science of Human Perfection: How Genes Became the Heart of American Medicine* (Yale University Press, 2012); Andrew J. Hogan, *Life Histories of Genetic Disease: Patterns and Prevention in Postwar Medical Genetics* (Johns Hopkins University Press, 2016); Soraya de Chadarevian, *Heredity Under the Microscope: Chromosomes and the Study of the Human Genome* (University of Chicago Press, 2020).

15. As Andrew Hogan explains, "aligning the late-nineteenth-century microbiological concept of one germ-one disease with the mid-twentieth-century molecular biology understanding of one gene-one protein, [Victor] McKusick proposed and defined the ideal model of medical genetics thinking as *one mutation-one disorder*" in 1966. Hogan, *Life Histories of Genetic Disease*, 16.

16. Hogan, *Life Histories of Genetic Disease*, 88.

17. Tim Friend, "The Chief of Genetic Detectives," *USA Today*, July 24, 1990.

18. Grob, *Testing Baby*; Vailly, *Birth of a Genetics Policy*; Timmermans and Buchbinder, *Saving Babies?*

19. See Kerem et al., "Genetic Analysis"; Riordan et al., "Cloning and Characterization of Complementary DNA"; Rommens et al., "Chromosome Walking and Jumping"; Koshland, "The Cystic Fibrosis Gene Story."

20. Gibson and Cooke, "A Test for Electrolytes in Sweat"; M. Shteinberg et al., "Cystic Fibrosis," *Lancet* 397, no. 10290 (2021), https://doi.org/10.1016/S0140-6736(20)32542-3. For more on genetic test results and "diagnostic protocols," see Daniel Navon, *Mobilizing Mutations: Human Genetics in the Age of Patient Advocacy* (University of Chicago Press, 2019).

21. Daniel J. Kevles, *In the Name of Eugenics: Genetics and the Uses of Human Heredity* (Knopf, 1985), 267; Hogan, *Life Histories of Genetic Disease*, chapter 2.; Chadarevian, *Heredity Under the Microscope*, 166; Navon, *Mobilizing Mutations*.

22. Paul Jacobs, "Gene Maps: A Guide to Body Defects," *Los Angeles Times*, June 3, 1983, 1. The scientist mentioned was Victor McKusick.

23. J. F. Gusella et al., "A Polymorphic DNA Marker Genetically Linked to Huntington's Disease," *Nature* 306, no. 5940 (1983), https://doi.org/10.1038/306234a0; L. C. Tsui et al., "Cystic Fibrosis Locus Defined by a Genetically Linked Polymorphic DNA Marker," *Science* 230, no. 4729 (1985), https://doi.org/10.1126/science.2997931; R. G. Knowlton et al., "A Polymorphic DNA Marker Linked to Cystic Fibrosis Is Located on Chromosome 7," *Nature* 318, no. 6044 (1985), https://doi.org/10.1038/318380a0; R. White et al., "A Closely Linked Genetic Marker for Cystic Fibrosis," *Nature* 318, no. 6044 (1985), https://doi.org/10.1038/318382a0; B. J. Wainwright et al., "Localization of Cystic Fibrosis Locus to Human Chromosome 7cen-Q22," *Nature* 318, no. 6044 (1985), https://doi.org/10.1038/318384a0; Helen Donis-Keller, interview with Mark Jones, Cambridge, Massachusetts, May 27, 2013, Oral History Transcript 0999, Science History Institute, Philadelphia. For more on efforts to create a "genetic linkage map of the human genome," see D. Botstein et al., "Construction of a Genetic Linkage Map in Man Using Restriction Fragment Length Polymorphisms," *American Journal of Human Genetics* 32, no. 3 (1980): 314, https://www.ncbi.nlm.nih.gov/pubmed/6247908. Comfort, *Science of Human Perfection*; Hogan, *Life Histories of Genetic Disease*; de Chadarevian, *Heredity Under the Microscope*; Robert M. Cook-Deegan, *The Gene Wars: Science, Politics, and the Human Genome* (W. W. Norton & Co., 1994), 29.

24. H. Pearson, "Human Genetics: One Gene, Twenty Years," *Nature* 460, no. 7252 (2009): 166, https://doi.org/10.1038/460164a.

25. "Gene That Causes Cystic Fibrosis Identified," *Commitment Special Edition: Cystic Fibrosis Foundation*, September, 1989, 1. For more on the work leading up to the gene discovery, see "The Search for the CF Gene: An Interview with Dr. Francis Collins," *Commitment: Cystic Fibrosis Foundation*, Summer, 1988, 3; Maya Pines, "Stalking a Lethal Gene," *Blazing a Genetic Trail: A Report from the Howard Hughes Medical Institute*, 1991, 18. Materials located at the Cystic Fibrosis Foundation headquarters in Bethesda, Maryland. P. N. Goodfellow, "Cystic Fibrosis: Steady Steps Lead to the Gene," *Nature* 341, no. 6238 (1989), https://doi.org/10.1038/341102a0; W. W. Grody, "Cystic Fibrosis: Molecular Diagnosis, Population Screening, and Public Policy," *Archives of Pathology and Laboratory Medicine* 123, no. 11 (1999): 1042, https://doi.org/10.5858/1999-123-1041-CF. "Finding the Burned Out Lightbulb:

The Identification of the Cystic Fibrosis Gene," speech given by Francis Collins, March 13, 1991, at the Congressional Biomedical Research Caucus, HGP-DO-052, news clippings, NHGRI Human Genome Project (HGP) Archive.

26. Pines, "Stalking a Lethal Gene," 19; Trivedi, *Breath from Salt*, chapter 25.

27. Pines, "Stalking a Lethal Gene," 19.

28. Richard Saltus, "Gene Discovery Fuels Hope for Cure of Cystic Fibrosis," *Boston Globe*, August 25, 1989, 8.

29. S. Chandrasekharan et al., "Impact of Gene Patents and Licensing Practices on Access to Genetic Testing for Cystic Fibrosis," *Genetics in Medicine* 12, no. 4, suppl. (2010): S194, https://doi.org/10.1097/GIM.0b013e3181d7cf7d; J. S. Sherkow and H. T. Greely, "The History of Patenting Genetic Material," *Annual Review of Genetics* 49 (2015), https://doi.org/10.1146/annurev-genet-112414-054731.

30. Trivedi, *Breath from Salt*, 210.

31. For example, the CF Foundation put out a "Gene Discovery" memo to media representatives, including a press release for August 24 and a set of four short articles related to the discovery. Materials located at the CF Foundation headquarters in Bethesda. Jerry E. Bishop, "Scientists to Unveil Gene That Causes Cystic Fibrosis," *Wall Street Journal*, August 24, 1989.

32. Rommens et al., "Chromosome Walking and Jumping"; Riordan et al., "Cloning and Characterization of Complementary DNA"; Kerem et al., "Genetic Analysis"; Koshland, "The Cystic Fibrosis Gene Story," 1029.

33. For more on gene therapy for CF, see Wailoo and Pemberton, *Troubled Dream of Genetic Medicine*; Lindee and Mueller, "Genetic Medicine's Canary?"; Alan Stockdale, "Waiting for the Cure: Mapping the Social Relations of Human Gene Therapy Research," *Sociology of Health & Illness* 21, no. 5 (1999), https://doi.org/10.1111/1467-9566.00174.

34. Cystic Fibrosis Foundation, "Scientists Identify Cystic Fibrosis Gene and Defective Protein," news release, August 24, 1989, 1; "Interviews: 'Now We Know Where We're Going . . . ,' " *Commitment Special Edition: Cystic Fibrosis Foundation* (September 1989), 5 (newsletter). Italics in original. The Hospital for Sick Children, "Scientists Discover Cystic Fibrosis Gene," news release, August 24, 1989, 2, Materials located at the Cystic Fibrosis Foundation headquarters in Bethesda.

35. Richard Saltus, "Race Is On to Apply Discovery: Cystic Fibrosis Gene's First Payoff Likely To Be in Prevention, Not Treatment," *Boston Globe* August 28, 1989, 25.

36. Saltus, "Race Is On to Apply Discovery," 25.

37. Sue Wallace, "Scientists Raise Hopes for CF Cure," *Herald News*, September 5, 1989.

38. Wallace, "Scientists Raise Hopes."

39. Wallace, "Scientists Raise Hopes."

40. F. S. Collins, "Realizing the Dream of Molecularly Targeted Therapies for Cystic Fibrosis," *New England Journal of Medicine* 381, no. 19 (2019): 1864, https://doi.org/10.1056/NEJMe1911602.

41. Bronya J. B. Keats and Terry J. Hassold, "Recollections from 60 ASHG Meetings," *American Journal of Human Genetics* 87, no. 5 (2010): 586, https://doi.org/10.1016/j.ajhg.2010.10.011. Quoted in Carolyn Y. Johnson, "The Journey from Scientific Breakthrough to a Life-Changing Cystic Fibrosis Drug," *Washington Post*, April 19, 2020.

42. Stacey Freedenthal, "Patients React Cautiously to Breakthrough," *Boston Globe*, August 25, 1989, 8.

43. Freedenthal, "Patients React Cautiously to Breakthrough," 8.

44. Freedenthal, "Patients React Cautiously to Breakthrough," 8; Max Gates, "Gene-Tracking May Not Bring Cures," *Chicago Sun-Times*, September 24, 1989.

45. Gates, "Gene Tracking."

46. Gates, "Gene Tracking"; Cook-Deegan, *The Gene Wars*, 141, 177.

47. Cook-Deegan, *The Gene Wars*; Nelkin and Lindee, *The DNA Mystique*; Lindee, *Moments of Truth*.

48. Cook-Deegan, *The Gene Wars*.

49. C. Thomas Caskey, "DNA-Based Medicine: Prevention and Therapy," in *The Code of Codes: Scientific and Social Issues in the Human Genome Project*, ed. Kevles and Hood (Harvard University Press, 1992).

50. Nancy Wexler, "Clairvoyance and Caution: Repercussions from the Human Genome Project," in *The Code of Codes: Scientific and Social Issues in the Human Genome Project*, ed. Daniel Kevles and Leroy Hood (Harvard University Press, 1992), 211.

51. Duster, *Backdoor to Eugenics*; Rayna Rapp, *Testing Women, Testing the Fetus: The Social Impact of Amniocentesis in America* (Routledge, 1999); Alexandra Minna Stern, *Telling Genes: The Story of Genetic Counseling in America* (Johns Hopkins University Press, 2012); Rayna Rapp and Faye D. Ginsburg, "Enabling Disability: Rewriting Kindship, Reimagining Citizenship," *Public Culture* 13 (2001); Hogan, *Life Histories of Genetic Disease*; Comfort, *Science of Human Perfection*; Diane B. Paul, *Controlling Human Heredity, 1865 to the Present* (Humanities Press, 1995); Kevles, *In the Name of Eugenics*; Wendy Kline, *Building a Better Race: Gender, Sexuality, and Eugenics from the Turn of the Century to the Baby Boom* (University of California Press, 2001); Löwy, *Tangled Diagnoses*; T. Shakespeare, "Choices and Rights: Eugenics, Genetics and Disability Equality," *Disability & Society* 13, no. 5 (1998), https://doi.org/10.1080/09687599826452; Andrew J. Hogan, *Disability Dialogues: Advocacy, Science, and Prestige in Postwar Clinical Professions* (Johns Hopkins University Press, 2022); B. H. Lerner, "When Diseases Disappear—the Case of Familial Dysautonomia," *New England Journal of Medicine* 361, no. 17 (2009), https://doi.org/10.1056/NEJMp0809587; S. P. Tomlinson, "Genetic Testing for Cystic Fibrosis: A Personal Perspective," *Harvard Journal of Law & Technology* 11, no. 3 (1998), https://www.ncbi.nlm.nih.gov/pubmed/12731545. For a more recent account, see Sandy Sufian and Rosemarie Garland-Thomson, "The Dark Side of CRISPR," *Scientific American* (2021), https://www.scientificamerican.com/article/the-dark-side-of-crispr/.

52. Vickie L. Venne, "Counseling for Cystic Fibrosis: What Do I Do Today?," *Perspectives in Genetic Counseling* 12, no. 1 (1990): 1. For more on the history of genetic counseling, see Stern, *Telling Genes*; Hogan, *Disability Dialogues*.

53. Kerem et al., "Genetic Analysis." Other names for this mutation include deltaF508, c.1521_1523delCTT, p.Phe508del, and F508del; Lora J. H. Bean and V. M. Pratt, "Cystic Fibrosis," in *Molecular Pathology in Clinical Practice*, ed. Debra G. B. Leonard (Springer, 2016), https://doi.org/10.1007/978-3-319-19674-9.

54. Cystic Fibrosis Foundation, "CF Gene, Protein Identified," article included with press release, August 23, 1989, Located at the Cystic Fibrosis Foundation headquarters, Bethesda, Maryland; "Interviews: 'Now We Know Where We're Going,'" 4.

55. "Understanding the Discoveries: When a Gene Is Defective . . . ," *Commitment Special Edition: Cystic Fibrosis Foundation* (September 1989), 3.

56. Cystic Fibrosis Foundation, "CF Gene, Protein Identified"; The Hospital for Sick Children, "Scientists Discover Cystic Fibrosis Gene," 2.

57. The Hospital for Sick Children, "Scientists Discover Cystic Fibrosis Gene," 2; Kerem et al., "Genetic Analysis," 1079.

58. Saltus, "Race Is On to Apply Discovery," 26.

59. Sally Squires, "Genetic Testing for Cystic Fibrosis: About One in 20 Americans Has the Gene and Can Pass It to Their Children," *Washington Post*, October 31, 1989, F8.

60. Cook-Deegan, *The Gene Wars*, 243.

61. Squires, "Genetic Testing for Cystic Fibrosis," F8; David Stipp, "Cystic Fibrosis Test May Provide Boost for Emerging Genetic Testing Industry," *Wall Street Journal*, September 19, 1989, B6.

62. Squires, "Genetic Testing for Cystic Fibrosis," F8.

63. Goodfellow, "Cystic Fibrosis," 103.

64. Robert J. Beall to Nancy Wexler, October 24, 1989, box EJ-06, folder 25, Elke Jordan Papers, HisGP-EJ, NHGRI Human Genome Project (HGP) Archive.

65. Beall to Wexler, October 24, 1989.

66. John Ferguson and Elke Jordan, "Implications of the Availability of a Genetic Test for Cystic Fibrosis," November 2, 1989, box EJ-06, folder 25, Elke Jordan Papers, HisGP-EJ, NHGRI Human Genome Project Archive.

67. Peter Lanciano and Nan DuCharme, "Genzyme/Integrated Genetics Announces the Availability of a Direct Test for Cystic Fibrosis," *Business Wire*, November 7, 1989; Ricki Lewis, "Cystic Fibrosis: Tests, Treatments Improve Survival," *FDA Consumer* (1993): 26; Genzyme, *CFplus: Cystic Fibrosis Mutation Analysis*, (2006), 2; "Genzyme/Integrated Genetics Have a New Test for Cystic Fibrosis," *Applied Genetics News* 10, no. 5 (1989): 3; Mark Ratner, "Digesting Genzyme's Integrated Deal," *Nature Biotechnology* 7 (1989), https://doi.org/10.1038/nbt0689-544.

68. Lanciano and DuCharme, "Genzyme/Integrated Genetics Announces the Availability of a Direct Test for Cystic Fibrosis." For a description of a ΔF508 test developed by investigators at the Mayo Clinic, see G. L. Chong and S. N. Thibodeau,

"A Simple Assay for the Screening of the Cystic Fibrosis Allele in Carriers of the Phe508 Deletion Mutation," *Mayo Clinic Proceedings* 65, no. 8 (1990), https://doi.org/10.1016/s0025-6196(12)62719-0.

69. C. T. Caskey et al., "The American Society of Human Genetics Statement on Cystic Fibrosis Screening," *American Journal of Human Genetics* 46, no. 2 (1990): 393, https://www.ncbi.nlm.nih.gov/pubmed/2301404. While the statement was published in 1990, it was dated November 13, 1989. L. Roberts, "Cystic Fibrosis Pilot Projects Go Begging," *Science* 250, no. 4984 (1990): 1076, https://doi.org/10.1126/science.2251497; Grody, "Cystic Fibrosis"; Cook-Deegan, *The Gene Wars*, 243–46; Steve Sturdy, "Framing Utility: Regulatory Reform and Genetic Tests in the USA, 1989–2000," *Social Science and Medicine* 304 (2022), https://doi.org/10.1016/j.socscimed.2020.112924.

70. Caskey et al., "Statement on Cystic Fibrosis Screening," 393.

71. W. K. Lemna et al., "Mutation Analysis for Heterozygote Detection and the Prenatal Diagnosis of Cystic Fibrosis," *New England Journal of Medicine* 322, no. 5 (1990), https://doi.org/10.1056/NEJM199002013220503.

72. Lemna et al., "Mutation Analysis," 291, 293, 295; A. L. Beaudet, "Genetic Testing for Cystic Fibrosis," *Pediatric Clinics of North America* 39, no. 2 (1992): 216, https://doi.org/10.1016/s0031-3955(16)38292-x.

73. Lemna et al., "Mutation Analysis," 292.

74. Cystic Fibrosis Foundation, Patient Registry Annual Data Report 1999. Patient registry data from 1989 was included in the report, which was located at the Cystic Fibrosis Foundation headquarters in Bethesda, Maryland.

75. Roberts, *Fatal Invention*, chapter 4; Garcia, "The Misuse of Race"; Wailoo and Pemberton, *Troubled Dream of Genetic Medicine*; Wailoo, *Dying in the City of the Blues*; Tuchman, *Diabetes*; Koenig et al., *Revisiting Race*; Montoya, *Making the Mexican Diabetic*; Fullwiley, *Enculturated Gene*; Braun, *Breathing Race into the Machine*.

76. Wailoo and Pemberton, *Troubled Dream of Genetic Medicine*, 113; Alam et al., *Ordering the Human*; Hammonds and Herzig, *The Nature of Difference*.

77. Jerry E. Bishop, "New Cystic-Fibrosis Test for Carriers Raises Moral Issue," *Wall Street Journal*, February 1, 1990, B1. For more on concerns related to disability, eugenics, and financial considerations, see Paul R. Billings, "Mutation Analysis in Cystic Fibrosis," *New England Journal of Medicine* 323, no. 1 (1990), https://doi.org/10.1056/NEJM199007053230114.

78. Gina Kolata, "Rush Is on to Capitalize on Testing for Gene Causing Cystic Fibrosis," *New York Times*, February 6, 1990, C3; Pines, "Stalking a Lethal Gene," 22–23; Ruth Schwartz Cowan, *Heredity and Hope: The Case for Genetic Screening* (Harvard University Press, 2008), 165; Wailoo, *Dying in the City of the Blues*.

79. Beall and Keramidas, "The Role of a Voluntary Health Agency," 2. They went on to note that "while the incidence of CF is highest among Caucasians, there is still a significant incidence among other racial groups."

80. *Screening and Counseling for Genetic Conditions: A Report on the Ethical, Social, and Legal Implications of Genetic Screening, Counseling, and Education Programs*, President's Commission for the Study of Ethical Probelms in Medicine and Biomedical and Behavioral Research, US Government Printing Office, 1983, 95; Cook-Deegan, *The Gene Wars*, 257; Wailoo and Pemberton, *Troubled Dream of Genetic Medicine*; Alondra Nelson, *Body and Soul: The Black Panther Party and the Fight Against Medical Discrimination* (University of Minnesota Press, 2011).

81. Wailoo and Pemberton, *Troubled Dream of Genetic Medicine.*

82. R. Todd Erkel, "Finding the Tiger," *Pitt Magazine*, February, 1990, 47.

83. Kolata, "Rush Is On," C3.

84. Kolata, "Rush Is On," C3.

85. Kolata, "Rush Is On," C3.

86. Kolata, "Rush Is On," C3.

87. Kolata, "Rush Is On," C3.

88. Kolata, "Rush Is On," C3; "Draft Summary of Mapping and Sequencing the Human Genome, HGP-DO-005."

89. Michael Waldholz, "Cystic Fibrosis Gene Testing Nationwide Runs into Technical and Ethical Barriers," *Wall Street Journal*, March 7, 1990, B4; Larry Thompson, "Panel Favors Limiting Cystic Fibrosis Testing: Screening Can Identify Parents with Gene," *Washington Post*, March 6, 1990, A8; February 28, 1990 Agenda for NIH Workshop for Population Screening for the Cystic Fibrosis Gene for March 5–6, 1990, box EJ-14, folder 32, HisGP-EJ, Elke Jordan Papers, NHGRI Human Genome Project (HGP) Archive.

90. Waldholz, "Cystic Fibrosis Gene Testing," B4. Longer quote from the NIH Workshop on Population Screening for the Cystic Fibrosis Gene, March 6, 1990, box EJ-06, folder 25, HisGP-EJ, Elke Jordan Papers, NHGRI Human Genome Project (HGP) Archive, 2. Highlighting the uncertainty associated with the carrier test, Arthur Beaudet, committee cochair, "said the group opposes using it in general community screening programs now because 'the test isn't good enough.'" Thompson, "Panel Favors Limiting Cystic Fibrosis Testing," A8. In contrast to CF carrier screening, which failed to detect all carriers, the Sickledex test detected both sickle cell carriers and those with the disease (and a reflex electrophoresis test was needed as a second step to distinguish between these groups). Cowan, *Heredity and Hope*, 160.

91. Waldholz, "Cystic Fibrosis Gene Testing," B4.

92. Waldholz, "Cystic Fibrosis Gene Testing," B4.

93. Waldholz, "Cystic Fibrosis Gene Testing," B4.

94. Waldholz, "Cystic Fibrosis Gene Testing," B4.

95. Larry Thompson, "Cystic Fibrosis Tests: Are They Precise Enough?," *Washington Post*, March 13, 1990, 11.

96. Waldholz, "Cystic Fibrosis Gene Testing," B4. For more on concerns about CF carrier screening, see B. S. Wilfond and N. Fost, "The Cystic Fibrosis Gene:

Medical and Social Implications for Heterozygote Detection," *JAMA* 263, no. 20 (1990), https://www.ncbi.nlm.nih.gov/pubmed/2332921.

97. Pines, "Stalking a Lethal Gene"; Ron Grossman, "Patient, Study Thyself," *Chicago Tribune*, March 9, 1993.

98. Pines, "Stalking a Lethal Gene," 11.

99. Pines, "Stalking a Lethal Gene," 8.

100. Pines, "Stalking a Lethal Gene," 9.

101. Pines, "Stalking a Lethal Gene," 10.

102. Pines, "Stalking a Lethal Gene," 11.

103. Pines, "Stalking a Lethal Gene," 11.

104. *Barbara Walters Special*, "The Perfect Baby," aired July 18, 1990, on ABC-TV.

105. Pines, "Stalking a Lethal Gene," 11.

106. Pines, "Stalking a Lethal Gene," 11.

107. Pines, "Stalking a Lethal Gene," 11.

108. Pines, "Stalking a Lethal Gene," 11.

109. Tim Friend, "Cystic Fibrosis: Mass Testing Not in Near Future," *USA Today*, July 24, 1990.

110. L. C. Tsui, "The Spectrum of Cystic Fibrosis Mutations," *Trends in Genetics* 8, no. 11 (1992): 392, https://doi.org/10.1016/0168-9525(92)90301-j. Pines, "Stalking a Lethal Gene," 11. "What's Ahead in CF Basic Science?," *Commitment: Cystic Fibrosis Foundation*, July, 1991, 5. For more on the consortium, see Lap-Chee Tsui to Arthur Beaudet, Francis Collins, Bob Williamson, and Michel Goossens, December 15, 1992, HGP-DO-053, NHGRI Human Genome Project (HGP) Archive.

111. Natalie Angier, "Regional Split in Cystic Fibrosis," *New York Times*, July 24, 1990.

112. The workshop took place in September 1990. Eric T. Juengst to James Watson, August 24, 1990, HGP-DO-046, NHGRI Human Genome Project (HGP) Archive. The working group was chaired by Nancy Wexler, and group members were Jonathan Beckwith, Robert Cook-Deegan, Patricia King, Victor McKusick, Robert F. Murray Jr., and Thomas H. Murray. The twelve additional participants were Arthur Beaudet, Barbara Bowles, Francis S. Collins, Norman Fost, Carol A. Heimer, Michael Kaback, Katherine Klinger, Loretta Kopelman, Jane Mackta, Marianne Schwartz, Doris Tulcin, and Robert Williamson. NIH and DOE staff included Benjamin Barnhardt, Bettie Graham, Elke Jordan, Eric Juengst, James Watson, and Michael Yelsey.

113. "Workshop on the Introduction of New Genetic Tests," draft report, ELSI Working Group Workshop, September 10, 1990, HGP-DO-046, NHGRI Human Genome Project (HGP) Archive; National Center for Human Genome Research, Program on the Ethical, Legal, and Social Implications of Human Genome Research, Progress Highlights, undated, circa 1991, ELSI Program Activities Report, 1990–1992, HGP-DO-022 NHGRI Human Genome Project (HGP) Archive.

114. NIH-DOE Joint Working Group on Ethical, Legal, and Social Implications of Human Genome Research FY 1991 Activities, HGP-DO-022, ELSI Program Activities Report, 1990–1992, NHGRI Human Genome Project (HGP) Archive; Department of Health and Human Services, Public Health Service, National Institutes of Health, National Center for Human Genome Research, "The Ethical, Legal, and Social Implications of Human Genome Research: Preparing for the Responsible Use of New Genetic Knowledge," William Raub (acting NIH director), report on ELSI program, January 1991, HGP-DO-045, NHGRI Human Genome Project (HGP) Archive; Genzyme, *CFplus: Cystic Fibrosis Mutation Analysis*, 2; F. Gilbert, "Is Population Screening for Cystic Fibrosis Appropriate Now?," *American Journal of Human Genetics* 46, no. 2 (1990): 394, https://www.ncbi.nlm.nih.gov/pubmed/1967902; Roberts, "Pilot Projects," 1077; Office of Technology Assessment, US Congress, *Cystic Fibrosis and DNA Tests: Implications of Carrier Screening*, OTA-BA-532, US Government Printing Office, 1992, 160–62; Roberts, "Pilot Projects," 1077.

115. Beaudet, "Genetic Testing," 216. The mutation count is based on Cystic Fibrosis Genetic Analysis Consortium data from May 1991. "What's Ahead in CF Basic Science?," 5.

116. William Booth, "Genetic Screening for Cystic Fibrosis Provokes Anxious Debate," *Washington Post*, August 10, 1991, A3. Quote by Norman Fost. Consistent with this claim, Orrie Friedman, the founder and chairman of Collaborative Research, a company that Tsui had collaborated with in the 1980s, noted that at least six companies, including his, were carrying out "reasonably aggressive marketing."

117. Booth, "Genetic Screening," A3.

118. Office of Technology Assessment, US Congress, "Genetic Counseling and Cystic Fibrosis Carrier Screening: Results of a Survey—Background Paper," OTA-BP-BA-97, Government Printing Office, September 1992, 2.

119. "Genetic Counseling and Cystic Fibrosis Carrier Screening," 17. Along those lines, another genetic counselor in New York argued that "withholding this knowledge . . . appears to be unjustified, harmful and possibly an invasion of the inherent right to know." "CF Carrier Testing: An Obligation to Disclose," *Perspectives in Genetic Counseling: Newsletter of the National Society of Genetic Counselors, Inc.* 14, no. 4 (1991/92): 4.

120. Consensus Report: Ad Hoc Committee on Cystic Fibrosis Carrier Screening, American Society of Human Genetics, February 11, 1992, HGP-DO-032, NHGRI Human Genome Project (HGP) Archive; Robert Steinbrook, "The Promise and Perils of Genetic Screening," *Los Angeles Times*, November 1, 1993, A12.

121. T. Shoshani et al., "Association of a Nonsense Mutation (W1282X), the Most Common Mutation in the Ashkenazi Jewish Cystic Fibrosis Patients in Israel, with Presentation of Severe Disease," *American Journal of Human Genetics* 50, no. 1 (1992): 222, https://www.ncbi.nlm.nih.gov/pubmed/1370365. For more about Kerem's work, see Trivedi, *Breath from Salt*, 212–13.

122. Genzyme, *CFplus: Cystic Fibrosis Mutation Analysis*, 2.

123. Genzyme, *CFplus: Cystic Fibrosis Mutation Analysis*, 2; Eric Juengst and Elizabeth Thomson, Summary from the Planning Meeting of the Cystic Fibrosis Studies Consortium (CFSC), November 1–2, 1991, National Institutes of Health, HGP-DO-058, NHGRI Human Genome Project (HGP) Archive.

124. Robert Cooke, "A Deadly Gene's Surprise," *Newsday (Suffolk Edition)*, August 17, 1993, 58.

125. Integrated Genetics, Cystic Fibrosis DNA Testing, 1994; Genzyme, *CFplus: Cystic Fibrosis Mutation Analysis*, 2. For reference to the seventy-mutation test, see Bettina C. Hilman, "Sweat Test vs Genetic Testing for Cystic Fibrosis," *Laboratory Medicine* 28, no. 7 (1997): 433; Genzyme Genetics, *Cystic Fibrosis DNA Testing*, 1997, pamphlet located at the Cystic Fibrosis Foundation headquarters in Bethesda. For more on genetic tests for CF and other diseases, see Nelkin and Tancredi, *Dangerous Diagnostics*.

126. Steven Epstein, *Inclusion: The Politics of Difference in Medical Research* (University of Chicago Press, 2007).

127. Duana Fullwiley, "Race and Genetics: Attempts to Define the Relationship," *BioSocieties* 2 (2007): 236; Fullwiley, *Enculturated Gene*; Catherine Bliss, *Race Decoded: The Genomic Fight for Social Justice* (Stanford University Press, 2012); Sandra Soo-Jin Lee, "Racial Realism and the Discourse of Responsibility for Health Disparities in a Genomic Age," in *Revisiting Race in a Genomic Age*, ed. Barbara Koenig, Sandra Soo-Jin Lee, and Sarah Richardson (Rutgers University Press, 2008), 351; Alam et al., *Ordering the Human*.

128. W. W. Grody et al., "Diversity of Cystic Fibrosis Mutation-Screening Practices," *American Journal of Human Genetics* 62, no. 5 (1998): 1252, https://doi.org/10.1086/301842.

129. National Institutes of Health, Consensus Development Conference Statement, Genetic Testing for Cystic Fibrosis, April 14–16, 1997, HGP-DO-052, NHGRI Human Genome Project (HGP) Archive. The consensus statement was available on the NIH website on April 17, 1997, and a slightly modified version was published in 1999. "Genetic Testing for Cystic Fibrosis. National Institutes of Health Consensus Development Conference Statement on Genetic Testing for Cystic Fibrosis," *Archives of Internal Medicine* 159, no. 14 (1999), https://doi.org/10.1001/archinte.159.14.1529.

130. NIH Consensus Development Conference Statement, 1997. Furthermore, conference participants "recommended that population-based CF screening be offered to all pregnant couples and those contemplating pregnancy in a program to be phased in over time." Grody et al., "Diversity of Cystic Fibrosis Mutation-Screening Practices," 1253; Chandrasekharan et al., "Impact of Gene Patents," S197.

131. Epstein, *Inclusion*; Alam et al., *Ordering the Human*, 16; Stuart Hall et al., *Selected Writings on Race and Difference* (Duke University Press, 2021); Lee, "Racial Realism."

132. Grody et al., "Diversity of Cystic Fibrosis Mutation-Screening Practices," 1252, 1253. According to Bean and Pratt, "there was no standardization of CF testing among laboratories and no commercially available reagents or kits" in 1997. Bean and Pratt, "Cystic Fibrosis," 191. In October 1997, the NIH convened a workshop to review the Consensus Conference recommendations and consider their implementation. M. T. Mennuti et al., "Screening for Cystic Fibrosis Carrier State," *Obstetrics & Gynecology* 93, no. 3 (1999), https://doi.org/10.1016/S0029-7844(98)00443-8. By the fall of 1999, the National Society of Genetic Counselors proposed a revised CF carrier testing position statement yet noted that "no recommendation is made about whether CF carrier testing programs should target all ethnic groups or only those with high carrier rates of detectable mutations." Anne Spencer, "CF Position Statement Revision Considered," *Perspectives in Genetic Counseling* 21, no. 3 (1999): 3.

133. NIH Consensus Development Conference Statement, 1997. As stakeholders continued to contemplate the ideal makeup of CF mutation panels and who should be targeted for carrier screening, the Genzyme panel expanded to eighty-six mutations in November 1999. The additional Genzyme mutations were "added for African Americans, Caucasians and Hispanics," resulting in an increased detection rate "to 75% for African Americans." Genzyme, *CFplus: Cystic Fibrosis Mutation Analysis*, 2, 3. For more on the search for CF mutations in Black individuals in the time leading up to this expanded test, see M. Macek Jr. et al., "Identification of Common Cystic Fibrosis Mutations in African-Americans with Cystic Fibrosis Increases the Detection Rate to 75%," *American Journal of Human Genetics* 60, no. 5 (1997), https://www.ncbi.nlm.nih.gov/pubmed/9150159. Genzyme Genetics, *Cystic Fibrosis DNA Testing*, 1997. For reference to the seventy-mutation test, see Hilman, "Sweat Test vs Genetic Testing for Cystic Fibrosis," 433.

134. W. W. Grody et al., "Laboratory Standards and Guidelines for Population-Based Cystic Fibrosis Carrier Screening," *Genetics in Medicine* 3, no. 2 (2001): 150, https://doi.org/10.1097/00125817-200103000-00010. For more on deliberations in the years before the recommendation of the "pan-ethnic" panel, see Draft Report 10/14/98, Preconceptional and Prenatal Carrier Screening for Cystic Fibrosis Provider Guidelines, Developed by the Provider Guidelines Working Group, located in the NHGRI Human Genome Project (HGP) Archive, American College of Obstetricians and Gynecologists, Cystic Fibrosis, 1998–1999, mixed materials, HGP-DO-057; "Confidential Draft Preconceptional and Prenatal Carrier Screening for Cystic Fibrosis," October 17, 1998, HGP-DO-057, American College of Obstetricians and Gynecologists (ACOG), Cystic Fibrosis, 1998–1999, mixed materials, NHGRI Human Genome Project (HGP) Archive; Recommendations of the Laboratory Standards Committee, ACMG Working Group on Cystic Fibrosis Screening fax, February 17, 1999, HGP-DO-057, American College of Obstetricians and Gynecologists (ACOG), Cystic Fibrosis, 1998–1999, mixed materials, NHGRI Human Genome Project (HGP) Archive.

135. Grody et al., "Laboratory Standards and Guidelines," 149.

136. Grody et al., "Laboratory Standards and Guidelines," 149; Chandrasekharan et al., "Impact of Gene Patents," S197; Genzyme, *CFplus: Cystic Fibrosis Mutation Analysis*, 3.

137. Grody et al., "Laboratory Standards and Guidelines," 150. Emphasis added within quote. E. A. Sugarman et al., "*CFTR* Mutation Distribution Among U.S. Hispanic and African American Individuals: Evaluation in Cystic Fibrosis Patient and Carrier Screening Populations," *Genetics in Medicine* 6, no. 5 (2004): 392, https://doi.org/10.1097/01.gim.0000139503.22088.66.

138. Grody et al., "Laboratory Standards and Guidelines," 151.

139. "Update on Carrier Screening for Cystic Fibrosis, ACOG Committee Opinion No. 486, American College of Obstetricians and Gynecologists," *Obstetrics & Gynecology* 117, no. 4 (2011): 1, https://doi.org/10.1097/AOG.0b013e31821922c2; American College of Obstetricians and Gynecologists, "Cystic Fibrosis Carrier Testing: The Decision Is Yours," 2001, 5. Document provided by Debra Maloney-Evans and Peter Evans. See also https://web.archive.org/web/20021017210616/http://www.acog.org/from_home/wellness/cf001.htm. American College of Obstetricians and Gynecologists, "Ob-Gyns Offering Large-Scale Cystic Fibrosis Screening: Represents First Major Change from the Human Genome Project," news release, December 12, 2001, https://web.archive.org/web/20021015101656/http://www.acog.org/from_home/publications/press_releases/nr12-12-01-2.cfm.

140. J. L. Deignan et al., "*CFTR* Variant Testing: A Technical Standard of the American College of Medical Genetics and Genomics (ACMG)," *Genetics in Medicine* 22, no. 8 (2020): 1288, https://doi.org/10.1038/s41436-020-0822-5.

141. Shari Roan, "A First for Genetic Testing," *Los Angeles Times*, November 26, 2001.

142. F. Gilbert, "Cystic Fibrosis Carrier Screening: Steps in the Development of a Mutation Panel," *Genetic Testing* 5, no. 3 (2001): 224, https://doi.org/10.1089/10906570152742272.; C. M. Strom et al., "Cystic Fibrosis Screening Using the College Panel: Platform Comparison and Lessons Learned from the First 20,000 Samples," *Genetics in Medicine* 4, no. 4 (2002), https://doi.org/10.1097/00125817-200207000-00007; Aaron Zitner, "Lost in Translation," *Los Angeles Times*, May 12, 2003.

143. R. A. Heim et al., "Improved Detection of Cystic Fibrosis Mutations in the Heterogeneous U.S. Population Using an Expanded, Pan-Ethnic Mutation Panel," *Genetics in Medicine* 3, no. 3 (2001): 168, https://doi.org/10.1097/00125817-200105000-00004.

144. Sugarman et al., "*CFTR* Mutation Distribution," 399.

145. Sugarman et al., "*CFTR* Mutation Distribution," 399.

146. Palomaki et al., "Clinical Sensitivity of Prenatal Screening," 405.

147. Palomaki et al., "Clinical Sensitivity of Prenatal Screening," 405. Epstein, *Inclusion*; Roberts, *Fatal Invention*.

148. Palomaki et al., "Clinical Sensitivity of Prenatal Screening," 413.

149. Zitner, "Lost in Translation," D12.

150. "Update on Carrier Screening for Cystic Fibrosis, ACOG Committee Opinion No. 325, American College of Obstetricians and Gynecologists," *Obstetrics & Gynecology* 106, no. 6 (2005), https://doi.org/10.1097/00006250-200512000-00055.

151. "ACOG Committee Opinion No. 325," 1465, 1466. Emphasis added.

152. "ACOG Committee Opinion No. 325," 1466. However, ACOG noted that "it is the physician's responsibility to interpret the results based on the patient's ethnicity."

153. "ACOG Committee Opinion No. 325," 1467. Emphasis added. Furthermore, the later 2011 ACOG update reiterated that "it is reasonable . . . to offer CF carrier screening to all patients." However, in recognition of the diagnostic uncertainty inherent in the carrier screening test, ACOG also stressed that "screening is most efficacious in the non-Hispanic white and Ashkenazi Jewish populations." "ACOG Committee Opinion No. 486," 1, 3.

154. Genzyme, *CFplus: Cystic Fibrosis Mutation Analysis*, 1, 3. M. S. Watson et al., "Cystic Fibrosis Population Carrier Screening: 2004 Revision of American College of Medical Genetics Mutation Panel," *Genetics in Medicine* 6, no. 5 (2004): 388, https://doi.org/10.1097/01.gim.0000139506.11694.7c. Even though updated data provided evidence that six additional mutations met the 0.1 percent threshold for inclusion, the ACMG did not recommend that these be added to the revised panel because the "incremental gain" did not outweigh the "potential increase in cost and errors." Anthropologist Duana Fullwiley documents a similar situation faced by researchers involved in studies of single nucleotide polymorphisms. Fullwiley, "Race and Genetics," 229–30.

155. W. W. Grody et al., "The Cystic Fibrosis Mutation 'Arms Race': When Less Is More," *Genetics in Medicine* 9, no. 11 (2007): 742, 743, https://doi.org/10.1097/gim.0b013e318159a331.

156. Grody et al., "Arms Race," 740; Watson et al., "Cystic Fibrosis Population Carrier Screening"; "ACOG Committee Opinion No. 486," 2.

157. Grody et al., "Arms Race," 740.

158. Grody et al., "Arms Race," 742.

159. Grody et al., "Arms Race," 742.

160. Grody et al., "Arms Race," 742.

161. Grody et al., "Arms Race," 743.

162. "Genzyme Launches Cystic Fibrosis Gene Sequencing Test," *Technology Networks: Applied Sciences*, November 2, 2006, https://www.technologynetworks.com/applied-sciences/news/genzyme-launches-cystic-fibrosis-gene-sequencing-test-196159.

163. Grody et al., "Arms Race," 743.

164. Grody et al., "Arms Race," 743.

165. G. R. Cutting, "Cystic Fibrosis Genetics: From Molecular Understanding to Clinical Application," *Nature Reviews Genetics* 16, no. 1 (2015), https://doi.org/10.1038/nrg3849. For more on CFTR2, see Cutting, "Annotating DNA Variants," 8; P. R. Sosnay et al., "Defining the Disease Liability of Variants in the Cystic Fibrosis Transmembrane Conductance Regulator Gene," *Nature Genetics* 45, no. 10 (2013), https://doi.org/10.1038/ng.2745. See the CFTR2 website, https://cftr2.org.

166. R. Pabary et al., "Highlights of the North American Cystic Fibrosis Conference 2011," *Journal of the Royal Society of Medicine* 105, suppl. 2 (2012), https://doi.org/10.1258/jrsm.2012.12s002.

167. Cutting, "Annotating DNA Variants," 5. For more on CF gene sequencing, see D. S. Grosu et al., "Clinical Investigational Studies for Validation of a Next-Generation Sequencing in Vitro Diagnostic Device for Cystic Fibrosis Testing," *Expert Review of Molecular Diagnostics* 14, no. 5 (2014), https://doi.org/10.1586/14737159.2014.916618. For more on variants of uncertain significance, see A. Hedgecoe et al., "Reflexive Standardization and the Resolution of Uncertainty in the Genomics Clinic," *Social Studies of Science* 53, no. 3 (2023), https://doi.org/10.1177/03063127231154863.

168. K. A. Beauchamp et al., "Sequencing as a First-Line Methodology for Cystic Fibrosis Carrier Screening," *Genetics in Medicine* 21, no. 11 (2019), https://doi.org/10.1038/s41436-019-0525-y.

169. Deignan et al., "*CFTR* Variant Testing," 1290.

170. Deignan et al., "*CFTR* Variant Testing," 1290.

171. J. L. Deignan et al., "Updated Recommendations for *CFTR* Carrier Screening: A Position Statement of the American College of Medical Genetics and Genomics (ACMG)," *Genetics in Medicine* 25, no. 8 (2023): 2, https://doi.org/10.1016/j.gim.2023.100867.

172. Deignan et al., "Updated Recommendations," 7. To make this determination, they looked to two iterations of the Genome Aggregation Database, gnomAD v2.1.1 and gnomAD v3.1.2. As the ACMG made clear, the updated recommendations were specific to carrier screening and "do not apply to *CFTR* variant testing for diagnosis or newborn screening."

173. See the CFTR2 website (https://cftr2.org) for an updated list.

174. A. Shenoy et al., "Cystic Fibrosis Newborn Screening," *Clinics in Perinatology* 52, no. 3 (2025), https://doi.org/10.1016/j.clp.2025.06.004; LaBonte, "Addressing Uncertainty"; Meghan E. McGarry et al., "Detection of Disease-Causing *CFTR* Variants in State Newborn Screening Programs," *Pediatric Pulmonology* 58, no. 2 (2023), https://doi.org/10.1002/ppul.26209. For more on uncertainty in disease classification, including CF, see F. A. Miller et al., "Ruling In and Ruling Out: Implications of Molecular Genetic Diagnoses for Disease Classification," *Social Science & Medicine* 61, no. 12 (2005), https://doi.org/10.1016/j.socscimed.2005.04.043; F. A. Miller et al., "Redefining Disease? The Nosologic Implications of Molecular Genetic Knowledge," *Perspectives in Biology and Medicine* 49, no. 1 (2006), https://doi.org/10.1353/pbm.2006.0012.

175. M. R. Rehani et al., "Variation in Cystic Fibrosis Newborn Screening Algorithms in the United States," *Pediatric Pulmonology* 58, no. 3 (2023), https://doi.org/10.1002/ppul.26279; Farrell, "50 Years of Cystic Fibrosis Newborn Screening."

176. Accounts of the number of mutations tested at this time vary. Sciortino et al., "Diagnostic Transitions"; McGarry et al., "Improved Detection of Cystic Fibrosis"; Rehani et al., "Variation in Cystic Fibrosis Newborn Screening Algorithms."

177. Rehani et al., "Variation in Cystic Fibrosis Newborn Screening Algorithms."

178. M. E. McGarry et al., "Cystic Fibrosis Newborn Screening: A Systematic Review-Driven Consensus Guideline from the United States Cystic Fibrosis Foundation," *International Journal of Neonatal Screening* 11, no. 2 (2025), https://doi.org/10.3390/ijns11020024.

179. McGarry et al., "Cystic Fibrosis Newborn Screening," 7.

180. McGarry et al., "Cystic Fibrosis Newborn Screening," 7.

181. McGarry et al., "Cystic Fibrosis Newborn Screening," 2.

182. Farrell, "50 Years of Cystic Fibrosis Newborn Screening"; Rehani et al., "Variation in Cystic Fibrosis Newborn Screening Algorithms."

183. McGarry et al., "Cystic Fibrosis Newborn Screening," 13; A. Tluczek et al., "When the Cystic Fibrosis Label Does Not Fit: A Modified Uncertainty Theory," *Qualitative Health Research* 20, no. 2 (2010), https://doi.org/10.1177/1049732309356285; R. B. Parad and A. M. Comeau, "Diagnostic Dilemmas Resulting from the Immunoreactive Trypsinogen/DNA Cystic Fibrosis Newborn Screening Algorithm," *Journal of Pediatrics* 147, no. 3, suppl. (2005), https://doi.org/10.1016/j.jpeds.2005.08.017.

184. McGarry et al., "Cystic Fibrosis Newborn Screening," 13.

185. US Food and Drug Administration, "FDA Approves New Breakthrough Therapy for Cystic Fibrosis," 2019, https://www.fda.gov/news-events/press-announcements/fda-approves-new-breakthrough-therapy-cystic-fibrosis.

186. "Our Venture Philanthropy Model," Cystic Fibrosis Foundation, https://www.cff.org/about-us/our-venture-philanthropy-model; Robert Steven Kaplan and Sophie Hood, "Bob Beall at the Cystic Fibrosis Foundation," Harvard Business School Case 409–107, April 2009 (revised October 2010).

187. Gates, "Gene Tracking."

188. A. Mullard, "Reshma Kewalramani," *Nature Reviews Drug Discovery* 18, no. 12 (2019), https://doi.org/10.1038/d41573-019-00194-6; Carolyn Y. Johnson, "Long-Awaited Cystic Fibrosis Drug Could Turn Deadly Disease into a Manageable Condition," *Washington Post*, October 31, 2019, https://www.washingtonpost.com/health/2019/10/31/long-awaited-cystic-fibrosis-drug-could-turn-deadly-disease-into-manageable-condition/.

189. Johnson, "Long-Awaited Cystic Fibrosis Drug." For Francis Collins's perspective on Trikafta, including his email exchange with Jenny McGlincy, see Francis Collins, "Dare to Dream: The Long Road to Targeted Therapies for Cystic Fibrosis," *NIH Director's Blog* (blog), October 31, 2019, https://directorsblog.nih.gov/2019/10/31/dare-to-dream-the-long-road-to-targeted-therapies-for-cystic-fibrosis/.

190. Johnson, "Long-Awaited Cystic Fibrosis Drug."

191. Julie Desch, oral history interview with the author, May 11, 2020.

192. Desch, interview. Another adult with CF, Robyn Petras, explained how "Trikafta gave me such peace, when I got COVID, that I knew I could beat it. I would've been very sick. The timing is divine, with the release of that drug." Robyn Petras, oral history interview with the author, May 4, 2020.

193. Stephanie Nolen and Rebecca Robbins, "The Drug Is a 'Miracle' but These Families Can't Get It," *New York Times*, February 7, 2023, https://www.nytimes.com/2023/02/07/health/cystic-fibrosis-drug-trikafta.html; J. L. Taylor-Cousar et al., "CFTR Modulator Therapy: Transforming the Landscape of Clinical Care in Cystic Fibrosis," *Lancet* 402, no. 10408 (2023), https://doi.org/10.1016/s0140-6736(23)01609-4.

194. Andrew Joseph, "'We're Still Waiting,'" *Boston Globe*, February 11, 2019, C3.

195. Kevin Davies, "Laying the Foundation for Cystic Fibrosis Therapy: An Interview with Michael Boyle," Human Gene Therapy, 31, no. 17–18 (2020): 918, https://doi.org/10.1089/hum.2020.29134.int; Collins, "Dare to Dream: The Long Road to Targeted Therapies for Cystic Fibrosis," *NIH Director's Blog* (blog), October 31, 2019, https://directorsblog.nih.gov/2019/10/31/dare-to-dream-the-long-road-to-targeted-therapies-for-cystic-fibrosis/.

196. E. Kramer-Golinkoff et al., "A Survey: Understanding the Health and Perspectives of People with CF Not Benefiting from CFTR Modulators," *Pediatric Pulmonology* 57, no. 5 (2022): 1258, https://doi.org/10.1002/ppul.25859; Manojna Maddipatla and Carl O'Donnell, "Vertex Prices Cystic Fibrosis Combo Treatment at $311,000-Per-Year," *Reuters*, October 21, 2019, https://www.reuters.com/article/us-vertex-pharms-fda/vertex-prices-cystic-fibrosis-combo-treatment-at-311000-per-year-idUSKBN1X024U.

197. Cambrey White, "The New Normal, a Miracle, & Information About the OC Great Strides Walk," *Rowling with the Punches* (blog), March 18, 2022, https://rowlingwiththepunches.blogspot.com/2022/03/the-new-normal-miracle-information.html.

198. Cambrey White, "Coming Together to Advocate for Our Sons," *Cystic Fibrosis Foundation CF Community Blog* (blog), May 17, 2023, https://www.cff.org/community-posts/2023-05/coming-together-advocate-our-sons.

199. White, "Rowland's Mutations." While Rowland has one mutation that may qualify him for modulator therapy in the future if laboratory studies of his nasal cells demonstrate drug efficacy, such studies are time-consuming and expensive and may still require specific insurance approval for coverage. White, "Rowland's Mutations"; Cambrey White, "Next Steps," *Rowling with the Punches* (blog), February 16, 2022, https://rowlingwiththepunches.blogspot.com/2022/02/next-steps.html; Cambrey White, "Summer Health Update 2022," *Rowling with the Punches* (blog), September 18, 2022, https://rowlingwiththepunches.blogspot.com/2022/09/summer-health-update-2022.html.

200. M. E. McGarry et al., "Left Behind: The Potential Impact of CFTR Modulators on Racial and Ethnic Disparities in Cystic Fibrosis," *Paediatric Respiratory Reviews* 42 (2022): 37, https://doi.org/10.1016/j.prrv.2021.12.001.

201. Roberts, *Fatal Invention*; Alan Toth, "Minority Patients Miss out on Life-Saving Cystic Fibrosis Drugs Due to Genetic Test Limitations," University of California, San Francisco, February 4, 2021, https://www.ucsf.edu/news/2021/02/419721/minority-patients-miss-out-life-saving-cystic-fibrosis-drugs-due-genetic-test.

Chapter Five

An earlier version of this chapter was originally published as Michelle LaBonte, "Diagnostic Uncertainty, Microbes, and the Isolation of People with Cystic Fibrosis," *Journal of the History of Medicine and Allied Sciences* 77, no. 2 (2022), https://doi.org/10.1093/jhmas/jrab056.

1. Michelle Patrovani, "Life with CF Prepared My Family for Covid-19: How One Disease Helps Train Us for Another," *Medium*, April 3, 2020, https://michelleapatrovani.medium.com/life-with-cf-prepared-my-family-for-covid-19-fb5ad883eb7d. "WHO Director-General's Opening Remarks at the Media Briefing on Covid-19," news release, March 11, 2020, https://www.who.int/dg/speeches/detail/who-director-general-s-opening-remarks-at-the-media-briefing-on-covid-19---11-march-2020.

2. Paul Quinton, oral history interview with the author, May 13, 2020; P. M. Quinton, "Chloride Impermeability in Cystic Fibrosis," *Nature* 301, no. 5899 (1983), https://doi.org/10.1038/301421a0.

3. Michael Boyle, "For Some, Social Distancing Is the Norm," *Medium*, March 31, 2020, https://medium.com/@MichaelBoyleMD/for-some-social-distancing-is-the-norm-bc87a597dcf8.

4. Boyle, "For Some, Social Distancing Is the Norm."

5. Andersen, "Cystic Fibrosis of the Pancreas," 370–71; Andersen and Hodges, "Celiac Syndrome: V."

6. "Sweating Is Clue to Deadly Child's Malady," 4; "A C/F Child Is in Your Class: A Teachers' Guide to Cystic Fibrosis," 1965, National Cystic Fibrosis Research Foundation, Collection AC12, box 2, cystic fibrosis folder, Boston Children's Hospital Archives. This effort to "decouple" a disease from a contagion was also seen in the case of cancer. Scheffler, *A Contagious Cause*, 35.

7. Andersen, "Cystic Fibrosis of the Pancreas"; Cystic Fibrosis Foundation, Patient Registry Annual Data Report, 2019, 72.

8. P. Rabinow, "Artificiality and Enlightenment: From Sociobiology to Biosociality," in *Incorporations*, ed. Jonathan Crary and Sanford Kwinter (Zone Books, 1992).

9. John V. Van Cleve and Barry A. Crouch, *A Place of Their Own: Creating the Deaf Community in America* (Gallaudet University Press, 1989); Wilson, *Living*

with Polio; Steven Epstein, *Impure Science: AIDS, Activism, and the Politics of Knowledge* (University of California Press, 1996); Douglas C. Baynton, *Forbidden Signs: American Culture and the Campaign Against Sign Language* (University of Chicago Press, 1996); Susan Burch, *Signs of Resistance: American Deaf Cultural History, 1900 to World War II* (New York University Press, 2002); Nicole Newnham and Jim LeBrecht, *Crip Camp: A Disability Revolution*, Netflix, 2020.

10. Isabel Stenzel Byrnes and Anabel Stenzel, *The Power of Two: A Twin Triumph over Cystic Fibrosis* (University of Missouri Press, 2007), 150.

11. For a discussion of conceptions of infectious versus chronic disease, see Allan M. Brandt, "Behavior, Disease, and Health in the Twentieth-Century United States: The Moral Valence of Individual Risk," in *Morality and Health*, ed. Allan M. Brandt and Paul Rozin (Routledge, 1997), 53–77.

12. For more on the relationship between clinical medicine and laboratory science, see Cunningham, "Transforming Plague"; Steve Sturdy, "Looking for Trouble: Medical Science and Clinical Practice in the Historiography of Modern Medicine," *Social History of Medicine* 24, no. 3 (2011), https://doi.org/10.1093/shm/hkq106; Rosemary Wall, *Bacteria in Britain, 1880–1939* (Pickering & Chatto, 2013).

13. Margaret B. Mearns et al., "Bacterial Flora of Respiratory Tract in Patients with Cystic Fibrosis, 1950–71," *Archives of Disease in Childhood* 47, no. 256 (1972), https://doi.org/10.1136/adc.47.256.902. Dorothy Andersen noted in 1938 that *S. aureus* was the "usual bacteriological agent" in lung disease detected on autopsy. Andersen, "Cystic Fibrosis of the Pancreas," 381.

14. G. Nolan et al., "Antibiotic Prophylaxis in Cystic Fibrosis: Inhaled Cephaloridine as an Adjunct to Oral Cloxacillin," *Journal of Pediatrics* 101, no. 4 (1982), https://doi.org/10.1016/S0022-3476(82)80726-9; Podolsky, *Pneumonia Before Antibiotics*; Podolsky, *The Antibiotic Era*.

15. Peter H. Gilligan, "Microbiology of Airway Disease in Patients with Cystic Fibrosis," *Clinical Microbiology Reviews* 4, no. 1 (1991): 37, https://doi.org/10.1128/cmr.4.1.35. However, there was debate about whether antibiotic use directly led to *P. aeruginosa* emergence.

16. David F. Welch, "Clinical Microbiology of Cystic Fibrosis," *Clinical Microbiology Newsletter* 6, no. 6 (1984).

17. Walter H. Burkholder, "Sour Skin, a Bacterial Rot of Onion Bulbs," *Phytopathology* 40 (1950).

18. Grace Mary Ederer and John M. Matsen, "Colonization and Infection with *Pseudomonas cepacia*," *Journal of Infectious Diseases* 125, no. 6 (1972): 617, https://doi.org/10.1093/infdis/125.6.613; William R. Jarvis, "Nosocomial Outbreaks: The Centers for Disease Control's Hospital Infections Program Experience, 1980–1990. Epidemiology Branch, Hospital Infections Program," *American Journal of Medicine* 91, no. 3B (1991), https://doi.org/10.1016/0002-9343(91)90352-x.

19. Ederer and Matsen, "Colonization and Infection with *Pseudomonas cepacia*," 617. The exact date is unknown, as Ederer and Matsen analyzed patient samples from January 1, 1968, to December 31, 1969, and pooled all results.

20. Marvin D. Lough et al., "Ten Years' Experience with a Camp for Children with Pulmonary Diseases," *Respiratory Care* 22, no. 8 (1977), http://www.ncbi.nlm.nih.gov/pubmed/10314876; J. Karen Scott, "Cystic Fibrosis—Camp Couchiching . . . Four Summers," *The Canadian Nurse* 73, no. 6 (1977), http://www.ncbi.nlm.nih.gov/pubmed/872069; Christie and Tansey, *Cystic Fibrosis. Wellcome Witnesses*.

21. According to a child who attended a CF camp in Canada in the mid-1970s, "I don't get depressed as much after being with kids with CF" because "I know other kids go through the same things as I do." Scott, "Camp Couchiching," 17.

22. Byrnes and Stenzel, *The Power of Two*, 51. In addition, twelve-year-old Robert Burtch pointed out in 1990 that CF camp "makes you feel normal, like you don't have the disease." Lisa Wright, "Hope Runs High in Summer as Young Campers Fight for Life," *Toronto Star*, August 13, 1990, A6.

23. Bruce Kalman Rubin and Douglas W. Geiger, "Pulmonary Function, Nutrition, and Self-Concept in Cystic Fibrosis Summer Campers," *Chest* 100, no. 3 (1991), https://doi.org/10.1378/chest.100.3.649; Ted A. Kaplan et al., "Impact of CF Summer Camp," *Clinical Pediatrics* 31, no. 3 (1992), https://doi.org/10.1177/000992289203100307. While the vast majority of accounts of CF camps are positive, not all campers found camps to be beneficial. For example, one father recalled years later that his son Kevin did not enjoy CF camp and instead found it to be "just a constant reminder that he was sick." Hendon, *It's Been a Good Life, Dad*, 27; Wilson, *Living with Polio*.

24. Christie and Tansey, *Cystic Fibrosis. Wellcome Witnesses*, 34. Quote by Professor John Dodge, referring to a CF camp that took place in South Wales. For more on the history of *P. cepacia* in people with CF, see James Littlewood, "*Burkholderia cepacia* Complex and Some Similar Organisms," https://cysticfibrosis.online/burkholderia-cepacia-complex-history.

25. Beryl J. Rosenstein and David E. Hall, "Pneumonia and Septicemia Due to *Pseudomonas cepacia* in a Patient with Cystic Fibrosis," *Johns Hopkins Medical Journal* 147, no. 5 (1980), http://www.ncbi.nlm.nih.gov/pubmed/7441939; Clare Randall, "The Problem of *Pseudomonas cepacia* in a Hospital," *Canadian Journal of Public Health* 71, no. 2 (1980), http://www.ncbi.nlm.nih.gov/pubmed/7388734; R. S. Baltimore et al., "Occurrence of Nonfermentative Gram-Negative Rods Other Than *Pseudomonas aeruginosa* in the Respiratory Tract of Children with Cystic Fibrosis," *Helvetica Paediatrica Acta* 37, no. 6 (1982), http://www.ncbi.nlm.nih.gov/pubmed/6820015.

26. J. R. Govan et al., "*Burkholderia cepacia*: Medical, Taxonomic and Ecological Issues," *Journal of Medical Microbiology* 45, no. 6 (1996): 397, https://doi.org/10.1099/00222615-45-6-395.

27. A. Isles et al., "*Pseudomonas cepacia* Infection in Cystic Fibrosis: An Emerging Problem," *Journal of Pediatrics* 104, no. 2 (1984): 208, https://doi.org/10.1016/s0022-3476(84)80993-2.

28. Govan et al., "*Burkholderia cepacia*," 395.

29. Isles et al., "*Pseudomonas cepacia* Infection," 208.

30. Isles et al., "*Pseudomonas cepacia* Infection," 209.

31. Lourdes R. Laraya-Cuasay et al., "*Pseudomonas cepacia* in the Respiratory Flora of Patients with Cystic Fibrosis (CF)," *Pediatric Research* 11, no. 4 (1977): 502, https://doi.org/10.1203/00006450-197704000-00792. Although CDC epidemiologists pointed out that "its significance was unknown" at the time, the SCHC cases are often referred to as the first reported cluster of *P. cepacia* infection in people with CF. O. C. Tablan et al., "The Epidemiology of *Pseudomonas cepacia* in Patients with Cystic Fibrosis," *European Journal of Epidemiology* 3, no. 4 (1987): 336, https://doi.org/10.1007/BF00145642.

32. John LiPuma, oral history interview with the author, April 19, 2016; Daniel Schidlow, oral history interview with the author, June 16, 2016.

33. Ofelia C. Tablan et al., "*Pseudomonas cepacia* Colonization in Patients with Cystic Fibrosis: Risk Factors and Clinical Outcome," *Journal of Pediatrics* 107, no. 3 (1985), https://doi.org/10.1016/S0022-3476(85)80511-4.

34. Tablan et al., "*Pseudomonas cepacia* Colonization," 382; Peter H. Gilligan and Daniel V. Shidlow, "The Role of *Pseudomonas cepacia* in Pulmonary Disease of Cystic Fibrosis Patients," *Clinical Microbiology Newsletter* 6, no. 6 (1984): 43, https://doi.org/10.1016/S0196-4399(84)80048-3.

35. Bernard Boxerbaum and Jeffrey D. Klinger, "*Pseudomonas cepacia* Bacteremia in Cystic Fibrosis," *Pediatric Research* 18 (1984), https://doi.org/10.1203/00006450-198404001-01059. While the hospital is now referred to as Rainbow Babies & Children's, in 1984 it was referred to as Rainbow Babies and Childrens. M. J. Thomassen et al., "*Pseudomonas cepacia* Colonization Among Patients with Cystic Fibrosis. A New Opportunist," *American Review of Respiratory Disease* 131, no. 5 (1985): 795, https://doi.org/10.1164/arrd.1985.131.5.791.

36. Thomassen et al., "*Pseudomonas cepacia* Colonization."

37. Ofelia C. Tablan et al., "Colonization of the Respiratory Tract with *Pseudomonas cepacia* in Cystic Fibrosis. Risk Factors and Outcomes," *Chest* 91, no. 4 (1987), https://doi.org/10.1378/chest.91.4.527.

38. M. J. Thomassen et al., "*Pseudomonas cepacia*: Decrease in Colonization in Patients with Cystic Fibrosis," *American Review of Respiratory Disease* 134, no. 4 (1986): 669, https://doi.org/10.1164/arrd.1986.134.4.669.

39. Alice Prince, "*Pseudomonas cepacia* in Cystic Fibrosis Patients," *American Review of Respiratory Disease* 134, no. 4 (1986): 644, https://doi.org/10.1164/arrd.1986.134.4.644.

40. Tablan et al., "Epidemiology of *Pseudomonas cepacia*," 339. For more on the history of the Epidemic Intelligence Service, see Stephen B. Thacker et al., "Epidemic Intelligence Service of the Centers for Disease Control and Prevention: 50 Years of Training and Service in Applied Epidemiology," *American Journal of Epidemiology* 154, no. 11 (2001), https://doi.org/10.1093/aje/154.11.985.

41. Thomassen et al., "*Pseudomonas cepacia*."

42. Tablan et al., "Epidemiology of *Pseudomonas cepacia*," 339.

43. C. S. Rabkin et al., "Current Status of *Pseudomonas cepacia* Typing Systems," *European Journal of Epidemiology* 3, no. 4 (1987), https://doi.org/10.1007/BF00145643.

44. Terrence L. Stull et al., "A Broad-Spectrum Probe for Molecular Epidemiology of Bacteria: Ribosomal RNA," *Journal of Infectious Diseases* 157, no. 2 (1988), https://doi.org/10.1093/infdis/157.2.280.

45. John J. LiPuma et al., "Molecular Epidemiology of *Pseudomonas cepacia* (Pc) in Patients with Cystic Fibrosis (CF)," *Pediatric Research* 21, no. 4 (1987), https://doi.org/10.1203/00006450-198704010-00547; LiPuma, interview; Stull et al., "Broad-Spectrum Probe"; John J. LiPuma et al., "Ribotype Analysis of *Pseudomonas cepacia* from Cystic Fibrosis Treatment Centers," *Journal of Pediatrics* 113, no. 5 (1988), https://doi.org/10.1016/S0022-3476(88)80018-0.

46. John J. LiPuma et al., "Person-to-Person Transmission of *Pseudomonas cepacia* Between Patients with Cystic Fibrosis," *Lancet* 336, no. 8723 (1990), https://doi.org/10.1016/0140-6736(90)92571-X.

47. Schidlow, interview; LiPuma et al., "Person-to-Person Transmission of Pseudomonas cepacia," 1095; Loretta A. Carson et al., "Proceedings of the Third Decennial International Conference on Nosocomial Infections: Isoenzyme Analysis of *Pseudomonas cepacia* as an Epidemiological Tool," *American Journal of Medicine* 91 (1991): 253S, https://doi.org/10.1016/0002-9343(91)90377-a.

48. R. Honicky et al., "*Pseudomonas cepacia* at Summer Camps for Persons with Cystic Fibrosis," *Morbidity and Mortality Weekly Report* 42, no. 23 (1993), http://www.ncbi.nlm.nih.gov/pubmed/7684813; Robert C. Stern to Giantonio Cazzola and Gianni Mastella, January 30, 1993. Copy of letter provided to Michelle LaBonte by Dr. Robert Stern. This form of contact tracing of summer camp attendees within the CF community, which includes a small fraction of the population, was logistically different from contact tracing in the setting of an infectious disease that a whole population would in theory be susceptible to.

49. David A. Pegues et al., "Acquisition of *Pseudomonas cepacia* at Summer Camps for Patients with Cystic Fibrosis. Summer Camp Study Group," *Journal of Pediatrics* 124, no. 5, part 1 (1994), https://doi.org/10.1016/s0022-3476(05)81357-5; Joanna L Burns and Jean M Keller, "Camping for Youth with Chronic Illnesses," *Camping Magazine* 67, no. 1 (1994); Sarah Walters and E. Grace Smith, "*Pseudomonas cepacia* in Cystic Fibrosis: Transmissibility and Its Implications," *Lancet* 342, no. 8862 (1993), https://doi.org/10.1016/0140-6736(93)91875-M.

50. A number of *P. cepacia* infections in UK hospitals were linked to contact with patients in North America. E. J. Simmonds et al., "*Pseudomonas cepacia*: A New Pathogen in Patients with Cystic Fibrosis Referred to a Large Centre in the United Kingdom," *Archives of Disease in Childhood* 65, no. 8 (1990), https://doi.org/10.1136/adc.65.8.874. L. Millar-Jones et al., "Transmission of *Pseudomonas cepacia* among Cystic Fibrosis Patients," *Lancet* 340, no. 8817 (1992), https://doi.org/10.1016/0140-6736(92)91817-r; John R. Govan et al., "Evidence for Transmission

of *Pseudomonas cepacia* by Social Contact in Cystic Fibrosis," *Lancet* 342, no. 8862 (1993), https://doi.org/10.1016/0140-6736(93)91881-l.

51. Schidlow, interview. For an account of the experience of alienation and difference in the setting of a diagnosis, see Goffman, *Stigma*.

52. Burkholder, "Sour Skin."

53. Schidlow, interview.

54. Helen Branswell, "Forced into Isolation: Bacteria That Rot Onions Turning Some People with CF into Modern Day Lepers," *Canadian Press*, December 4, 2002.

55. Branswell, "Forced into Isolation." Just like those with leprosy, many *P. cepacia*–infected people with CF felt stigmatized and questioned "the necessity of mandatory isolation." Heather Varughese John, "Translating Leprosy: The Expert and the Public in Stanley Stein's Anti-Stigmatization Campaigns, 1931–60," *Journal of the History of Medicine and Allied Sciences* 68, no. 4 (2013): 669, https://doi.org/10.1093/jhmas/jrs018; Rod Edmond, *Leprosy and Empire: A Medical and Cultural History* (Cambridge University Press, 2006); Michelle Therese Moran, *Colonizing Leprosy: Imperialism and the Politics of Public Health in the United States* (University of North Carolina Press, 2007).

56. Branswell, "Forced into Isolation."

57. Cystic Fibrosis Foundation, "Microbiology and Infectious Disease in Cystic Fibrosis," Consensus Conferences: Concepts in Care, Appendix VIII, 1994. Document provided by Sarah Hempstead at the Cystic Fibrosis Foundation.

58. Katrina Miles, "Bacterium Keeps a Disease's Victims Apart: For a Few Cystic Fibrosis Patients, a Bug Spells Isolation from Other Sufferers," *Philadelphia Inquirer*, August 10, 1995.

59. Miles, "Bacterium Keeps a Disease's Victims Apart." For an account of the history of quarantine as an approach to prevent the spread of disease, see Howard Markel, *Quarantine!: East European Jewish Immigrants and the New York City Epidemics of 1892* (Johns Hopkins University Press, 1999). Scholars have examined the impact of the separation of children from their parents in the hospital setting, yet those with *P. cepacia* (and later all people with CF) faced separation from others with CF during hospital stays and outside of the hospital setting. For more on child separation from parents during hospitalization, see Daniel J. Wilson, "Psychological Trauma and Its Treatment in the Polio Epidemics," *Bulletin of the History of Medicine* 82, no. 4 (2008), https://doi.org/10.1353/bhm.0.0119; David Wright, *SickKids: The History of the Hospital for Sick Children* (University of Toronto Press, 2016), chapter 8.

60. Miles, "Bacterium Keeps a Disease's Victims Apart."

61. Miles, "Bacterium Keeps a Disease's Victims Apart."

62. Govan et al., "*Burkholderia cepacia*," 397.

63. Microbiologists played a key role in the development of infection control protocols in response to an outbreak of *Staphylococcus aureus* strain 80/81 in the

1950s in hospital nurseries. See Kathryn Hillier, "Babies and Bacteria: Phage Typing, Bacteriologists, and the Birth of Infection Control," *Bulletin of the History of Medicine* 80, no. 4 (2006), https://doi.org/10.1353/bhm.2006.0130.

64. Welch, "Clinical Microbiology of Cystic Fibrosis," 41.

65. On the concept of the healthy carrier, see Nancy Tomes, *The Gospel of Germs: Men, Women, and the Microbe in American Life* (Harvard University Press, 1998), 92–93; Judith Walzer Leavitt, *Typhoid Mary: Captive to the Public's Health* (Beacon Press, 1996); Hammonds, *Childhood's Deadly Scourge*. On the changing conceptions of germ theory over time and in different locations, see Nancy J. Tomes and John Harley Warner, "Introduction to Special Issue on Rethinking the Reception of the Germ Theory of Disease: Comparative Perspectives," *Journal of the History of Medicine and Allied Sciences* 52, no. 1 (1997), https://doi.org/10.1093/jhmas/52.1.7; Brandt, "Behavior, Disease, and Health."

66. Furthermore, the detection of a microbe has not always been synonymous with the diagnosis of disease. With the advent of bacteriological diagnosis of diphtheria, there was a shift from defining diphtheria by symptoms (a clinical diagnosis) to defining it based on the detection of the microbe in the laboratory. See Hammonds, *Childhood's Deadly Scourge*, chapter 2.

67. For an earlier example of the challenge of microbe detection in samples from people with symptomatic typhoid fever in late nineteenth century England, see Jacob Steere-Williams, *The Filth Disease: Typhoid Fever and the Practices of Epidemiology in Victorian England* (University of Rochester Press, 2021).

68. Burkholder, "Sour Skin."

69. Burkholder, "Sour Skin," 115.

70. Burkholder, "Sour Skin," 115, 116. On the role of the laboratory in "translating" or linking a microbe to a disease, see Bruno Latour, *The Pasteurization of France* (Harvard University Press, 1988). For more on Koch and bacteriology, see Thomas D. Brock, *Robert Koch: A Life in Medicine and Bacteriology* (ASM Press, 1999); Christoph Gradmann, *Laboratory Disease: Robert Koch's Medical Bacteriology* (Johns Hopkins University Press, 2009).

71. Burkholder, "Sour Skin," 115.

72. Gilligan and Shidlow, "The Role of *Pseudomonas cepacia*," 43. Even though Koch, Pasteur, and others thought of bacteria as "natural kinds," they were not able to distinguish the kinds by observing differences in size and shape but instead needed to focus on "what these cells did." As such, "variable responses to media became central in defining species." Christopher Hamlin, "Bacteriology as a Cultural System: Analysis and Its Discontents," *History of Science* 49, no. 164 (2011): 273, https://doi.org/10.1177/007327531104900303. Furthermore, as Maureen O'Malley notes, the advent of the "pure culture method" aided investigators in the challenging task of attempting to classify microorganisms. Maureen O'Malley, *Philosophy of Microbiology* (Cambridge University Press, 2014), 69.

73. Gilligan and Shidlow, "The Role of *Pseudomonas cepacia*," 43.

74. Gilligan and Shidlow, "The Role of *Pseudomonas cepacia*," 43.

75. Peter H. Gilligan et al., "Isolation Medium for the Recovery of *Pseudomonas cepacia* from Respiratory Secretions of Patients with Cystic Fibrosis," *Journal of Clinical Microbiology* 22, no. 1 (1985), https://doi.org/10.1128/jcm.22.1.5-8.1985.

76. Gilligan et al., "Isolation Medium," 5.

77. David F. Welch et al., "Selective and Differential Medium for Recovery of *Pseudomonas cepacia* from the Respiratory Tracts of Patients with Cystic Fibrosis," *Journal of Clinical Microbiology* 25, no. 9 (1987), https://doi.org/10.1128/jcm.25.9.1730-1734.1987.

78. Cynthia Black-Payne et al., "Comparison of Two Selective Media Developed to Isolate *Pseudomonas cepacia* from Patients with Cystic Fibrosis," *Diagnostic Microbiology and Infectious Disease* 6, no. 4 (1987), https://doi.org/10.1016/0732-8893(87)90175-1.

79. Ofelia C. Tablan et al., "Laboratory Proficiency Test Results on Use of Selective Media for Isolating *Pseudomonas cepacia* from Simulated Sputum Specimens of Patients with Cystic Fibrosis," *Journal of Clinical Microbiology* 25, no. 3 (1987), https://doi.org/10.1128/jcm.25.3.485-487.1987.

80. Tablan et al., "Laboratory Proficiency Test Results."

81. Tablan et al., "Epidemiology of *Pseudomonas cepacia*"; Karin L. McGowan, "The Microbiology Associated with Cystic Fibrosis," *Clinical Microbiology Newsletter* 10, no. 2 (1988): 10.

82. L. A. Carson et al., "Comparative Evaluation of Selective Media for Isolation of *Pseudomonas cepacia* from Cystic Fibrosis Patients and Environmental Sources," *Journal of Clinical Microbiology* 26, no. 10 (1988), https://doi.org/10.1128/jcm.26.10.2096-2100.1988.

83. Carson et al., "Comparative Evaluation of Selective Media." *P. cepacia* medium (PCM) appears to be the same as the PC medium described by Gilligan and colleagues above.

84. Carson et al., "Comparative Evaluation of Selective Media," 2100.

85. J. J. Kilbane et al., "Biodegradation of 2,4,5-Trichlorophenoxyacetic Acid by a Pure Culture of *Pseudomonas cepacia*," *Applied and Environmental Microbiology* 44, no. 1 (1982), https://doi.org/10.1128/aem.44.1.72-78.1982.

86. Mueller, "Impact of Transmissible Microbes."

87. Cystic Fibrosis Foundation, "Microbiology and Infectious Disease in Cystic Fibrosis."

88. Deborah A. Henry et al., "Identification of *Burkholderia cepacia* Isolates from Patients with Cystic Fibrosis and Use of a Simple New Selective Medium," *Journal of Clinical Microbiology* 35, no. 3 (1997): 618, https://doi.org/10.1128/jcm.35.3.614-619.1997.

89. Henry et al., "Identification of *Burkholderia cepacia* Isolates," 614.

90. Tom Coenye et al., "Taxonomy and Identification of the *Burkholderia cepacia* Complex," *Journal of Clinical Microbiology* 39, no. 10 (2001): 3427, https://doi.org/10.1128/JCM.39.10.3427-3436.2001.

91. Coenye et al., "Taxonomy and Identification of the Burkholderia cepacia Complex," 3433.

92. Robert Stern, oral history interview with the author, June 9, 2016.

93. Stern, interview. In the context of Lyme disease diagnostics, Aronowitz notes that "many patients test positive in some laboratories and negative in others." Aronowitz, "Lyme Disease," 99.

94. D. L. Smith et al., "Epidemic of *Pseudomonas cepacia* in an Adult Cystic Fibrosis Unit: Evidence of Person-to-Person Transmission," *Journal of Clinical Microbiology* 31, no. 11 (1993), https://doi.org/10.1128/jcm.31.11.3017-3022.1993.

95. Smith et al., "Epidemic of *Pseudomonas cepacia*."

96. Peter Vandamme and Peter Dawyndt, "Classification and Identification of the *Burkholderia cepacia* Complex: Past, Present and Future," *Systematic and Applied Microbiology* 34, no. 2 (2011): 87, https://doi.org/10.1016/j.syapm.2010.10.002. By the 1990s, *P. cepacia* had been reclassified as part of the *B. cepacia* complex as described below.

97. LiPuma, interview.

98. As Christopher Hamlin notes, efforts at bacterial taxonomy weren't as valued during Koch's time because linking a microbe to a disease was prioritized. Hamlin, "Bacteriology as a Cultural System," 280. Just as Lorraine Daston argues that "wonder was . . . the maker of scientific objects" in the late sixteenth century and the seventeenth century, the medical relevance of *P. cepacia* (and corresponding efforts to trace its spread) prompted it to become an object of intensive scientific investigation in the 1990s. Lorraine Daston, "What Can Be a Scientific Object? Reflections on Monsters and Meteors," *Bulletin of the American Academy of Arts and Sciences* 52, no. 2 (1998): 50, https://doi.org/10.2307/3824838.

99. LiPuma, interview.

100. As Ritvo notes, organisms such as the kangaroo and the platypus were difficult to classify using the taxonomic systems that were in place at the time they were identified. Harriet Ritvo, *The Platypus and the Mermaid and Other Figments of the Classifying Imagination* (Harvard University Press, 1997). Noting that many scholars have emphasized the dominance of genetic over naturalist classification systems, Sommerlund argues that the two systems can coexist in the setting of a microbial ecology laboratory. Julie Sommerlund, "Classifying Microorganisms: The Multiplicity of Classifications and Research Practices in Molecular Microbial Ecology," *Social Studies of Science* 36, no. 6 (2006), https://www.jstor.org/stable/25474488. Helmreich highlights how the identification of lateral gene transfer caused microbiologists to rethink the tree of life and view it more as a web and called into question the species category in microbiology. Stefan Helmreich, *Alien Ocean: Anthropological Voyages in Microbial Seas* (University of California Press, 2009). For more on lateral gene transfer and the species concept, see O'Malley, *Philosophy of Microbiology*, chapter 3. For an account of Koch's views on the classification of bacteria, see Pauline M. H. Mazumdar, *Species and Specificity: An Interpretation of the History of Immunology* (Cambridge University Press, 1995);

Evan Hepler-Smith, "'Just as the Structural Formula Does': Names, Diagrams, and the Structure of Organic Chemistry at the 1892 Geneva Nomenclature Congress," *Ambix* 62, no. 1 (2015), https://doi.org/10.1179/1745823414Y.0000000006.

101. Burkholder, "Sour Skin."

102. Burkholder, "Sour Skin," 117. As O'Malley notes, "early in the official history of microbial classification, distinctions between Gram-negative and Gram-positive cells were made on the basis of staining techniques developed in the late nineteenth century." O'Malley, *Philosophy of Microbiology*, 58.

103. Burkholder, "Sour Skin," 117.

104. Burkholder, "Sour Skin."

105. R. Y. Stanier et al., "The Aerobic Pseudomonads: A Taxonomic Study," *Journal of General Microbiology* 43, no. 2 (1966): 247, https://doi.org/10.1099/00221287-43-2-159; Valguard Jonsson, "Proposal of a New Species *Pseudomonas kingii*," *International Journal of Systematic Bacteriology* 20, no. 3 (1970): 255, https://doi.org/10.1099/00207713-20-3-255; R. W. Ballard et al., "Taxonomy of the Aerobic Pseudomonads: *Pseudomonas cepacia, P. marginata, P. alliicola* and *P. caryophylli*," *Journal of General Microbiology* 60, no. 2 (1970), https://doi.org/10.1099/00221287-60-2-199. J. J. S. Snell et al., "Identification of *Pseudomonas cepacia* Burkholder and Its Synonymy with *Pseudomonas kingii* Jonsson," *International Journal of Systematic Bacteriology* 22, no. 3 (1972), https://doi.org/10.1099/00207713-22-3-127. Sally B. Samuels et al., "The Fatty Acids of *Pseudomonas multivorans* (*Pseudomonas cepacia*) and *Pseudomonas kingii*," *Journal of General Microbiology* 74, no. 2 (1973), https://doi.org/10.1099/00221287-74-2-275.

106. As Meerwijk notes, visualizations of pathogens such as bacteria have been key to defining and legitimizing a disease. See Maurits Bastiaan Meerwijk, "Viral Imagery of Dengue Fever in the Age of Bacteriology," *Isis* 111, no. 2 (2020), https://doi.org/10.1086/708927.

107. Vandamme and Dawyndt, "Classification and Identification of the Burkholderia cepacia Complex," 87.

108. N. J. Palleroni et al., "Nucleic Acid Homologies in the Genus Pseudomonas," *International Journal of Systematic Bacteriology* 23, no. 4 (1973): 337, https://doi.org/10.1099/00207713-23-4-333.

109. The five groups were determined by hybridization of rRNA to DNA.

110. Palleroni et al., "Nucleic Acid Homologies in the Genus *Pseudomonas*," 337.

111. In 1981, Palleroni and Holmes revived the name *P. cepacia*, which had not been included on the approved list of bacterial species names in 1980. N. J. Palleroni and B. Holmes, "*Pseudomonas cepacia* sp. nov., nom. rev.," *International Journal of Systematic Bacteriology* 31, no. 4 (1981), https://doi.org/10.1099/00207713-31-4-479.

112. E. Yabuuchi et al., "Proposal of *Burkholderia* gen. nov. and Transfer of Seven Species of the Genus *Pseudomonas* Homology Group II to the New Genus, with the Type Species *Burkholderia cepacia* (Palleroni and Holmes 1981) comb. nov.," *Micro-*

biology and Immunology 36, no. 12 (1992), https://doi.org/10.1111/j.1348-0421.1992.tb02129.x.

113. Yabuuchi et al., "Proposal of *Burkholderia*," 1268.

114. Vandamme and Dawyndt, "Classification and Identification of the *Burkholderia cepacia* Complex." 88. *B. cepacia* isolate variation was attributed to distinct strains of microbes, in contrast to the cyclogenic theories of bacterial variation expressed in the early twentieth century. Olga Amsterdamska, "Stabilizing Instability: The Controversy over Cyclogenic Theories of Bacterial Variation During the Interwar Period," *Journal of the History of Biology* 24, no. 2 (1991), https://doi.org/10.1007/BF00209429; William C. Summers, "From Culture as Organism to Organism as Cell: Historical Origins of Bacterial Genetics," *Journal of the History of Biology* 24, no. 2 (1991), https://doi.org/10.1007/BF00209428. For more on the history of conceptions of bacterial variation, see J. Andrew Mendelsohn, "'Like All That Lives': Biology, Medicine and Bacteria in the Age of Pasteur and Koch," *History and Philosophy of the Life Sciences* 24, no. 1 (2002), https://doi.org/10.1080/03919710210001714293; Olga Amsterdamska, "Achieving Disbelief: Thought Styles, Microbial Variation, and American and British Epidemiology, 1900–1940," *Studies in History and Philosophy of Biological and Biomedical Sciences* 35 (2004), https://doi.org/10.1016/j.shpsc.2004.06.001. For an account of variation in bacterial metabolism, see Robert E. Kohler, "Innovation in Normal Science. Bacterial Physiology," *Isis* 76, no. 282 (1985), https://doi.org/10.1086/353798.

115. Vandamme and Dawyndt, "Classification and Identification of the *Burkholderia cepacia* Complex." 88.

116. P. Gilligan, "Report on the Consensus Document for Microbiology and Infectious Diseases in Cystic Fibrosis," *Clinical Microbiology Newsletter* 18, no. 11 (1996): 84.

117. Govan et al., "*Burkholderia cepacia*," 400.

118. Since new species names could not be designated in the absence of clearly distinct phenotypic features, they used the "recently introduced" term *genomovar* to "denote phenotypically similar but genotypically distinct groups of strains." In other words, genomovar was the term used to designate a microbe that was possibly a distinct species, but one that had not necessarily been given species status. While two of the genomovars were assigned formal species names at that time, the other three were designated by roman numerals. P. Vandamme et al., "Occurrence of Multiple Genomovars of *Burkholderia cepacia* in Cystic Fibrosis Patients and Proposal of *Burkholderia multivorans* sp. nov.," *International Journal of Systematic Bacteriology* 47, no. 4 (1997): 1188, https://doi.org/10.1099/00207713-47-4-1188.

119. Vandamme et al., "Occurrence of Multiple Genomovars," 1198.

120. T. Coenye et al., "*Burkholderia cepacia* Genomovar VI, a New Member of the *Burkholderia cepacia* Complex Isolated from Cystic Fibrosis Patients," *International Journal of Systematic and Evolutionary Microbiology* 51, part 2 (2001), https://doi.org/10.1099/00207713-51-2-271.

121. The term *species* is used instead of genomovar for simplicity. J. J. LiPuma et al., "Disproportionate Distribution of *Burkholderia cepacia* Complex Species and Transmissibility Markers in Cystic Fibrosis," *American Journal of Respiratory and Critical Care Medicine* 164, no. 1 (2001), https://doi.org/10.1164/ajrccm.164.1.2011153. D. P. Speert et al., "Epidemiology of *Burkholderia cepacia* Complex in Patients with Cystic Fibrosis, Canada," *Emerging Infectious Diseases* 8, no. 2 (2002), https://doi.org/10.3201/eid0802.010163.

122. Peter Vandamme et al., "*Burkholderia anthina* sp. nov. and *Burkholderia pyrrocinia*, Two Additional *Burkholderia cepacia* Complex Bacteria, May Confound Results of New Molecular Diagnostic Tools," *FEMS Immunology and Medical Microbiology* 33, no. 2 (2002): 143, https://doi.org/10.1111/j.1574-695X.2002.tb00584.x; John J. Lipuma, "Preventing *Burkholderia cepacia* Complex Infection in Cystic Fibrosis: Is There a Middle Ground?," *Journal of Pediatrics* 141, no. 4 (2002), https://doi.org/10.1067/mpd.2002.128892.

123. LiPuma, interview.

124. John LiPuma, "Update on Burkholderia Nomenclature and Resistance," *Clinical Microbiology Newsletter* 29, no. 9 (2007); Leo Eberl and Peter Vandamme, "Members of the Genus Burkholderia: Good and Bad Guys," *F1000 Research* 5 (2016), https://doi.org/10.12688/f1000research.8221.1.

125. John J. LiPuma, "The Changing Microbial Epidemiology in Cystic Fibrosis," *Clinical Microbiology Reviews* 23, no. 2 (2010), https://doi.org/10.1128/CMR.00068-09.

126. Pablo Martina et al., "*Burkholderia puraquae* sp. nov., a Novel Species of the *Burkholderia cepacia* Complex Isolated from Hospital Settings and Agricultural Soils," *International Journal of Systematic and Evolutionary Microbiology* 68, no. 1 (2018), https://doi.org/10.1099/ijsem.0.002293.

127. LiPuma, interview. For a powerful account by a young woman who had CF and was also infected with *B. cenocepacia*, see Mallory Smith, *Salt in My Soul: An Unfinished Life* (Spiegel & Grau, 2019).

128. LiPuma, interview.

129. Lisa Saiman and Jane Siegel, "Infection Control in Cystic Fibrosis," *Clinical Microbiology Reviews* 17, no. 1 (2004), https://doi.org/10.1128/cmr.17.1.57-71.2004. As noted in the report, "while *P. aeruginosa* is the most clinically significant pathogen in patients with CF, more is known about the transmission of *B. cepacia* complex," which "serves as a prototype for infection control issues in patients with CF," 60.

130. Lisa Saiman et al., "Infection Control Recommendations for Patients with Cystic Fibrosis: Microbiology, Important Pathogens, and Infection Control Practices to Prevent Patient-to-Patient Transmission," *Infection Control and Hospital Epidemiology* 24, no. 5, suppl. (2003): S7, https://doi.org/10.1086/503485.

131. Saiman et al., "Infection Control Recommendations," S7. Segregation practices were also deemed unsafe for those with confirmed *B. cepacia* complex infections.

132. Saiman et al., "Infection Control Recommendations," S10.

133. LiPuma, interview.

134. LiPuma, interview. For an account from a person with CF, see Kayla Rachlin Small, "The Steep Price of Our Forbidden Kiss," *New York Times*, March 16, 2008, http://www.nytimes.com/2008/03/16/fashion/16love.html?_r=1.

135. The most prevalent microbe in people diagnosed with CF in the US in 2013 was *S. aureus*, followed by *P. aeruginosa*, MRSA, MDR-PA, *H. influenzae*, *S. maltophilia*, *A. xylosoxidans*, and *B. cepacia* complex. In contrast, the most prevalent microbe in the CF population in 1988 was *P. aeruginosa*, followed by *S. aureus*, *H. influenzae*, and *B. cepacia* complex microorganisms. It was and continues to be common for people with CF to test positive for multiple microbes. The 2013 CFF guidelines recommended that people with CF "receive four microbiological cultures" each year, a recommendation followed by 52 percent of people with CF. Cystic Fibrosis Foundation, Patient Registry Annual Data Report, 2013, 12. Report provided by Christina Pietrasanta at the Cystic Fibrosis Foundation.

136. Lisa Saiman et al., "Infection Prevention and Control Guideline for Cystic Fibrosis: 2013 Update," *Infection Control and Hospital Epidemiology* 35 (2014): S3, S4, https://doi.org/10.1086/676882. As noted in the report, "For decades, person-to-person transmission of *Burkholderia* spp. has been described, while person-to-person transmission of *P. aeruginosa* has been increasingly recognized in CF centers worldwide," S28. Concern about antibiotic resistance of other microbes in people with CF is also noted.

137. Saiman et al., "Infection Prevention and Control Guideline 2013," S4.

138. James C. Cunningham and Lynn M. Taussig, *An Introduction to Cystic Fibrosis for Patients and Their Families*, 6th ed., Cystic Fibrosis Foundation, 2013, 109. Document provided by Christina Pietrasanta at the Cystic Fibrosis Foundation.

139. Julie Desch, "When the CFF Gets It Wrong," *Sick and Happy* (blog), August 27, 2013, http://www.sickandhappy.com/when-the-cff-gets-it-wrong/#comments.

140. Desch, "When the CFF Gets It Wrong." Freedom has had different meanings over time and in various contexts. In the case of Mary Mallon, freedom meant the ability to choose one's place of residence, without confinement to an island; with *cepacia*, as Desch notes, freedom meant the ability to choose what types of risks to expose oneself to, including the ability to gather with other people with CF. For more on conceptions of freedom in the setting of infectious disease, see Graham Mooney, *Intrusive Interventions: Public Health, Domestic Space, and Infectious Disease Surveillance in England, 1840–1914* (University of Rochester Press, 2015); Leavitt, *Typhoid Mary*.

141. E. E. Andrews et al., "The Evolution of Disability Language: Choosing Terms to Describe Disability," *Disability and Health Journal* 15, no. 3 (2022): 2, https://doi.org/10.1016/j.dhjo.2022.101328.

142. Desch, "When the CFF Gets It Wrong." Quotes in the previous sentence are from people who responded to Desch's blog post. For an example of someone

who supported the foundation's guidelines, see the comment by Erin on August 28, 2013.

143. Manu Jain et al., "Point: Does the Risk of Cross Infection Warrant Exclusion of Adults with Cystic Fibrosis from Cystic Fibrosis Foundation Events? Yes," *Chest* 145, no. 4 (2014): 678, https://doi.org/10.1378/chest.13-2404.

144. Jain et al., "Point: Yes," 679.

145. Steven L. Shepherd et al., "Counterpoint: Does the Risk of Cross Infection Warrant Exclusion of Adults with Cystic Fibrosis from Cystic Fibrosis Foundation Events? No," *Chest* 145, no. 4 (2014): 681, https://doi.org/10.1378/chest.13-2406.

146. Shepherd et al., "Counterpoint: No," 682.

147. Shepherd et al., "Counterpoint: No," 682. There are important parallels between the CF case and efforts to keep Deaf persons apart in the form of marriage restrictions and the promotion of integration through oralism, yet the two cases are distinct in terms of the reasons why separation was promoted. As Jaipreet Virdi notes, "the Deaf were expected to give up their separate community . . . and absorb values that reflected the vision of 'normal' America," whereas in the CF case, instead of the goal of assimilation, those in leadership positions favored infection control guidelines that called for the separation of people with CF to reduce the mortality and morbidity of those with CF. Virdi, *Hearing Happiness*, 12.

148. Manu Jain et al., "Rebuttal from Dr Jain et al," *Chest* 145, no. 4 (2014): 683, https://doi.org/10.1378/chest.13-2405.

149. Steven L. Shepherd et al., "Rebuttal from Mr Shepherd et al," *Chest* 145, no. 4 (2014): 685, https://doi.org/10.1378/chest.13-2407.

150. Shepherd et al., "Rebuttal." See the supplemental audio material. The podcast was hosted by D. Kyle Hogarth. Shepherd pointed to Cystic Fibrosis Research, Inc., as a model for how to safely allow more than one person with CF to attend meetings in person.

151. Daniela J. Lamas, "Cystic Fibrosis Patients Losing a Connection," *Boston Globe*, November 18, 2013, https://www.bostonglobe.com/lifestyle/health-wellness/2013/11/18/cystic-fibrosis-patients-losing-connection/vl06v1Je4DiI5CLjNLMrMP/story.html.

152. Quinton, interview. A person with CF was able to attend the 2015 North American Cystic Fibrosis Conference as a "robot," or a "tablet on wheels." Danielle Lowe, "Creating a Meaningful Virtual Community," *Cystic Fibrosis Foundation CF Community Blog* (blog), October 21, 2015, https://www.cff.org/CF-Community-Blog/Posts/2015/Creating-a-Meaningful-Virtual-Community/.

153. Erin Evans, oral history interview with the author, May 14, 2020.

154. Peter Evans and Debra Maloney-Evans, oral history interview with the author, May 20, 2020. Erin's mother, Debra Maloney-Evans, did not feel the same sense of loss following the implementation of infection control guidelines because she found the "interactions with families . . . very upsetting because so many of the kids were so much sicker than Erin."

155. S. and S., interview.

156. The CF Foundation has supported BreatheCon, an online community for CF adults to "connect, learn, share, and inspire each other." "BreatheCon: A Virtual Conference for Adults with CF," https://www.cff.org/For-Caregivers/For-Clinicians/Network-News/Fall-2016/BreatheCon-A-Virtual-Conference-for-Adults-With-CF/.

157. Cystic Fibrosis Foundation, "Microbiology and Infectious Disease in Cystic Fibrosis," 1.

158. Cystic Fibrosis Foundation, "Microbiology and Infectious Disease in Cystic Fibrosis," 1.

159. Eric Sorscher, oral history interview with the author, April 23, 2019.

160. Jeff Truesdell, "Wife in Real-Life Fault in Our Stars Couple Opens up About Their Heartbreaking Love Story: 'He Was My Other Half,' " *People*, September 20, 2016, https://people.com/celebrity/wife-in-real-life-fault-in-our-stars-couple-shares-their-love-story/. While some individuals with CF have met through online communities for people with the disease, that was not the case for Katie and Dalton. Instead, Dalton's mother (a pediatric nurse) and Katie had a mutual connection on Facebook, and Katie found Dalton through his mother's Facebook page.

161. Truesdell, "Wife in Real-Life Fault in Our Stars Couple."

162. "Husband of Real Fault in Our Stars Couple Has Died," *Newser.com*, September 19, 2016.

163. Elizabeth Cohen, " 'Fault in Our Stars' Couple: Katie Prager Dies," *CNN.com*, September 23, 2016, http://www.cnn.com/2016/09/22/health/cystic-fibrosis-katie-prager-death/.

164. The existence of online communities likely facilitated debates about in-person contact between people with CF in the context of Katie and Dalton Prager. On the use of social media by people with CF, and the role of online communities, see Margaret Anne Faust, "The Use of Social Media and the Impact of Support on the Well-Being of Adult Cystic Fibrosis Patients" (master's thesis, University of South Carolina, Columbia, 2014).

165. Gunnar Esiason, "Cystic Fibrosis and 'the Fault in Our Stars,' " *Own It* (blog), September 22, 2016, http://www.gunnaresiason.com/cystic-fibrosis-fault-stars/. It appears that Dalton Prager had *B. multivorans* for seventeen years before passing away. See comments by Dalton's mother, Sandy Renee Strauser, in the comments section of the blog post.

166. Esiason, "Cystic Fibrosis and 'the Fault in Our Stars.' "

167. In a 2020 interview, Esiason expanded on this "public health issue," noting that "whereas people may think that their behaviors are limited to their experience or exposure between one another, it's really more broadly impactful because they're also going to the same CF clinics that we all go to." Gunnar Esiason, oral history interview with the author, May 27, 2020.

168. Gunnar Esiason, "Cystic Fibrosis and 'the Fault in Our Stars.'" See the comments section.

169. Desch, interview.

Epilogue

Some of the material in this chapter was originally published in Michelle Lynne LaBonte, "Addressing Uncertainty: The Emergence of the CRMS/CFSPID Diagnostic Category Following Newborn Screening for Cystic Fibrosis," *OBM Genetics* 5, no. 3 (2021), https://doi.org/10.21926/obm.genet.2103139.

1. Michelle Mastrianni, "Reading Palms: Aquagenic Wrinkling and a Late CF Diagnosis," April 5, 2021, https://www.youtube.com/watch?v=VeHjClIp4TQ; Michelle Mastrianni, oral history interview with the author, October 21, 2021.

2. Mastrianni, "Reading Palms."

3. This skin condition was also described to Michelle as aquagenic keratoderma.

4. Mastrianni, "Reading Palms."

5. Mastrianni, "Reading Palms."

6. K. A. Katz et al., "Aquagenic Wrinkling of the Palms in Patients with Cystic Fibrosis Homozygous for the ΔF508 *CFTR* Mutation," *Archives of Dermatology* 141, no. 5 (2005), https://doi.org/10.1001/archderm.141.5.621; L. C. Stewart et al., "Aquagenic Palmar Wrinkling as a Presenting Feature of Cystic Fibrosis Gene Dysfunction," *Clinical and Experimental Dermatology* 34, no. 8 (2009), https://doi.org/10.1111/j.1365-2230.2009.03357.x; L. M. Arkin et al., "High Prevalence of Aquagenic Wrinkling of the Palms in Patients with Cystic Fibrosis and Association with Measurable Increases in Transepidermal Water Loss," *Pediatric Dermatology* 29, no. 5 (2012), https://doi.org/10.1111/j.1525-1470.2011.01708.x; L. Weibel and R. Spinas, "Images in Clinical Medicine. Aquagenic Wrinkling of Palms in Cystic Fibrosis," *New England Journal of Medicine* 366, no. 21 (2012), https://doi.org/10.1056/NEJMicm1103833; J. M. Thomas et al., "Aquagenic Wrinkling of the Palms: A Diagnostic Clue to Cystic Fibrosis Carrier Status and Non-Classic Disease," *Lancet* 389, no. 10071 (2017), https://doi.org/10.1016/S0140-6736(16)31636-1; H. Kaiser et al., "Aquagenic Wrinkling of the Palms in Patients with Cystic Fibrosis," *British Journal of Dermatology* 179, no. 2 (2018), https://doi.org/10.1111/bjd.16448; G. R. Paul et al., "Aquagenic Wrinkling in Children under Two Years of Age: Could This Be a Potential Clinical Referral Tool for Cystic Fibrosis Among Non-Screened Populations?," *Journal of Cystic Fibrosis* 20, no. 5 (2021), https://doi.org/10.1016/j.jcf.2021.04.002.

7. Mastrianni, interview. For more on the history of sweat chloride cutoff values, see P. M. Farrell et al., "Diagnosis of Cystic Fibrosis: Consensus Guidelines from the Cystic Fibrosis Foundation," *Journal of Pediatrics* 181S (2017), https://doi.org/10.1016/j.jpeds.2016.09.064; Farrell and Koscik, "Sweat Chloride Concentrations."

8. Mastrianni, interview.

9. Mastrianni, interview.

10. C. Bombieri et al., "Recommendations for the Classification of Diseases as CFTR-Related Disorders," *Journal of Cystic Fibrosis* 10, suppl. 2 (2011), https://doi.org/10.1016/S1569-1993(11)60014-3. Later definitions of CFTR-RD would allow for disease manifestations in more than one organ system. I. Sermet-Gaudelus et al., "ECFS Standards of Care on CFTR-Related Disorders: Diagnostic Criteria of *CFTR* Dysfunction," *Journal of Cystic Fibrosis* 21, no. 6 (2022), https://doi.org/10.1016/j.jcf.2022.09.005. For more on diagnosis and management of CFTR-RD, see N. J. Simmonds et al., "ECFS Standards of Care on CFTR-Related Disorders: Identification and Care of the Disorders," *Journal of Cystic Fibrosis* 23, no. 4 (2024), https://doi.org/10.1016/j.jcf.2024.03.008.

11. Investigators in France suggested in 2016 that aquagenic wrinkling might be considered a CFTR-RD, defined as a "clinical entity associated with *CFTR* dysfunction that does not fulfil the diagnostic criteria for CF." C. Cabrol et al., "Aquagenic Palmoplantar Keratoderma as a CFTR-Related Disorder," *Acta Dermato-Venereologica* 96, no. 6 (2016): 848, https://doi.org/10.2340/00015555-2424. The investigators used the term *aquagenic palmoplantar keratoderma* (APK). For more on APK as a CFTR-RD, see C. Raynal et al., "*CFTR* Gene Variants: A Predisposition Factor to Aquagenic Palmoplantar Keratoderma," *British Journal of Dermatology* 181, no. 5 (2019): 1098, https://doi.org/10.1111/bjd.18162.

12. Parad and Comeau, "Diagnostic Dilemmas"; S. J. Mayell et al., "A European Consensus for the Evaluation and Management of Infants with an Equivocal Diagnosis Following Newborn Screening for Cystic Fibrosis," *Journal of Cystic Fibrosis* 8, no. 1 (2009), https://doi.org/10.1016/j.jcf.2008.09.005; D. Borowitz et al., "Cystic Fibrosis Foundation Practice Guidelines for the Management of Infants with Cystic Fibrosis Transmembrane Conductance Regulator-Related Metabolic Syndrome during the First Two Years of Life and Beyond," *Journal of Pediatrics* 155, no. 6, suppl. (2009), https://doi.org/10.1016/j.jpeds.2009.09.003.

13. Clement L. Ren et al., "Clinical Outcomes in Infants with Cystic Fibrosis Transmembrane Conductance Regulator (CFTR) Related Metabolic Syndrome," *Pediatric Pulmonology* 46, no. 11 (2011), https://doi.org/10.1002/ppul.21475; A. Munck et al., "Cystic Fibrosis Screen Positive, Inconclusive Diagnosis (CFSPID): A New Designation and Management Recommendations for Infants with an Inconclusive Diagnosis Following Newborn Screening," *Journal of Cystic Fibrosis* 14, no. 6 (2015), https://doi.org/10.1016/j.jcf.2015.01.001; K. W. Southern et al., "Inconclusive Diagnosis after a Positive Newborn Bloodspot Screening Result for Cystic Fibrosis: Clarification of the Harmonised International Definition," *Journal of Cystic Fibrosis* 18, no. 6 (2019), https://doi.org/10.1016/j.jcf.2019.04.010; Danieli Salinas, oral history interview with the author, July 14, 2021. For more on uncertainty following CF newborn screening, see Grob, *Testing Baby*; Vailly, *Birth of a Genetics Policy*.

14. J. Barben et al., "Updated Guidance on the Management of Children with Cystic Fibrosis Transmembrane Conductance Regulator-Related Metabolic Syndrome/Cystic Fibrosis Screen Positive, Inconclusive Diagnosis (CRMS/CFSPID)," *Journal of Cystic Fibrosis* (2020), https://doi.org/10.1016/j.jcf.2020.11.006; Danieli B Salinas et al., "Gradual Increase in Sweat Chloride Concentration Is Associated with a Higher Risk of CRMS/CFSPID to CF Reclassification," *Pediatric Pulmonology* 58, no. 4 (2023), https://doi.org/10.1002/ppul.26296; Vito Terlizzi et al., "Biochemical and Genetic Tools to Predict the Progression to Cystic Fibrosis in CRMS/CFSPID Subjects: A Systematic Review," *Paediatric Respiratory Reviews* 51 (2024), https://doi.org/10.1016/j.prrv.2024.01.001.

15. H. Levy et al., "Refining the Continuum of CFTR-Associated Disorders in the Era of Newborn Screening," *Clinical Genetics* 89, no. 5 (2016), https://doi.org/10.1111/cge.12711. This assertion is reminiscent of Barton Childs' suggestion that we think of "an unbroken continuity in the expression of disease" as opposed to the existence of specific disease entities in the context of genetic disease more generally. Childs, *Genetic Medicine*, 224.

16. Mastrianni, interview. It is possible that her parents were tested to confirm that each of Michelle's mutations was on a different copy of the CF gene, as opposed to her having two mutations on a single allele.

17. Mastrianni, "Reading Palms."

18. Greene, *Prescribing by Numbers*; Aronowitz, *Unnatural History*; Aronowitz, *Risky Medicine*.

19. In response to expanded newborn screening, Timmermans and Buchbinder note that "the adoption of new screening technologies has generated diagnostic uncertainty about the nature of screening targets, making it unclear not only whether a newborn will develop a disease but also what the condition actually is." Timmermans and Buchbinder, "Patients-in-Waiting," 408. As Michelle explained, "I was relieved at the second appointment that they said, 'okay, we're diagnosing you [with CF],' because I didn't want to be in this limbo state. I'm still in a limbo state, but I didn't want to be in a limbo state with the diagnosis." Mastrianni, interview. For more on this topic, see Aronowitz, *Risky Medicine*; Robert A. Aronowitz, "The Converged Experience of Risk and Disease," *Milbank Quarterly* 87, no. 2 (2009), https://doi.org/10.1111/j.1468-0009.2009.00563.x; Greene, *Prescribing by Numbers*.

20. Mastrianni, "Reading Palms."

21. Álvaro La Parra-Pérez, "Living in the Gray Area," *Cystic Fibrosis Foundation CF Community Blog* (blog), January 19, 2023, https://www.cff.org/community-posts/2023-01/living-gray-area.

22. F. Johnson et al., "Psychological Impact on Parents of an Inconclusive Diagnosis Following Newborn Bloodspot Screening for Cystic Fibrosis: A Qualitative Study," *International Journal of Neonatal Screening* 5, no. 2 (2019): 9, https://doi.org/10.3390/ijns5020023.

23. F. Boardman and C. Clark, "'We're Kind of Like Genetic Nomads': Parents' Experiences of Biographical Disruption and Uncertainty Following in/Conclusive Results from Newborn Cystic Fibrosis Screening," *Social Science & Medicine* 301 (2022): 4–5, https://doi.org/10.1016/j.socscimed.2022.114972.

24. For another account of uncertainty following newborn screening for CF, see Faye Johnson et al., "Receiving Results of Uncertain Clinical Relevance from Population Genetic Screening: Systematic Review & Meta-Synthesis of Qualitative Research," *European Journal of Human Genetics* 30, no. 5 (2022), https://doi.org/10.1038/s41431-022-01054-5.

25. Karen Raraigh, "Beyond CF: A Spectrum of CFTR Variation & CFTR-Opathies." The session was later made accessible on YouTube by the Cystic Fibrosis Foundation: https://www.youtube.com/watch?v=W9BjniFZWb0. Investigators have also pointed to modifier genes and environmental factors to explain the range of phenotypes associated with CF.

26. Douglas B. Hornick, "Are CF Carriers at Increased Risk for a Broad Range of CF-Related Conditions?," North American Cystic Fibrosis Conference, 2020, DG03: Beyond CF: A Spectrum of CFTR Variation & CFTR-opathies.

27. Hornick, "Are CF Carriers at Increased Risk."

28. Hornick, "Are CF Carriers at Increased Risk."

29. Miller et al., "Cystic Fibrosis Carriers"; Y. Colak et al., "Morbidity and Mortality in Carriers of the Cystic Fibrosis Mutation *CFTR* Phe508del in the General Population," *European Respiratory Journal* 56, no. 3 (2020), https://doi.org/10.1183/13993003.00558-2020. For a discussion of earlier studies, see Bombieri et al., "Recommendations for the Classification of Diseases as CFTR-Related Disorders"; P. M. Farrell, "Setting a New Standard in Cystic Fibrosis Newborn Screening Illustrates Controversial Issues as New Data Emerge," *European Journal of Human Genetics* 28, no. 10 (2020), https://doi.org/10.1038/s41431-020-0690-0. For reference to "heterozygote disadvantage" in the 1970s, before the CF gene was identified, see Wailoo, "Inventing the Heterozygote," reference 31. In 2000, Anne Kerr noted that "consideration might also be given to the notion that CF carriers might not always be asymptomatic, despite the obvious concerns that this might raise about discrimination." Kerr, "(Re)Constructing Genetic Disease," 870. Paul di Sant'Agnese also reflected on the possibility of symptomatic "heterozygous cases" in 1956. Paul A. di Sant'Agnese, application for research grant to the National Cystic Fibrosis Research Foundation, July 10, 1956, Joseph Stokes, Jr. Papers: Series II. Organizations, Foundations and Conferences, box 109, National Cystic Fibrosis Research Foundation 1955–1959 folder, section 11: Detailed Outline of Research Program, 1, American Philosophical Society archives.

30. See the introduction for a quote from my gastroenterologist outlining this assumption on May 8, 2001.

31. Miller et al., "Cystic Fibrosis Carriers," 1622. While the researchers estimated that approximately 0.3–0.6 percent of those identified as carriers in their

study were in fact misclassified, they pointed out that more than 15 percent of the carriers in the study would have needed to be misclassified to alter their findings for most of the health conditions examined. Furthermore, when they excluded CF carriers who appeared to have gotten sweat or genetic testing because of suspected CF, their results still demonstrated an increased prevalence of most CF-associated health conditions in carriers. The authors did note that "for some of the rare conditions that would likely lead to suspicion of CF," including pancreatic steatorrhea, "statistical significance fell below a 0.05% threshold with the reduced cohort," yet "most results remained significant," 21 (appendix). The authors also expected that some individuals in their control cohort were actually carriers who had not been detected.

32. Miller et al., "Cystic Fibrosis Carriers," 1626.

33. Polgreen and Comellas, "Clinical Phenotypes of Cystic Fibrosis Carriers."

34. Miller et al., "Cystic Fibrosis Carriers," 1626.

35. P. E. Bratcher and P. L. Zeitlin, "Expanding CFTR Modulator Testing to Carriers of CFTR Variants," *Annals of the American Thoracic Society* 18, no. 11 (2021), https://doi.org/10.1513/AnnalsATS.202011-1397PS. Bratcher and Zeitlin also suggested that CF carriers of rare variants be used to test new CFTR modulators. P. M. Farrell et al., "Challenging the Dogma of the Healthy Heterozygote: Implications for Newborn Screening Policies and Practices," *Molecular Genetics and Metabolism* 134, no. 1–2 (2021), https://doi.org/10.1016/j.ymgme.2021.08.008; C. Martin and P. R. Burgel, "Carriers of a Single *CFTR* Mutation Are Asymptomatic: An Evolving Dogma?," *European Respiratory Journal* 56, no. 3 (2020), https://doi.org/10.1183/13993003.02645-2020.

36. Fisman, "Cystic Fibrosis Heterozygosity." Fisman also pointed out that the study by Miller and colleagues is "forcing us to rethink the relationship between heterozygosity and burden of disease," and it "should flag the emerging likelihood that common genetic variants will be linked to elevated risk of disease occurrence, as genetic testing data, and genomic sequencing data, become more widely available," 2741.

37. For more on newborn screening for CF, see Grob, *Testing Baby*; J. Vailly, "Genetic Screening as a Technique of Government: The Case of Neonatal Screening for Cystic Fibrosis in France," *Social Science & Medicine* 63, no. 12 (2006), https://doi.org/10.1016/j.socscimed.2006.07.025; J. Vailly, "The Expansion of Abnormality and the Biomedical Norm: Neonatal Screening, Prenatal Diagnosis and Cystic Fibrosis in France," *Social Science & Medicine* 66, no. 12 (2008), https://doi.org/10.1016/j.socscimed.2008.02.010; Vailly, *Birth of a Genetics Policy*; M. H. Farrell et al., "Vulnerable Child Syndrome and Newborn Screening Carrier Results for Cystic Fibrosis or Sickle Cell," *Journal of Pediatrics* 224 (2020), https://doi.org/10.1016/j.jpeds.2020.03.042. Noting that carrier status increases the risk of vulnerable child syndrome, Farrell and colleagues cautioned that "the impact of raising concerns about future health risks in the newborn period requires careful

follow up and additional study." Farrell et al., "Challenging the Dogma of the Healthy Heterozygote," 17.

38. Farrell et al., "Challenging the Dogma of the Healthy Heterozygote," 15. Italics in original. In other words, instead of using genetic information for diagnostic purposes, they note that it could be used in the context of CF for the assessment of risk of CF-related health conditions.

39. As Farrell and colleagues note, it may be possible to "potentially compare genomic data to reference tables, and eventually . . . obtain risk percentages derived from research using epidemiologic, biochemical, and clinical methods." Farrell et al., "Challenging the Dogma of the Healthy Heterozygote," 15.

40. Aronowitz, *Risky Medicine.*

41. Polgreen and Comellas, "Clinical Phenotypes of Cystic Fibrosis Carriers."

42. Louisa Flintoft, "Disease Genetics: A Mendelian Code for Complex Disease," *Nature Reviews Genetics* 14, no. 11 (2013), https://doi.org/10.1038/nrg3599.

43. Fisman, "Cystic Fibrosis Heterozygosity." As Daniel Navon notes, "Increasingly, many geneticists are starting to question the very notion of 'carrier genes' and 'incomplete penetrance' altogether." Navon, *Mobilizing Mutations*, 272. For a discussion of clinical phenotypes in female carriers of fragile X, see Hogan, *Life Histories of Genetic Disease*, 45. For more on disease manifestations in heterozygotes, see A. R. Barton et al., "A Spectrum of Recessiveness Among Mendelian Disease Variants in UK Biobank," *American Journal of Human Genetics* 109, no. 7 (2022), https://doi.org/10.1016/j.ajhg.2022.05.008; Seulki Song et al., "Systematic Analysis of Mendelian Disease-Associated Gene Variants Reveals New Classes of Cancer-Predisposing Genes," *Genome Medicine* 15, no. 1 (2023), https://doi.org/10.1186/s13073-023-01252-w; Anita Slomski, "Sickle Cell Trait Associated with Kidney Failure and Covid-19 Death," *JAMA* 328, no. 5 (2022), https://doi.org/10.1001/jama.2022.11938.

44. Zeng et al., "Diseases Common in Persons with Cystic Fibrosis among *CFTR* Heterozygotes," 1021. As the authors noted, "we found no statistically significant associations of diseases and conditions with *CFTR* heterozygotes overall and across genetic ancestral populations."

45. L. D. Richter et al., "Beyond Carrier Status: *CFTR* Heterozygosity as an Overlooked Clinical Risk Factor for Pancreatitis," *Clinical Genetics* (2025), https://doi.org/10.1111/cge.14780.

46. Basu Biswajit et al., "The Future of Cystic Fibrosis Care: Exploring AI's Impact on Detection and Therapy," *Current Respiratory Medicine Reviews* 20, no. 4 (2024), https://doi.org/10.2174/011573398X283365240208195944; Gina Kolata, "A.I. Chatbots Defeated Doctors at Diagnosing Illness," *New York Times*, November 17, 2024.

47. Reuben, "Learning Diagnostic Restraint"; Rosenbaum, "Living Unlabeled"; Simpkin and Schwartzstein, "Tolerating Uncertainty"; A. Kelly and R. S. Panush, "Diagnostic Uncertainty and Epistemologic Humility," *Clinical Rheumatology* 36,

no. 6 (2017), https://doi.org/10.1007/s10067-017-3631-8. As sociologist Annemarie Jutel notes, some physicians have even suggested that "obsession with diagnosis is an antithesis to patient-centred care." Jutel, "Uncertainty and the Inconvenient Facts of Diagnosis," 5.

48. Maram Khazen et al., "Developing a Framework and Electronic Tool for Communicating Diagnostic Uncertainty in Primary Care: A Qualitative Study," *JAMA Network Open* 6, no. 3 (2023), https://doi.org/10.1001/jamanetworkopen.2023.2218; Badar Patel et al., "Navigating Uncertainty in Clinical Practice: A Structured Approach," *Journal of General Internal Medicine* 39, no. 5 (2024), https://doi.org/10.1007/s11606-023-08596-4; Neha Bansal Etherington et al., "Implementation of a Curriculum on Communicating Diagnostic Uncertainty for Clerkship-Level Medical Students: A Pseudorandomized and Controlled Study," *Diagnosis* 12, no. 3 (2025), https://doi.org/doi:10.1515/dx-2025-0006.

49. Amos Etsy, "Navigating the Uncertainties of Medicine," *Harvard Medicine*, Summer 2024, https://magazine.hms.harvard.edu/articles/navigating-uncertainties-medicine.

50. Etsy, "Navigating the Uncertainties of Medicine."

Index

Page numbers in italics refer to figures.